Obstetrics
by Ten Teachers

Obstetrics
by Ten Teachers

18th Edition

Edited by

Philip N. Baker BMed(Sci) BM BS DM FRCOG
Professor of Maternal and Fetal Health,
Director of the Maternal and Fetal Health Research Centre,
Consultant Obstetrician, St Mary's Hospital,
University of Manchester, Manchester, UK

This book owes a great debt to Professor Stuart Campbell and Dr Christoph Lees,
editors of the seventeenth edition of this book. They presided over, and were intimately
involved in, the comprehensive revision of what had become a rather old-fashioned book,
bringing it fully up-to-date in the year 2000, and were responsible for introducing many
of the concepts and features on which this edition has built.

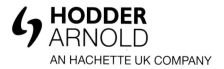

HODDER
ARNOLD

AN HACHETTE UK COMPANY

First published in Great Britain in 1917 as *Midwifery*
Eleventh edition published in 1966 as *Obstetrics*
Seventeenth edition published in 2000
This eighteenth edition published in 2006 by
Hodder Arnold, an imprint of Hodder Education,
an Hachette UK Company,
338 Euston Road, London NW1 3BH

www.hoddereducation.com

British Library Cataloguing in Publication Data
A catalogue record for this book is available from the British Library

Library of Congress Cataloging-in-Publication Data
A catalog record for this book is available from the Library of Congress

ISBN 978 0 340 81665 3
ISBN 978 0 340 81666 0 (International Student's Edition, restricted teritorial availability)

6 7 8 9 10

Commissioning Editors; Georgina Bentliff and Clare Christian
Development Editor: Heather Smith
Project Editor: Wendy Rooke
Production Controller: Jane Lawrence
Cover Design: Amina Dudhia

Typeset in Minion 9.5/12 pts by Charon Tec Pvt. Ltd, Chennai, India
www.charontec.com
Printed and bound in India by Replika Press Pvt. Ltd

What do you think about this book? Or any other Hodder Arnold title?
Please visit our website at www.hoddereducation.com

This book is dedicated to my younger daughter, Sara

Contents

The Ten Teachers

Philip N. Baker BMed(Sci) BM BS DM FRCOG
Professor of Maternal and Fetal Health, Director of
the Maternal and Fetal Health Research Centre,
Consultant Obstetrician, St Mary's Hospital,
University of Manchester, Manchester, UK

Ian Johnson BSc MB BS DM FRCOG
Professor of Obstetrics and Gynaecology, Faculty of
Medicine and Health Sciences, University of
Nottingham, Nottingham, UK

Griffith Jones MRCOG FRCSC
Obstetrician and Gynaecologist, Winchester,
Ontario, and Assistant Professor, Division of
Maternal–Fetal Medicine, University of Ottawa,
Ottawa, Canada

Lucy Kean MA DM MRCOG
Consultant Obstetrician and Sub-specialist in Fetal
and Maternal Medicine, Department of Obstetrics,
City Hospital, Nottingham, UK

Louise C. Kenny MBChB(Hons) MRCOG PhD
Clinical Lecturer, Maternal and Fetal Health
Research Centre, St Mary's Hospital, University of
Manchester, Manchester, UK

Gary Mires MBChB MD FRCOG ILTM
Reader and Consultant Obstetrician,
University of Dundee,
Ninewells Hospital and Medical School,
Dundee, UK

Alec McEwan BA BM BCh MRCOG
Subspecialty Trainee in Fetal and Maternal Medicine,
Queen's Medical Centre, Nottingham, UK

Catherine Nelson-Piercy MA FRCP
Consultant Obstetric Physician, Guy's and St
Thomas' Hospitals, London, UK

Janet M. Rennie MA MD FRCP FRCPCH DCH
Consultant and Senior Lecturer in Neonatal
Medicine, Elizabeth Garrett Anderson and Obstetric
Hospital, University College London Hospitals,
London, UK

Abdul H. Sultan MBChB MRCOG MD
Consultant Obstetrician and Gynaecologist,
Mayday University Hospital, Surrey, UK

(In addition, Dr Phillip Hay, one of the ten teachers
contributing to the companion Gynaecology text,
has prepared the chapter on Perinatal infections.)

Acknowledgements

The editor and the publishers would also like to thank the contributors to the previous edition who have not been directly involved in the preparation of this 18th edition:

Stuart Campbell
James Drife
William Dunlop
Jason Gardosi
Donald Gibb
J.G. Grudzinskas
Kevin Harrington
Des Holden
Richard Johanson

Christoph Lees
Kypros Nicolaides
Margaret R. Oates
Michael Robson
Neil Sebire
E. Malcolm Symonds
Basky Thilaganathan
J. Guy Thorpe-Beeston

Preface

Obstetrics by Ten Teachers is the oldest and most respected English language textbook on the subject; like previous editors, I fully appreciate the responsibility to ensure its continuing success.

The first edition was published as *Midwifery by Ten Teachers* in 1917, and was edited under the direction of Comyns Berkley (Obstetric and Gynaecological Surgeon to the Middlesex Hospital). The aims of the book as detailed in the preface to the first edition still pertain today:

> *This book is frankly written for students preparing for their final examination, and in the hope that it will prove useful to them afterwards, and to others who have passed beyond the stage of examination.*

The 17th edition incorporated extensive revisions to the previous edition, and much credit must go to the previous editors, Stuart Campbell and Christoph Lees, for their diligent efforts. For this 18th edition I have reverted to the tradition of utilizing the collective efforts of ten teachers of repute. The ten teachers teach in medical schools that vary markedly in the philosophy and structure of their courses. Some adopt a wholly problem-based approach, while others adopt a more traditional 'subject-based' curriculum. All of the ten teachers have an active involvement in both undergraduate and postgraduate teaching, and all have previously written extensively within their areas of expertise. Some of the contributors, such as Gary Mires and Ian Johnson, have been at the forefront of innovations in undergraduate teaching, and have been heavily involved in developing the structure of courses and curricula. In contrast, other teachers are at earlier stages in their career: Louise Kenny and Alec McEwan are clinical lecturers, closely involved in the day-to-day tutoring of students. The extensive and diverse experience of our ten teachers should maximize the relevance of the text to today's medical students.

The content of this 18th edition differs markedly from that of the first edition, in which three chapters were devoted to 'the toxins of pregnancy'. Although the structure of the 17th edition has been largely retained, many of the chapters have been considerably revised by our ten teachers. Throughout the textbook I have endeavoured to continue the previous editors' efforts to incorporate clinically relevant material.

Finally, I echo the previous editors in hoping that this book will enthuse a new generation of obstetricians to make pregnancy and childbirth an even safer and more fulfilling experience.

Philip N. Baker
2006

Commonly used abbreviations

ABC	airway, breathing and circulation	ECV	external cephalic version
AC	abdominal circumference	EDD	estimated date of delivery
ACE	angiotensin-converting enzyme	EEG	electroencephalogram
ACTH	adrenocorticotrophic hormone	EFM	external fetal monitoring
AED	anti-epileptic drug	EFW	estimated fetal weight
AF	amniotic fluid	EGF	epidermal growth factor
AFI	amniotic fluid index	ELISA	enzyme-linked immunosorbent assay
AFP	alpha-fetoprotein	ERPC	evacuation of retained products of conception
AIDS	acquired immunodeficiency syndrome		
AP	antero-posterior	ESR	erythrocyte sedimentation rate
APCR	activated protein C resistance	ET	embryo transfer
APH	antepartum haemorrhage	FBS	fetal blood sampling
APS	antiphospholipid syndrome	FDP	fibrin degradation product
APTT	activated partial thromboplastin time	FEV_1	forced expiratory volume in 1 second
ARM	artificial rupture of membranes	fFN	fetal fibronectin
AT	antithrombin	FFO	'failed forceps outside'
BMI	body mass index	FISH	fluorescence in-situ hybridization
BPD	biparietal diameter	FL	femur length
bpm	beats per minute	FM	fetal movements
BV	bacterial vaginosis	FSE	fetal scalp electrode
CBG	cortisol-binding globulin	FSH	follicle-stimulating hormone
CDC	Communicable Disease Center	FT3	free tri-iodothyronine
CDH	congenital diaphragmatic hernia	FT4	free thyroxine
CEMACH	Confidential Enquiry into Maternal and Child Health	FTA	fluorescent treponemal antibody (test)
		G	gravida
CEMD	Confidential Enquiry into Maternal Death	GBS	group B *Streptococcus*
CESDI	Confidential Enquiry into Stillbirths and Deaths in Infancy	GDM	gestational diabetes mellitus
		GMH-IVH	germinal matrix-intraventricular haemorrhage
CHD	congenital heart defect		
CMV	cytomegalovirus	GnRH	gonadotrophin-releasing hormone
CNST	Clinical Negligence Scheme for Trusts	G6PD	glucose 6-phosphate dehydrogenase
CPD	cephalo-pelvic disproportion	GP	general practitioner
CRF	corticotrophin-releasing factor	GTN	glyceryl trinitrate
CRH	corticotrophin-releasing hormone	HAART	highly active antiretroviral therapy
CRL	crown–rump length	Hb	haemoglobin
CRM	clinical risk management	HBeAg	hepatitis B e antigen
CS	Caesarean section	HBsAg	hepatitis B surface antigen
CSF	cerebrospinal fluid	HC	head circumference
CT	computerized tomography	hCG	human chorionic gonadotrophin
CTG	cardiotocograph	HDN	haemolytic disease of the newborn
CVA	cerebrovascular accident	HELLP	haemolysis, elevation of liver enzymes and low platelets
CVP	central venous pressure		
CVS	chorionic villus sampling	hGH	human growth hormone
DCDA	dichorionic diamniotic	HIE	hypoxic–ischaemic encephalopathy
DDH	developmental dysplasia of the hip	HIV	human immunodeficiency virus
DHEA	dihydroepiandrosterone	hPL	human placental lactogen
DIC	disseminated intravascular coagulation	HPV	human papillomavirus
2,3-DPG	2,3-diphosphoglycerate	HSV	herpes simplex virus
DVT	deep vein thrombosis	HTLV-1	human T-cell leukaemia virus
ECG	electrocardiograph	HVS	high vaginal swab
ECM	extracellular matrix	IDDM	insulin-dependent diabetes mellitus
ECT	electroconvulsive therapy	Ig	immunoglobulin

IGF	insulin-like growth factor		PMR	perinatal mortality rate
IOL	induction of labour		PPH	postpartum haemorrhage
ITP	autoimmune thrombocytopenic purpura		PPHN	persistent pulmonary hypertension of the newborn
IUGR	intrauterine growth restriction		PPIH	proteinuric pregnancy-induced hypertension (pre-eclampsia)
IVF	in-vitro fertilization			
IVH	intraventricular haemorrhage		PROM	preterm prelabour rupture of membranes
LFT	liver function test		PTH	parathyroid hormone
LH	luteinizing hormone		PTU	propylthiouracil
LIF	leukaemia inhibitory factor		PVL	periventricular leukomalacia
LLETZ	large loop excision of the transformation zone		RCOG	Royal College of Obstetricians and Gynaecologists
LMP	last menstrual period		RDS	respiratory distress syndrome
LSCS	lower segment Caesarean section		REM	rapid eye movement (sleep)
MAS	meconium aspiration syndrome		Rh	rhesus
MCDA	monochorionic diamniotic		RI	resistance index
MCMA	monochorionic monoamniotic		SCBU	special care baby unit
M, C & S	microscopy, culture and sensitivities		SFH	symphysis–fundal height
MCV	mean corpuscular volume		SGA	small for gestational age
MMR	maternal mortality rate		SLE	systemic lupus erythematosus
MRI	magnetic resonance imaging		SROM	spontaneous rupture of membranes
MROP	manual removal of placenta		SSRI	selective serotonin reuptake inhibitor
MSLC	Maternity Services Liaison Committee		STOP	suction termination of pregnancy
MSU	midstream specimen of urine		SVD	spontaneous vaginal delivery
NAD	nothing abnormal detected		T3	tri-iodothyronine
NCT	National Childbirth Trust		T4	thyroxine
NEC	necrotizing enterocolitis		TENS	transcutaneous electrical nerve stimulation
NHS	National Health Service		TNF-α	tumour necrosis factor-alpha
NICE	National Institute for Clinical Excellence		TOP	termination of pregnancy
NIDDM	non-insulin-dependent diabetes mellitus		TORCH	toxoplasmosis, rubella, cytomegalovirus, herpes
NND	neonatal death			
NNU	neonatal unit		TOS	trial of scar
NSAID	non-steroidal anti-inflammatory drug		TPHA	*Treponema pallidum* haemagglutination assay
NTD	neural tube defect			
OA	occipito-anterior		TPN	total parenteral nutrition
OFD	occipito-frontal diameter		TRH	thyrotrophin-releasing hormone
OP	occipito-posterior		TSH	thyroid-stimulating hormone
OT	occipito-transverse		TTN	transient tachypnoea of the newborn
P	para		TTTS	twin-to-twin transfusion syndrome
PAPP-A	pregnancy-associated plasma protein		USS	ultrasound scan
PCA	patient-controlled analgesia		UTI	urinary tract infection
PCR	polymerase chain reaction		VBAC	vaginal birth after Caesarean
PE	pulmonary embolus		VDRL	Venereal Diseases Research Laboratory (test)
PEP	polymorphic eruption of pregnancy			
PG	prostaglandin		VE	vaginal examination
PGD	pre-implantation genetic diagnosis		VZIG	varicella zoster immune globulin
PI	pulsatility index		WHO	World Health Organization
PID	pelvic inflammatory disease		WR	Wasserman reaction
PIH	pregnancy-induced hypertension			

Obstetric history taking and examination

OVERVIEW

Taking a history and performing an obstetric examination are quite different from their medical and surgical equivalents. Not only will the type of questions change with gestation but also so will the purpose of the examination. The history will often cover physiology, pathology and psychology and must always be sought with care and sensitivity.

Etiquette in taking a history

Patients expect doctors and students to be well presented and appearances do have an enormous impact on patients, so make sure that your appearance is suitable before you enter the room.

When meeting a patient for the first time, always introduce yourself; tell the patient who you are and say why you have come to see them. If you are a medical student, some patients will decide that they do not wish to talk to you. This may be for many reasons and, if your involvement in their care is declined, accept without questioning.

Some areas of the obstetric history cover subjects that are intensely private. In occasional cases there may be events recorded in the notes that are not known by other family members, such as previous terminations of pregnancy. It is vital that the history taker is sensitive to each individual situation and does not simply follow a formula to get all the facts right.

Some women will wish another person to be present if the doctor or student is male, even just to take a history, and this wish should be respected.

Where to begin

The amount of detail required must be tailored to the purpose of the visit. At a booking visit, the history must be thorough and meticulously recorded. Once this baseline information is established, many women find it tedious to go over all this information again. Before starting, ask yourself what you need to achieve. In late pregnancy, women will be attending the antenatal clinic for a particular reason. It is certainly acceptable to ask why the patient has attended in the opening discussion. For some women it will be a routine visit (usually performed by the midwife or general practitioner), others are attending because there is or has been a problem.

Make sure that the patient is comfortable (usually seated but occasionally sitting on a bed).

It is important to establish some very general facts when taking a history. Asking for the patient's age or date of birth and whether this is a first pregnancy are usually safe opening questions.

At this stage you can also establish whether a woman is working and, if so, what she does.

Dating the pregnancy

Pregnancy is dated from the last menstrual period (LMP), not the date of conception. The median duration of pregnancy is 280 days (40 weeks) and this gives the estimated date of delivery (EDD). This assumes that:
- the cycle length is 28 days,
- ovulation occurs generally on the 14th day of the cycle,
- the cycle was a normal cycle (i.e. not straight after stopping the oral contraceptive pill or soon after a previous pregnancy).

The EDD is calculated by taking the date of the LMP, counting forward by 9 months and adding 7 days. If the cycle is longer than 28 days, add the difference between the cycle length and 28, to compensate.

In most antenatal clinics, there are pregnancy calculators (wheels) that do this for you (Fig. 1.1). It is worth noting that pregnancy-calculating wheels do differ a little and may give dates that are a day or two different from those previously calculated. Whilst this should not make much difference, it is an area that often causes heated discussion in the antenatal clinic. Term is actually defined as 37–42 weeks and so the estimated time of delivery should ideally be defined as a range of dates rather than a fixed date, but women have been highly resistant to this idea and generally do want a specific date.

Almost all women who undergo antenatal care in the UK will have an ultrasound scan in the late first trimester or early second trimester. The purposes of this scan are to establish dates, to ensure that the pregnancy is ongoing and to determine the number of fetuses. If performed before 20 weeks, the ultrasound scan can be used for dating the pregnancy. After this time, the variability in growth rates of different fetuses makes it unsuitable for use in defining dates. It has been shown that ultrasound-defined dates are more accurate than those based on a certain LMP and reduce the need for post-dates induction of labour.

Figure 1.1 Gestation calculator.

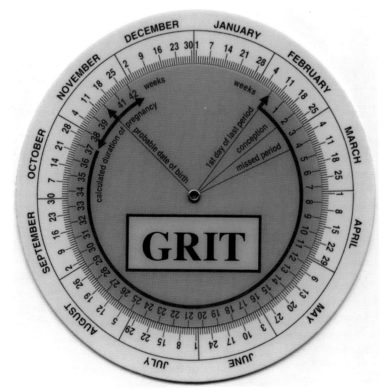

This may be because the actual time of ovulation in any cycle is much less fixed than was previously thought. In most units, however, the LMP date is used if it is within a week of the scan date.

In late pregnancy, many women will have long forgotten their LMP date, but will know exactly when their EDD is, and it is therefore more straightforward to ask this.

Taking the history

Social history

Some aspects of history taking require considerable sensitivity, and the social history is one such area. There are important facts to establish, but in many cases these can come out at various different parts of the history and some can almost be part of normal conversation. It is important to have a list of things to establish in your mind. It is here more than anywhere that some local knowledge is helpful, as much can be gained from knowing where the patient lives. However, be careful not to jump to conclusions, as these can often be wrong.

The following facts demonstrate why a social history is important.

- Women in social class 9 (includes all unemployed women) had a maternal mortality rate of 135 compared to a rate of 2.9 for women in social class 1 in the last Confidential Enquiry into Maternal Deaths 1997–1999 (CEMD).
- Social exclusion was seen in 18 out of 19 deaths in women under 20 in the last CEMD (one homeless teenager froze to death in a front garden).
- Domestic violence was reported in 12 per cent of the 378 women whose deaths were reported in 1997–1999.
- Married women are more likely to request amniocentesis after a high-risk Down's syndrome screening result than unmarried women. Husbands clearly have a strong voice in decision making.
- If a woman is unmarried, her partner cannot provide consent for a post mortem after stillbirth.

Enquiry about domestic violence is extremely difficult. It is recommended that all women are seen on their own at least once during pregnancy, so that they can discuss this, if needed, away from an abusive partner. This is not always easy to accomplish. If you happen to be the person to whom this information is given, you must ensure that it is passed on to the relevant team, as this may be the only opportunity the woman has to disclose it. Sometimes younger women find medical students and young doctors much easier to talk to. Be aware of this.

Smoking, alcohol and illicit drug intake also form part of the social history. Smoking causes a reduction in birth weight in a dose-dependent way. It also increases the risk of miscarriage, stillbirth and neonatal death. There are interventions that can be offered to women who are still smoking in pregnancy, but the likelihood of success is not high. New research is investigating the use of nicotine replacement, which may help some women.

Alcohol is probably not harmful in small amounts (less than one drink per day). Binge drinking is particularly harmful and can lead to a constellation of features in the baby known as fetal alcohol syndrome.

Enquiry about illicit drug taking is more difficult. Approximately 0.5–1 per cent of women continue to take illicit drugs during pregnancy. Be careful not to make assumptions. During the booking visit, the midwife should directly enquire about drug taking. If it is seen as part of the long list of routine questions asked at this visit, it is perceived as less threatening. However, sometimes this information comes to light at other times. Cocaine and crack cocaine are the most harmful of the illicit drugs taken, but all have some effects on the pregnancy, and all have financial implications.

By the time you have finished your history and examination you should know the following facts that are important in the social history:

- whether the patient is married or single and what sort of support she has at home (remember that married women whose only support is a working husband may be very isolated after the birth of a baby),
- generally whether there is a stable income coming into the house,
- what sort of housing the patient occupies (e.g. a flat with lots of stairs and no lift may be problematic),
- whether the woman works and for how long she is planning to work during the pregnancy,
- whether the woman smokes/drinks or uses drugs,
- if there are any other features that may be important.

Previous obstetric history

Past obstetric history is one of the most important aspects of establishing risk in the current pregnancy. It is helpful to list the pregnancies in date order and to discover what the outcome was in each pregnancy.

The features that are likely to have impact on future pregnancies include:

- recurrent miscarriage (increased risk of miscarriage, intrauterine growth restriction (IUGR)),
- preterm delivery (increased risk of preterm delivery),
- early-onset pre-eclampsia (increased risk of pre-eclampsia/IUGR),
- abruption (increased risk of recurrence),
- congenital abnormality (recurrence risk depends on type of abnormality),
- macrosomic baby (may be related to gestational diabetes),
- IUGR (increased recurrence),
- unexplained stillbirth (increased risk of gestational diabetes).

The method of delivery for any previous births must be recorded, as this can have implications for planning in the current pregnancy, particularly if there has been previous Caesarean section, difficult vaginal delivery, postpartum haemorrhage or significant perineal trauma.

When you have noted all the pregnancies, you can convert this into the obstetric shorthand of parity. This is often confusing. Remember that:

- *gravida* is the total number of pregnancies regardless of how they ended,
- *parity* is the number of live births at any gestation or stillbirths after 24 weeks.

In terms of parity, therefore, twins count as 2. Thus a woman at 12 weeks in this pregnancy who has never had a pregnancy before is gravida 1, parity 0. If she delivers twins and comes back next time at 12 weeks, she will be gravida 2, parity 2 (twins). A woman who has had six miscarriages and is pregnant again with only one live baby born at 25 weeks will be gravida 8, parity 1.

The other shorthand you may see is where the parity is recorded as parity then the number of pregnancies that did not result in live birth or stillbirth after 24 weeks. The above cases would thus be defined as: para 0^{+0}, para 2^{+0} (twins), para 1^{+6}.

However, when presenting a history, it is much easier to describe exactly what has happened, e.g. 'Mrs Jones is in her eighth pregnancy. She has had six miscarriages at gestations of 8–12 weeks and one spontaneous delivery of a live baby boy at 25 weeks. Baby Tom is now 2 years old and healthy.'

Past gynaecological history

The regularity of periods is important in dating pregnancy (as above). Women with very long cycles may have a condition known as polycystic ovarian syndrome. This is a complex endocrine condition and its relevance here is that some women with this condition have increased insulin resistance and a higher risk for the development of gestational diabetes.

Contraceptive history can be relevant if conception has occurred soon after stopping the combined oral contraceptive pill or depot progesterone preparations, as, again, this makes dating more difficult. Also, some women will conceive with an intrauterine device still in situ. This carries an increase in the risk of miscarriage.

Previous episodes of pelvic inflammatory disease increase the risk for ectopic pregnancy. This is only of relevance in early pregnancy. However, it is important to establish that any infections have been adequately treated and that the partner was also treated.

The date of the last cervical smear should be noted. Every year a small number of women are diagnosed as having cervical cancer in pregnancy, and it is recognized that late diagnosis is more common around the time of pregnancy because smears are deferred. If a smear is due, it can be taken in the first trimester. It is important to record that the woman is pregnant, as the slides can be difficult to assess without this knowledge. It is also important that smears are not deferred in women who are at increased risk of cervical disease (e.g. previous cervical smear abnormality or very overdue smear). Gently taking a smear in the first trimester does not cause miscarriage and women should be reassured about this. Remember that if it is deferred at this point, it may be nearly a year before the opportunity arises again. If there has been irregular bleeding, the cervix should at least be examined to ensure that there are no obvious lesions present.

If a woman has undergone treatment for cervical changes, this should be noted. Knife cone biopsy is associated with an increased risk for both cervical incompetence (weakness) and stenosis (leading to preterm delivery and dystocia in labour respectively). There is no convincing risk associated with large loop excision of the transformation zone (LLETZ); however, women who have needed more than one excision are likely to have a much shorter cervix, which does increase the risk for second and early third trimester delivery.

Previous ectopic pregnancy increases the risk of recurrence to 1 in 10. It is also important to know the site of the ectopic and how it was managed. The implications of a straightforward salpingectomy for an ampullary ectopic are much less than those after a complex operation for a cornual ectopic. Women who have had an ectopic pregnancy should be offered an early ultrasound scan to establish the site of any future pregnancies.

Recurrent miscarriage may be associated with a number of problems. Antiphospholipid syndrome increases the risk of further pregnancy loss, IUGR and pre-eclampsia. Balanced translocations can occasionally lead to congenital abnormality, and cervical incompetence can predispose to late second and early third trimester delivery. Also, women need a great deal of support during pregnancy if they have experienced recurrent pregnancy losses.

Multiple previous first trimester terminations of pregnancy potentially increase the risk of preterm delivery, possibly secondary to cervical weakness. Sometimes information regarding these must be sensitively recorded. Some women do not wish this to be recorded in their hand-held notes.

Previous gynaecological surgery is important, especially if it involved the uterus, as this can have potential sequelae for delivery. In addition, the presence of pelvic masses such as ovarian cysts and fibroids should be noted. These may impact on delivery and may also pose some problems during pregnancy.

A previous history of subfertility is also important. The CEMD 1997–1999 showed that the maternal mortality rate for women who had undergone in-vitro fertilization (IVF) was estimated at 48 per 10 000 IVF pregnancies. Donor egg or sperm use is associated with an increased risk of pre-eclampsia. The rate of preterm delivery is higher in assisted conception pregnancies, even after the higher rate of multiple pregnancies has been taken into account. Women who have undergone fertility treatment are often older and generally need increased psychological support during pregnancy.

Legally, you should not write down in notes that a pregnancy is conceived by IVF or donor egg or sperm unless you have written permission from the patient. It is obviously a difficult area, as there is an increased risk of problems to the mother in these pregnancies and therefore the knowledge is important. Generally, if the patient has told you herself that the pregnancy was an assisted conception, it is reasonable to state that in your presentation.

CASE HISTORY

Miss C is a 24-year-old woman in her third pregnancy. She has presented to the admissions unit with watery vaginal discharge for 12 hours. She has an estimated date of delivery of 28th August, which was confirmed by ultrasound at 12 weeks' gestation, making her 28 weeks and 4 days pregnant.

The watery loss was a sudden gush of fluid that occurred when she was sitting at her desk at work. She has continued to leak clear fluid since then. The baby has been active and she feels generally well. She does not report any abdominal pain or tightenings.

The pregnancy has been uncomplicated until today. Screening for neural tube defects and Down's syndrome gave no cause for concern and the anomaly scan at 21 weeks was normal.

Miss C had a termination of pregnancy at 11 weeks in 2000 and a termination at 9 weeks in 2002. She is now in a stable relationship and this pregnancy was planned. Her smears are up to date.

Otherwise, Miss C is fit and well. She does not drink or smoke and has no known allergies. There is no family history of note.

On examination, her pulse is 90 beats per minute and there is a mild pyrexia of 37.7 °C. The symphysis–fundal height is 23 cm. There is mild uterine tenderness across the whole uterus. The presenting part is difficult to feel, but seems to be a cephalic presentation. A speculum examination has revealed clear liquor draining, with an external os that was closed on visual inspection. A digital examination has not been performed.

Blood has been taken for full blood count and C-reactive protein. An ultrasound has been requested urgently to confirm the presentation.

The clinical picture suggests premature rupture of membranes with developing chorioamnionitis.

Medical and surgical history

All pre-existing medical disease should be carefully noted and any associated drug history also recorded. The major pre-existing diseases that impact on pregnancy and their potential effects are shown in the box.

Major pre-existing diseases that impact on pregnancy

- Diabetes mellitus: macrosomia, IUGR, congenital abnormality, pre-eclampsia, stillbirth, neonatal hypoglycaemia.
- Hypertension: pre-eclampsia.
- Renal disease: worsening renal disease, pre-eclampsia, IUGR, preterm delivery.
- Epilepsy: increased fit frequency, congenital abnormality.
- Venous thromboembolic disease: increased risk during pregnancy; if associated thrombophilia, increased risk of pre-eclampsia, IUGR.
- Human immunodeficiency virus (HIV) infection: risk of mother-to-child transfer if untreated.
- Connective tissue diseases, e.g. systemic lupus erythematosus: pre-eclampsia, IUGR.
- Myasthenia gravis/myotonic dystrophy: fetal neurological effects and increased maternal muscular fatigue in labour.

Previous surgery should be noted. Occasionally surgery has been performed for conditions that may continue to be a problem during pregnancy, such as Crohn's disease. Rarely, complications from previous surgery, such as adhesional obstruction, present in pregnancy.

Psychiatric history is important to record. Deaths from psychiatric causes were the largest single category in the last CEMD, contributing to 12 per cent of all deaths. The enquiry recommended that enquiries about previous psychiatric history, its severity, care received and clinical presentation should be made in a systematic and sensitive way at the antenatal booking visit. A good question to lead into this is 'Have you ever suffered with your nerves?'. If women have had children before, you can ask whether they had problems with depression or 'the blues' after the births of any of them.

Drug history

It is vital to establish what drugs women have been taking for their condition and for what duration. You should also ask about over-the-counter medication and homeopathic/herbal remedies. In some cases, medication needs to be changed in pregnancy. For some women it may be possible to stop their medication completely for some or all of pregnancy (e.g. mild hypertension). Some women need to know that they must continue their medication (e.g. epilepsy, for which women often reduce their medication for fear of potential fetal effects, with detriment to their own health).

Family history

Family history is important if it can:
- impact on the health of the mother in pregnancy or afterwards,
- have implications for the fetus or baby.

Often, information is recorded under this title that can have no impact on the above, such as details about the paternal side that do not affect the mother or fetus.

Important areas are a maternal history of a first-degree relative (sibling or parent) with:
- diabetes (increased risk of gestational diabetes),
- thromboembolic disease (increased risk of thrombophilia, thrombosis),
- pre-eclampsia (increased risk of pre-eclampsia),
- psychotic psychiatric disorder (increased risk of puerperal psychosis).

For both parents, it is important to know about any family history of babies with congenital abnormality and any potential genetic problems, such as haemoglobinopathies. If any close family member has tuberculosis, the baby will be offered immunization after birth.

Finally, any known allergies should be recorded. If a woman gives a history of allergy, it is important to ask about how this was diagnosed and to explain the potential problems the allergy can cause.

Identifying risk

By the time you have finished the history, you will have a general idea of whether or not the pregnancy is likely to be uncomplicated. Of course, in primigravid women, the likelihood of later complications can be difficult to predict, but even here some features such as a strong family history of pre-eclampsia may be present.

Examination

Before moving on to examine the patient, it is important to be aware of what you are aiming to achieve. The examination should be directed at the presenting problem, if any, and the gestation. For instance, it is generally unnecessary to spend time defining the presentation at 32 weeks unless the presenting problem is threatened preterm labour.

Maternal weight and height

The measurement of weight at the initial examination is important to identify women who are significantly underweight or overweight. Women with a body mass index (BMI) [weight (kg)/height (m^2)] of <20 are at higher risk of fetal growth restriction and increased perinatal mortality. This is particularly the case if weight gain in pregnancy is poor. Repeated weighing of underweight women during pregnancy will identify that group of women at increased risk for adverse perinatal outcome due to poor weight gain. In the obese woman (BMI 30), the risks of gestational diabetes and hypertension are increased. Additionally, fetal assessment, both by palpation and ultrasound, is more difficult. Obesity is also associated with increased birth weight and a higher perinatal mortality rate.

In women of normal weight at booking, and in whom nutrition is of no concern, there is no need to repeat weight measurement in pregnancy.

Height should be measured at booking to assist with BMI assessment. Other than this, it is only relevant in pregnancy when fetal overgrowth or undergrowth is suspected, as customized charts have significant advantages in the case of very tall or short women, leading to more accurate diagnosis of growth restriction or macrosomia. Short women are significantly more likely to have problems in labour, but these are generally unpredictable during pregnancy. Shoe size is unhelpful when height is known. Height alone is the best indicator of potential problems in labour, but even this is not a useful predictor. On no account should you give women the impression that their labour will be unsuccessful because they are short. Were this always the case, the genes for being short would have disappeared from the population long ago.

Blood pressure evaluation

The first recording of blood pressure should be made as early as possible in pregnancy. Hypertension diagnosed for the first time in early pregnancy (blood pressure >140/90 mmHg on two separate occasions at least 4 hours apart) should prompt a search for underlying causes, i.e. renal, endocrine and collagen-vascular disease. Although 90 per cent of cases will be due to essential hypertension, this is a diagnosis of exclusion and can only be confidently made when other causes have been excluded. Blood pressure measurement is one of the few aspects of antenatal care that is truly beneficial. It should be performed at every visit.

Measure the blood pressure with the woman seated or semi-recumbent. Do not lie her in the left lateral position, as this will lead to under-reading of the blood pressure.

Use an appropriately sized cuff. The cuffs have markings to indicate how they should fit. Large women will need a larger cuff. Using one too small will overestimate blood pressure. If you are using an automated device and the blood pressure appears high, recheck it with a mercury sphygmomanometer if possible. If not available, use a hand-operated device that has been recently calibrated (every clinic should have one).

Convention is to use Korotkoff V (i.e. disappearance of sounds), as this is more reproducible than Korotkoff IV. Deflate the cuff slowly so that you can record the blood pressure to the nearest 2 mmHg. Do not round up or down.

Urinary examination

Screening of midstream urine for asymptomatic bacteriuria in pregnancy is of proven benefit. The risk of ascending urinary tract infection in pregnancy is much higher than in the non-pregnant state. Acute pyelonephritis increases the risk of pregnancy loss/premature labour, and is associated with considerable maternal morbidity. Additionally, persistent proteinuria or haematuria may be an indicator of underlying renal disease, prompting further investigation.

At repeat visits, urinalysis should be performed. This is the other beneficial aspect of antenatal care. If there is any proteinuria, a thorough evaluation with regard to a diagnosis of pre-eclampsia should be undertaken. A trace of protein is unlikely to be problematic in terms of pre-eclampsia, and may point to urinary tract infection. However, if even a trace of protein is seen persistently, further investigation should be undertaken.

General medical examination

In fit and healthy women presenting for a routine visit there is little benefit in a full formal physical examination. Where a woman presents with a problem, there may be a need to undertake a much more thorough physical examination.

Cardiovascular examination

Routine auscultation for maternal heart sounds in asymptomatic women with no cardiac history is unnecessary. Flow murmurs can be heard in approximately 80 per cent of women at the end of the first trimester. Studies suggest that only women coming from areas where rheumatic heart disease is prevalent and those with significant symptoms or a known history of heart murmur or heart disease need undergo cardiovascular examination during pregnancy.

Breast examination

Formal breast examination is also not necessary; self-examination is as reliable as a general physician examination in detecting breast masses. Women should, however, be encouraged to report new or suspicious lumps that develop and, where appropriate, full investigation should not be delayed because of pregnancy. The risk of a definite lump being cancer in the under 40s is approximately 5 per cent, and late-stage diagnosis is commoner in pregnancy because of delayed referral and investigation. Nipple examination is not a good indicator of problems with breastfeeding and there is no intervention that improves feeding success in women with nipple inversion.

Abdomen

To examine the abdomen of a pregnant woman, place her in a semi-recumbent position on a couch or bed.

Women in late pregnancy or with multiple pregnancies may not be able to lie very flat. Sometimes a pillow under one buttock to move the weight of the fetus a little to the right or left can help. Cover the woman's legs with a sheet and make sure she is comfortable before you start. Always have a chaperone with you to perform this examination.

Think about what you hope to achieve from the examination and ask about areas of tenderness before you start.

Inspection
- Assess the shape of the uterus and note any asymmetry.
- Look for fetal movements.
- Look for scars (women often forget to mention previous surgical procedures if they were performed long ago). The common areas to find scars are:
  - suprapubic (Caesarean section, laparotomy for ectopic pregnancy or ovarian masses),
  - sub-umbilical (laparoscopy),
  - right iliac fossa (appendicectomy),
  - right upper quadrant (cholycystectomy).
- Note any striae gravidarum or linea nigra (the faint brown line running from the umbilicus to the symphysis pubis) – not because they mean anything, but because obstetricians like to see that students notice these.

Palpation
Symphysis–fundal height measurement
First, measure the symphysis–fundal height (SFH). This will give you a clue regarding potential problems such as polyhydramnios, multiple pregnancy or growth restriction before you start to palpate.

Feel carefully for the top of the fundus. This is rarely in the midline. Make a mental note of where it is. Now feel very carefully and gently for the upper border of the symphysis pubis. Place the tape measure on the symphysis pubis and, with the centimetre marks face down, measure to the previously noted top of the fundus. Turn the tape measure over and read the measurement. Plot the measurement on a SFH chart – this will usually be present in the hand-held notes. Many clinicians believe that the fundal height in centimetres should be equal to the number of weeks of gestation. In fact, if plotted on a correctly derived chart, it is apparent that the fundal height is usually approximately 2 cm less than the number of weeks. It is always important to use the chart where one is available (Fig. 1.2). Encourage women to ask to have their abdomen measured rather than just palpated at every visit and for the results to be plotted on the chart.

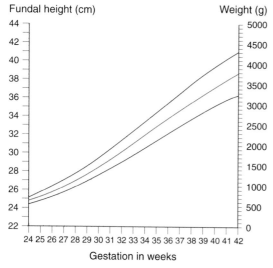

Figure 1.2 Customized symphysis–fundal height chart. (Courtesy of the West Midlands Perinatal Institute.)

Fetal lie, presentation and engagement

Before you start to palpate, you will have an idea about any potential problems. A large SFH raises the possibility of:

- macrosomia
- multiple pregnancy
- polyhydramnios.

Rarely, a twin is missed on ultrasound!

A small SFH could represent:

- IUGR
- oligohydramnios.

After you have measured the SFH, palpate to count the number of fetal poles (Fig. 1.3). A pole is a head or a bottom. If you can feel one or two, it is likely to be a singleton pregnancy. If you can feel three or four, a twin pregnancy is likely. Sometimes large fibroids can mimic a fetal pole; remember this if there is a history of fibroids.

Now you can assess the lie (Fig. 1.3d). This is only necessary as the likelihood of labour increases, i.e. after 34–36 weeks in an uncomplicated pregnancy.

If there is a pole over the pelvis, the lie is longitudinal regardless of whether the other pole is lying more to the left or right (Fig. 1.3b). An oblique lie is where the leading pole does not lie over the pelvis, but just to one side;

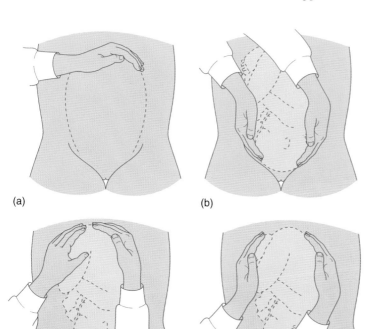

(a)

(b)

(c)

(d)

Figure 1.3 a–d Engagement of the fetal head in the maternal pelvic brim assessed. (a) Palpating the uterine fundus. (b) Assessing engagement of the fetal head. (c) and (d) Palpating fetal poles.

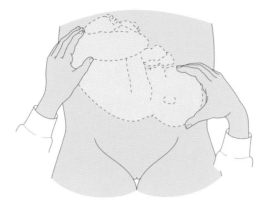

Figure 1.4 Abdominal palpation of the fetus lying transversely.

a transverse lie is where the fetus lies directly across the abdomen (Fig. 1.4). Once you have established that there is a pole over the pelvis, if the gestation is 34 weeks or more, you need to establish what the presentation is. It will be either cephalic (head down) or breech (bottom/feet down). Using a two-handed approach and watching the woman's face, gently feel for the presenting part (Fig. 1.3b). The head is generally much firmer than the bottom, although even in experienced hands it can sometimes be very difficult to tell. As you are feeling the presenting part in this way, assess whether it is engaged or not. If you can feel the whole of the fetal

head and it is easily movable, the head is likely to be 'free'. This equates to 5/5th palpable and is recorded as 5/5. As the head descends into the pelvis, less can be felt. When the head is no longer movable, it has 'engaged' and only 1/5th or 2/5th will be palpable (see Fig. 1.5). Do not use a one-handed technique, as this is much more uncomfortable for the woman.

Do not worry about trying to determine the fetal position (i.e. whether the fetal head is occipito-posterior, lateral or anterior). It makes no difference until labour begins, and even then is only of import-ance if progress in labour is slow. What is more, we do not often get it right, and women can be very troubled if told their baby is 'back to back'.

If the SFH is large and the fetal parts very difficult to feel, there may be polyhydramnios present. If the SFH is small and the fetal parts very easy to feel, oligohydramnios may be the problem.

Auscultation

If the fetus has been active during your examination, there is little need to auscultate the fetal heart, except that this is a ritual that mothers expect. If you are using a Pinard stethoscope, position it over the fetal shoulder (the *only* reason to assess the fetal position). Hearing the heart sounds with a Pinard takes a lot of practice. If you cannot hear the fetal heart, *never say*

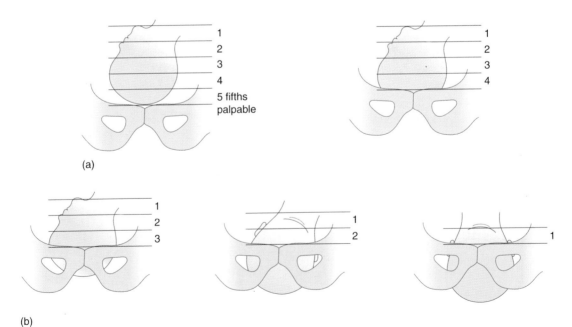

(a)

(b)

Figure 1.5 Palpation of the fetal head to assess engagement.

that you cannot detect a heart beat; always explain that a different method is needed and move on to use a hand-held Doppler device. If you have begun the process of listening to the fetal heart, you must proceed until you are confident that you have heard the heart. Hand-held Dopplers have the advantage that the mother can also hear the fetal heart. With twins, you must be confident that both have been heard.

Pelvic examination

Routine pelvic examination is not recommended. Given that as many as 18 per cent of women think that a pelvic examination can cause miscarriage, and at least 55 per cent find it an unpleasant experience, routine vaginal examination if ultrasound is planned has few advantages beyond the taking of a cervical smear. Consent must be sought and a female chaperone (nurse, midwife etc. – never a relative) present (regardless of the sex of the examiner). However, there are circumstances in which a vaginal examination is necessary (in most cases a speculum examination is all that is needed). These include:
- excessive or offensive discharge,
- vaginal bleeding (in the known absence of a placenta praevia),
- to perform a cervical smear,
- to confirm potential rupture of membranes.

A digital examination may be undertaken to perform a membrane sweep at term, prior to induction of labour.

The contraindications to digital examination are:
- known placenta praevia or vaginal bleeding when the placental site is unknown and the presenting part un-engaged,
- prelabour rupture of the membranes (increased risk of ascending infection).

Before commencing the examination, assemble everything you will need (swabs etc.) and ensure the light source works. Position the patient semi-recumbent with knees drawn up and ankles together. Ensure that the patient is adequately covered. If performing a speculum examination, a Cusco speculum is usually used (Fig. 1.6). Select an appropriate size.

Proceed as follows.
- Put on a pair of gloves.
- If the speculum is metal, warm it slightly under warm water first.

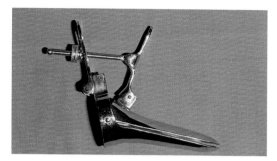
Figure 1.6 A Cusco speculum.

- Apply sterile lubricating gel or cream to the blades of the speculum. Do not use Hibitane cream if taking swabs for bacteriology.
- Gently part the labia.
- Introduce the speculum with the blades in the vertical plane.
- As the speculum is gently introduced, aiming towards the sacral promontory (i.e. slightly downward), rotate the speculum so that it comes to lie in the horizontal plane with the ratchet uppermost.
- The blades can then slowly be opened until the cervix is visualized. Sometimes minor adjustments need to be made at this stage.
- Assess the cervix and take any necessary samples.
- Gently close the blades and remove the speculum, reversing the manoeuvres needed to insert it. Take care not to catch the vaginal epithelium when removing the speculum.

A digital examination may be performed when an assessment of the cervix is required. This can provide information about the consistency and effacement of the cervix that is not obtainable from a speculum examination.

The patient should be positioned as before. Examining from the patient's right, two fingers of the gloved right hand are gently introduced into the vagina and advanced until the cervix is palpated. Prior to induction of labour, a full assessment of the Bishop's score can be made (Table 1.1).

Other aspects of the examination

In the presence of hypertension and in women with headache, fundoscopy should be performed. Signs of

Table 1.1 – Bishop score

	Score			
	0	1	2	3
Dilatation of cervix (cm)	0	1 or 2	3 or 4	5 or more
Consistency of cervix	Firm	Medium	Soft	–
Length of cervical canal (cm)	>2	2–1	1–0.5	<0.5
Position	Posterior	Central	Anterior	–
Station of presenting part (cm above ischial spine)	3	2	1 or 0	Below

chronic hypertension include silver-wiring and arterio-venous nipping. In severe pre-eclampsia and some intracranial conditions (space-occupying lesions, benign intracranial hypertension), papilloedema may be present.

Oedema of the extremities affects 80 per cent of term pregnancies. Its presence should be noted, but it is not a good indicator for pre-eclampsia as it is so common. To assess pre-tibial oedema, press reasonably firmly over the pre-tibial surface for 20 seconds. This can be very painful if there is excessive oedema, and when there is it is so obvious that testing for pitting is not necessary. More importantly, facial oedema should be commented upon.

When pre-eclampsia is suspected, the reflexes should be assessed. These are most easily checked at the ankle. The presence of more than three beats of clonus is pathological.

Presentation skills

Part of the art of taking a history and performing an examination is to be able to pass this information on to others in a clear and concise format. It is not necessary to give a full list of negative findings; it is enough to summarize negatives such as: there is no important medical, surgical or family history of note. Adapt your style of presentation to meet the situation. A very concise presentation is needed for a busy ward round. In an examination, a full and thorough

presentation may be required. Be very aware of giving sensitive information in a ward setting where other patients may be within hearing distance.

🔑 Key Points

- Always introduce yourself and say who you are.
- Make sure you are wearing your identity badge.
- Be courteous and gentle.
- Always ensure the patient is comfortable and warm.
- Always have a chaperone present when you examine patients.
- Tailor your history and examination to find the key information you need.
- Adapt to new findings as you go along.
- Present in a clear way.
- Be aware of giving sensitive information in a public setting.

History template

Demographic details

- Name
- Age
- Occupation
- Make a note of ethnic background
- Presenting complaint or reason for attending

This pregnancy

- Gestation, LMP or EDD
- Dates as calculated from ultrasound
- Single/multiple (chorionicity)
- Details of the presenting problem (if any) or reason for attendance (such as problems in a previous pregnancy)
- What action has been taken?
- Is there a plan for the rest of the pregnancy?
- What are the patient's main concerns?
- Have there been any other problems in this pregnancy?
- Has there been any bleeding, contractions or loss of fluid vaginally?

Ultrasound

- What scans have been performed?
- Why?
- Were any problems identified?

Past obstetric history

- List the previous pregnancies and their outcomes in order
- Gynaecological history
- Periods: regularity

Contraceptive history

- Previous infections and their treatment
- When was the last cervical smear? Was it normal? Have there ever been any that were abnormal? If yes, what treatment has been undertaken?
- Previous gynaecological surgery

Past medical and surgical history

- Relevant medical problems
- Any previous operations; type of anaesthetic used, any complications

Psychiatric history

- Postpartum blues or depression
- Depression unrelated to pregnancy
- Major psychiatric illness

Family history

- Diabetes, hypertension, genetic problems, psychiatric problems etc.

Social history

- Smoking/alcohol/drugs
- Marital status
- Occupation, partner's occupation
- Who is available to help at home?
- Are there any housing problems?

Drugs

- All medication including over-the-counter medication
- Folate supplementation

Allergies

- To what?
- What problems do they cause?

Modern maternity care

OVERVIEW

Modern maternity care has evolved over more than 100 years. Many of the changes have been driven by political and consumer pressure. Only recently has any good quality research been conducted into which aspects of care actually make a difference to women and their babies.

History of maternity care

The original impetus to address the health of mothers and children was driven by a lack of healthy recruits to fight in the Boer War. Up until this point, successive governments had paid little attention to maternal or child health. In 1929 the first government document stated a minimum standard for antenatal care that was so prescriptive in its recommendations that it is still practised in many regions, despite the lack of research to show that it is effective.

The introduction of the National Health Service Act of 1946 provided for maternity services to be available to all without cost. As part of these arrangements, a specified fee was paid to the general practitioner (GP) depending on whether he or she was on the obstetric list. This encouraged a large number of GPs to take an interest in maternity care, reversing the previous trend to leave this work to the midwives.

Antenatal care became perceived as beneficial, acceptable and available for all. This was reinforced by the finding that the perinatal death rate seemed to be inversely proportional to the number of antenatal visits. In 1963, the first perinatal mortality study showed that the perinatal mortality rate was lowest for those women attending between 10 and 24 times in pregnancy. This failed to take into account prematurity and poor education as reasons for decreased visits and increased mortality. However, antenatal care became established, and with increased professional contact came the drive to continue to improve outcomes with an emphasis on mortality (maternal and perinatal), without always establishing the need for or safety of all procedures or interventions for all women.

Even at this early time, the apportioning of antenatal care to different professionals was causing problems, with little communication between hospital and GP. It was not until the late 1950s that the idea of the co-operation card was devised. This allowed a continuous record to be held by the mother and improved communication between professionals.

The ability to see into the pregnant uterus in 1958 with ultrasound brought with it a revolution in antenatal care. This new intervention became quickly established and is now so much part of current antenatal care that the fact that its use in improving the outcome for low-risk women was never proven has been little questioned. Attending for the 'scan' has become such a social part of antenatal care that many surmise that it is for many women the sole reason for attending the hospital antenatal clinic.

The move towards hospital confinement began in the early 1950s. At this time, there were simply not the facilities to allow hospital confinement for all women, and 1 in 3 were planned home deliveries. The Cranbrook Report in 1959 recommended sufficient hospital maternity beds for 70 per cent of all confinements to take place in hospital, and the subsequent Peel Report (1970) recommended a bed available for every woman to deliver in hospital if she so wished.

The trend towards hospital confinement was not only led by obstetricians. Women themselves were pushing to at least be allowed the choice to deliver in hospital. By 1972, only 1 in 10 deliveries were planned for home, and the publication of the Social Services Committee report in (The Short Report 1980) led to further centralization of hospital confinement. It made a number of recommendations. Amongst these were:

> An increasing number of patients should be delivered in large units; selection of patients should be improved for smaller consultant units and isolated GP units; home deliveries should be phased out further.

> It should be mandatory that all pregnant women should be seen at least twice by a consultant obstetrician – preferably as soon as possible after the first visit to the GP in early pregnancy and again in late pregnancy.

This report and the subsequent reports Maternity Care in Action, Antenatal and Intrapartum Care, and Postnatal and Neonatal Care led to a policy of increasing centralization of units for delivery and consequently care. Thus home deliveries are now very infrequent events, with most regions reporting less than 2 per cent, the majority of these being unplanned.

The gradual decline in maternal and perinatal mortality was thought to be due in greater part to this move, although proof for this was lacking. Indeed, the decline in perinatal mortality was least in those years when hospitalization increased the most. As other new technologies became available, such as continuous fetal monitoring and the ability to induce labour, a change in practice began to establish these as the norm for most women. In England and Wales between 1966 and 1974, the induction rate rose from 12.7 per cent to 38.9 per cent.

The fact that these new technologies had not undergone thorough trials of benefit prior to introduction meant that benefit to the whole population of women was never established.

During the 1980s, with increasing consumer awareness, the unquestioning acceptance of unproven technologies was challenged. Women, led by the more vociferous groups such as the National Childbirth Trust (NCT), began to question not only the need for any intervention but also the need to come to the hospital at all. The professional bodies also began to question the effectiveness of antenatal care. The need to attend hospital as often as was occurring was debated and conclusions were drawn that the frequency, timing and effectiveness of antenatal visits are a form of care with an unknown effect which therefore requires further evaluation.

Once again in the early 1990s, the whole question of maternity care entered the political arena. The Winterton Committee heard evidence from all involved in maternity care on all sides:

> The Committee was stimulated into conducting the enquiry by its awareness of the fact that it was over a decade since the last major enquiry into maternity services by the Social Services Committee, and by hearing many voices saying that all was not well with the maternity services and that women had needs that were not being met.
> (House of Commons Select Committee, 1992)

The report culminated in a list of 98 conclusions and recommendations. The most important of which were:

> Given the absence of conclusive evidence, it is no longer acceptable that the pattern of maternity care provision should be driven by presumptions about the applicability of a medical model of care based on unproven assertions.

> We conclude that there is a strong desire among women for the provision of continuity of care and carer throughout pregnancy and childbirth, and that the majority of them regard midwives as the group best placed and equipped to provide this.

We are persuaded that the present imposition of a rigid pattern of frequent antenatal visits is not grounded in any good scientific base and that there is no evidence that such a pattern is medically necessary ... There is widespread agreement that this requires a more flexible system, which is based in the community, not in the hospital. The present system of shared care between the hospital and the community should, by and large, be abandoned. Hospitals are not the appropriate place to care for healthy women.

The Government set up an expert committee to review policy on maternity care and to make recommendations. This committee produced the document *Changing childbirth* (Department of Health, Report of the Expert Maternity Group, 1993), which essentially provided purchasers and providers with a number of action points aiming to improve choice, information and continuity for all women. It outlined a number of indicators of success to be achieved within 5 years:

- the carriage of hand-held notes by women,
- midwifery-led care in 30 per cent of pregnancies,
- a known midwife at delivery in 75 per cent of cases,
- a reduction in the number of antenatal visits for low-risk mothers.

Unfortunately, those targets which required significant financial input, such as the presence of a known midwife at 75 per cent of deliveries, have not been met. Nevertheless, this landmark report did provide a new impetus to examine the provision of maternity care in the UK and enshrine choice as a concept in maternity care.

Since *Changing childbirth*, a number of new initiatives and research have occurred.

Research into patterns of maternity care provision

The efficiency of antenatal care for mothers with problem-free pregnancies has been examined in much greater depth, with very interesting results. Comparisons between what was the 'standard' pattern of visits laid down in the 1929 document with a more flexible but reduced visit schedule show that women have outcomes as good as when seen more frequently, but have lower coping scores both antenatally and postnatally. In addition, many women prefer a rigid pattern of visits, as they feel nervous about scheduling their own appointments when they feel they need them.

Improved continuity of midwifery care has shown that midwives who care for women antenatally are less likely to perform episiotomy in labour, and that the women under their care undergo fewer inductions. They are also more likely to monitor the fetus intermittently. Women are more satisfied with most aspects of their care if they are cared for in a community setting. One interesting and reproducible finding has been that if 'low-risk' women attend the hospital as they would have done with traditional care shared between community midwife, GP and hospital consultant, they are significantly more likely to develop hypertension. This appears to be more than a labelling or 'white coat' hypertension problem, and the reasons for this finding remain unclear. This research has therefore confirmed that women with problem-free pregnancies are best managed in the community by midwives and GPs. The impact of this has been twofold. First, hospital antenatal clinics can concentrate time and expertise on those women who need it, and second, women cared for in the community should have better continuity at least for antenatal and postnatal care. One drawback that has been noticed, however, is that fewer GPs are interested in obstetrics, and minor problems of pregnancy, once the remit of GPs, are now devolving to hospitals.

First-class delivery

In 1997, the Audit Commission published the document *First class delivery: improving maternity services in England and Wales*. This reviewed the provision of maternity care in England and Wales and, very importantly, sent questionnaires to 3570 mothers. The recommendations of this document are that:

- trusts should:
  - ensure clinicians have access to good quality research and encourage development of guidelines and protocols,
  - improve the quality of written information, especially for antenatal screening and testing,
- commissioners should:
  - actively involve women in maternity services planning,
  - work closely with GPs,
  - take local users' views into account as well as cost.

A number of important organizations exist to help the above targets to be achieved. The ways in which various organizations have striven to meet these recommendations are discussed in the following sections.

Co-ordination of research: the Cochrane Collaboration (Fig. 2.1)

The study of the efficiency of pregnancy care has been revolutionized by the establishment of the Cochrane Collaboration. This has encouraged the evaluation of each aspect of antenatal care, and allowed each to be meticulously examined on the basis of the available trials. Concentrating particularly on the randomized controlled trial design, and using meta-analysis, obstetric practice has been scrutinized to an extent unique in medicine.

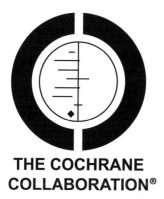

THE COCHRANE COLLABORATION®

Figure 2.1 The logo of the Cochrane Collaboration. (Reproduced with permission from the Cochrane Collaboration.)

The database originally grew from the publication of Archie Cochrane's *Effectiveness and efficiency: random reflections on health services* in 1972. The identification of controlled trials in perinatal medicine began in Cardiff in 1974. In 1978, the World Health Organization and English Department of Health funded work at the National Perinatal Epidemiology Unit, Oxford, UK, to assemble a register of controlled trials in perinatal medicine. Now the collaboration covers all branches of medicine. The findings are published in the Cochrane Library, which is free to access for all UK healthcare workers via the National Electronic Library for Health at www.nelh.nhs.uk. It is serially updated to keep up with published work and represents an enormous body of information available to the clinician.

Involvement of professional bodies and consumer groups in maternity care

Maternity care is considered so important that many clinical, political and consumer bodies are now involved in how it is provided.

National Institute for Clinical Excellence

As can be seen from the above, maternity care has been the subject of political debate for the last 100 years. More recently, attention has been paid to differences in standards of health care across the UK. The National Institute for Clinical Excellence (NICE) has begun to look at maternity care and has published three important guidelines. The first, on fetal monitoring in labour, was published in May 2001 and the second, on induction of labour, soon afterwards in June 2001. The third guideline on antenatal care was launched in October 2003. This is the first time antenatal care has been examined in detail since the original recommendations of the 1929 committee. This document should standardize the provision of care across the UK. There is a legal requirement for trusts to implement the recommendations in these guidelines, which can be seen on the NICE website (www.NICE.org.uk).

National Screening Committee

Screening has formed a part of antenatal care since its inception. Antenatal care is essentially screening in its widest form. However, screening for fetal disease has been implemented in a very haphazard way in the UK, often driven by single units and limited by funding issues. Currently there are marked countrywide discrepancies in:
- standards of ultrasound screening,
- tests offered for Down's syndrome screening,
- haemoglobinopathy screening.

The National Screening Committee is responsible for developing standards and strategies for the implementation of these. Already, nationwide screening for human immunodeficiency virus (HIV) has been implemented, with considerable benefits to babies born to infected mothers. Eventually all screening in pregnancy will be standardized across the National

Health Service (NHS), providing a more equitable standard of care.

The National Screening Committee has recently launched standards for screening for Down's syndrome. It has been instrumental in improvements in the quality of written information available to parents, has reduced duplication of effort and makes leaflets available to all trusts.

Royal College of Obstetricians and Gynaecologists

The Royal College of Obstetricians and Gynaecologists (RCOG) has many roles. These include developing guidelines, setting standards for the provision of care, training and revalidation, audit and research.

Guidelines and standards
The RCOG now has a large number of guidelines pertinent to pregnancy. Recent RCOG guidelines include the management of group B streptococcal carriage in pregnancy and the management of herpes simplex infection in pregnancy. These guidelines are accessible to all on the college website (www.rcog.org.uk). Standards have been set in areas such as the provision of maternity services and the quality of ultrasound examination in pregnancy.

Revalidation and continuing professional development
Revalidation of professionals is increasingly important. In order to be maintained on the General Medical Council Register, all doctors need to produce evidence that they are keeping up to date within their chosen specialty. Part of the revalidation process involves the co-ordination and documentation of education and professional developmental activity. The RCOG plays the major role in this important task. All practising obstetricians need to complete a 5-year cycle of education in order to be registered. The list of doctors whose educational programme is up to date is published by the college and available to the public.

Training
The college also has an important role in ensuring quality of training of doctors wishing to become consultants. It is recognized that with the limitations on working time that have come into force as a result of the European Working Time Directive, and a government initiative to limit total time in training, junior doctors now work many fewer hours than previously. Training is thus changing from an apprenticeship to a much more structured activity. The need to identify specific training areas has led to the development of special skills modules in obstetrics, which include labour ward management, maternal medicine and fetal medicine. Additionally there is a longer, 2–3-year, training scheme in maternal and fetal medicine, aimed at those who wish to train to become sub-specialists in this area. Only with improved time management and structured training can we allow trainees to become consultants with the requisite skills to deliver high quality care to mothers.

Confidential enquiries and audit
Another important role of the college is to co-ordinate national audit in conjunction with other bodies such as the Royal Colleges of Midwives, Paediatricians and Anaesthetists and NCT. The most recent audit, published by the RCOG Clinical Effectiveness Support Unit and entitled *The national sentinel Caesarean section audit report*, examined Caesarean sections across the UK. The audit came about as a result of concern regarding the increasing Caesarean section rate. It has provided interesting data for the trends in Caesarean section across the UK. The confidential enquiries are discussed in the next chapter.

Clinical Negligence Scheme for Trusts

Obstetrics is the highest litigation risk area in the NHS. It is estimated that the outstanding potential obstetric litigation bill is of the order of £200 million. As individual trusts cannot hope to meet the cost of huge settlements sometimes running into millions of pounds, an insurance scheme has been established. The Clinical Negligence Scheme for Trusts (CNST) was established by the NHS Executive in 1994 'to provide a means for Trusts to fund the costs of clinical negligence litigation and to encourage and support effective management of claims and risk'. The amount any individual trust has to pay to the scheme is graded from level 0 to 3. The insurance premium is discounted by 10 per cent for a level 1 trust, 20 per cent for level 2 and 30 per cent for level 3. In 2003, it was decided to assess obstetrics separately, as many trusts were failing on the obstetric standards only. The standards set by CNST are stringent. They cover:

- organization
- learning from experience

- communication
- clinical care
- documentation and note keeping
- clinical governance strategy
- staffing levels.

Trusts are assessed at least every 2 years. They can bring forward an assessment if they believe they have improved, as the financial implications of improved grading are great. This is the first time that improvements in maternity care have been linked to financial incentive, and measurable improvements in many units have been brought about as managers realize the importance of improving standards of care.

Consumer groups

There are now more consumer and support groups in existence than ever before. As well as providing support and advice for women, often at times of great need, they also allow women to have a louder voice in the planning and provision of maternity care. National consumer groups such as the NCT have representatives on many influential panels such as the National Screening Committee and RCOG working groups. At a local level, each trust should have a Maternity Services Liaison Committee (MSLC). When these committees work well, they can provide essential consumer input into service delivery at a local level. Consumers should make up at least one-third of the membership of the MSLCs. The influence of consumer groups can be huge: the recommendation that all women should have the right to deliver in hospital was essentially consumer led. Interestingly, it was this drive that led to the demise of many local units, the centralization of obstetric services and a huge reduction in the numbers of home deliveries, something that consumer groups are now trying

to reverse. Many groups have been criticized as being unrepresentative of the whole population. This will continue to be so, as disenfranchised groups are less able to co-ordinate themselves to be heard. However, many groups are making efforts to canvass the opinions of those rarely heard, such as teenagers and women who speak little or no English.

Choice is now being sought by consumers in a way never experienced before. *The national sentinel Caesarean section audit report* showed that maternal choice as a reason for Caesarean section is becoming increasingly common, a move driven, at least in part, by high-profile women choosing not to undergo labour with their first baby. Consumer groups will need to lead the way in deciding how far choice should be balanced against the financial constraints of a free-at-the-point-of-care health service. The guidelines on Caesarean section produced by NICE promote the ideal of Caesarean section for obstetric indications only, although they do not go as far as recommending that women's preferences be completely ignored.

✂ Key Points

- Maternity care will continue to be a political arena, as it has been for nearly 100 years.
- There is increasing public interest in the results of national audits such as the confidential enquiries (see next chapter) and *The national sentinel Caesarean section audit report*.
- Antenatal care is subject to national standards in a way never seen before.
- The need for trusts to reduce insurance costs is leading to improved standards of care across the UK.
- National guidelines now cover almost all aspects of maternity care and should lead to standardization of care across the UK.

Additional reading

Audit Commission for Local Health Authorities and the National Health Service in England and Wales. *First class delivery: improving maternity services in England and Wales*. London: HSMO, 1997.

CNST standards for maternity services: available online at www.nhsla.com

Cochrane Library: available online at www.nelh.nhs.uk

Department of Health. *Changing childbirth*. Report of the Expert Maternity Group. London: HMSO, 1993.

Royal College of Obstetricians and Gynaecologists Clinical Effectiveness Support Unit. *The national sentinel Caesarean section audit report*. London: RCOG Press, 2001.

Chapter 3

Maternal and perinatal mortality: the Confidential Enquiries

OVERVIEW

Worldwide, childbearing poses the major risk to the life of a woman. Whilst in developed countries it is assumed that childbirth is a safe process, for the majority of women in the world this is not the case. Without any health care whatsoever, 2 per cent of women will die during their pregnancy due to complications. Estimates from the World Health Organization (WHO) in 2001 suggest that complications during pregnancy and childbirth are responsible for the deaths of 515 000 women each year. For women in sub-Saharan Africa, the area of greatest mortality, the lifetime risk of dying as a result of childbirth is 1 in 13. In addition, for every mother who dies, as many as 30 will suffer injury and serious long-term complications.

Worldwide causes of maternal mortality

The major causes of death in pregnancy and the puerperium globally are shown in Figure 3.1.

Together, haemorrhage and infection account for almost half of all deaths. Deaths related to indirect causes are becoming more common, as human immunodeficiency virus (HIV) increases in prevalence.

The impact of care at various stages in pregnancy, labour and the puerperium has been assessed. Skilled attendance at birth was set as a benchmark for the improvement of maternal health care in 1999 by the United Nations, as it is becoming increasingly clear that skilled care at delivery is a major need, the commonest cause of maternal death being haemorrhage. Despite much effort, not all areas have improved the access to this level of care.

Figure 3.2 shows the trends in skilled care at delivery in 1990 and 2000 based on 51 countries with trend data.

As can be seen from Figure 3.3, only 53 per cent of women in developing countries have access to skilled

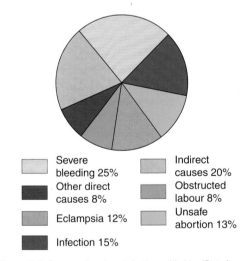

Figure 3.1 Causes of maternal death worldwide. (Data from the Safe Motherhood Project.)

- Severe bleeding 25%
- Other direct causes 8%
- Eclampsia 12%
- Infection 15%
- Indirect causes 20%
- Obstructed labour 8%
- Unsafe abortion 13%

health care in labour, and even fewer have access to postnatal care.

Interestingly, antenatal care itself can only reduce maternal mortality to a limited extent, though many

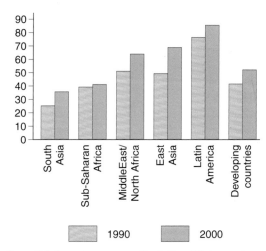

Figure 3.2 Percentage women attended by skilled carer at delivery, 1990–2000. (Source: UNICEF, 2001.)

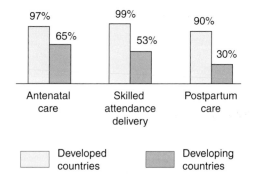

Figure 3.3 Access to skilled care during pregnancy, labour and the puerperium. (Source: Coverage of maternal care: A listing of available information, 4th edn. Geneva: WHO, 1997.)

of its interventions benefit the health of the baby. A WHO study has demonstrated that in the developing world, the ability of care to identify current risk is much more effective than trying to identify potential risk. This almost certainly stems from the fact that most women in developing countries are at some risk during pregnancy, due to intercurrent illness, anaemia or multiple previous pregnancies. Where no maternal risk is identified, it would appear that four antenatal visits are the most that is required during pregnancy. More care is needed for delivery and in the postpartum period than is currently provided in many areas.

As well as poor access to health care, the rapidly evolving acquired immunodeficiency syndrome (AIDS) epidemic is also hampering efforts to improve outcomes for both mothers and babies. In many areas of sub-Saharan Africa, 30 per cent of women of childbearing age are infected with HIV.

Any strategy for maternal mortality reduction in sub-Saharan Africa or South Asia today needs to take the rapidly evolving pandemic into account. In countries such as South Africa and Zambia, AIDS and related complications already contribute significantly to the indirect causes of maternal death (see Fig. 3.1).

A global initiative was launched at a conference held in Nairobi, Kenya, in 1987. Its aim was to draw the world's attention to the thousands of deaths and millions of serious illnesses that afflict women every year. The Nairobi conference was co-sponsored by a group of international agencies that founded the Safe Motherhood Interagency Group.

The aims of the Safe Motherhood Project are to improve access to health care. Safe motherhood can be achieved by providing high quality maternal health services to all women during pregnancy, childbirth and the postpartum period. The Safe Motherhood Project aims to provide:

- care by skilled health personnel before, during and after childbirth,
- emergency care for life-threatening obstetric complications,
- services to prevent and manage the complications of unsafe abortion,
- family planning to enable women to plan their pregnancies and prevent unwanted pregnancies,
- health education and services for adolescents,
- community education for women, their families and decision makers.

Working with this project, many other agencies, including the United Nations, have been assessing the impact of various schemes on maternal mortality. Unfortunately not all news is good, and in many areas few changes have been made (see Fig. 3.2).

Maternal and perinatal mortality in the UK

The death of a woman in childbirth is now a rare event in the UK. Although the safety of the mother is now taken for granted in this country, people are well aware that pregnancy carries risks for the baby's life. It is standard practice for each hospital to monitor the numbers of its stillbirths and neonatal deaths, and any change in the perinatal mortality rate is of local concern. Perinatal mortality is now also being examined on a nationwide basis in England, Wales and Northern Ireland, and new lessons are being learned about why babies die. Health improvement targets are now a national agenda, with the aim of reducing the numbers of teenage mothers with unplanned pregnancies and the rates of delivery of low-birth-weight babies.

Maternal and perinatal deaths in the UK are subject to confidential enquiry, conducted mainly by doctors and midwives. The confidential nature of the enquiries encourages openness amongst staff and allows investigators to obtain a clearer picture of what happened in a culture of 'low blame'. The reporting is anonymized before being seen by the regional assessors. By this means, recommendations for improvements in care can be made without direct identification of either the patient or hospital involved. The findings of the national confidential enquiries are made public in regular reports. The reporting of maternal and infant deaths is funded through the National Institute for Clinical Excellence (NICE) and is managed by a Consortium of Royal Colleges:

- Royal College of Obstetricians and Gynaecologists
- Royal College of Midwives
- Royal College of Paediatrics and Child Health
- Royal College of Pathologists
- Royal College of Anaesthetists
- Faculty of Public Health

and is called the Confidential Enquiry into Maternal and Child Health (CEMACH).

Maternal and perinatal mortality: the confidential enquiries

Maternal mortality

In order to make accurate historical or international comparisons, clear definitions are needed; deaths can be maternal, direct, indirect, late or fortuitous.

Definitions
- *Maternal death*: death of a woman while pregnant, or within 42 days of termination of pregnancy, from any cause related to, or aggravated by, the pregnancy or its management, but not from accidental or incidental causes.
- *Direct deaths*: resulting from obstetric complications of the pregnant state (pregnancy, labour and puerperium), from interventions, omissions, incorrect treatment or from a chain of events resulting from any of the above (e.g. death from major postpartum haemorrhage in a previously well woman).

- *Indirect deaths*: resulting from previous existing disease, or disease that developed during pregnancy and which was not due to direct obstetric causes, but which was aggravated by the physiologic effects of pregnancy that are due to direct or indirect maternal causes (e.g. death from a cardiac lesion, such as Ebstein's anomaly).
- *Late deaths*: occurring between 42 days and 1 year after abortion, miscarriage or delivery that are due to direct or indirect maternal causes.
- *Coincidental (fortuitous) deaths*: from unrelated causes that happen to occur in pregnancy or the puerperium (e.g. road traffic accidents).

Maternal mortality rate

This is defined in the UK as the number of deaths from obstetric causes per 100 000 maternities. 'Maternities' are the number of mothers delivered of registerable live births at any gestation or stillbirths of 24 weeks or later. The WHO definitions differ slightly, so care is needed when comparing figures.

Trends in the UK

The maternal mortality rate (MMR) in Britain has been recorded reliably since 1847, and its history over the last 150 years can be divided into three phases.

Phase 1

Throughout the period from 1847 until 1934, the rate remained virtually unchanged at around 400 per 100 000 or 1 in 250 births. Other indicators of public health, such as infant mortality, had begun to fall well before 1935 and the MMR may have been kept artificially high through neglect of asepsis and excessive use of forceps under chloroform anaesthesia by general practitioner obstetricians.

At the end of the First World War, one mother died for every 264 babies born alive, but over the next 14 years this figure rose to one mother dying for every 238 live births. In 1924, the first government report devoted specifically to maternal mortality was published. It was written by Janet Campbell, Senior Medical Officer to the newly created Ministry of Health. She felt that many maternal deaths were avoidable and conducted her own confidential enquiry into deaths. She investigated a sample of deaths from puerperal fever and found that in many cases antenatal care had been lacking, with only 48 of 256 women receiving any antenatal care at all. She found that if the quality of professional attendance in pregnancy, at delivery and postnatally was good, nearly all of the other likely causes of maternal mortality became of minor importance.

In 1929, the government produced a document covering the conduct and scope of antenatal clinics (Maternal Mortality Committee, Ministry of Health, 1929). This was so precise in its outline for antenatal care that the pattern of visits set is still practised in many regions today. In fact, there was little empirical evidence to support the timing or scope of these visits, and the document was based on a survey of what was happening at those clinics already established.

Phase 2

A dramatic fall in maternal mortality occurred between 1935 and 1985, when the MMR halved every decade (Fig. 3.4). This fall is often seen as part of a general improvement in public health, but the timing suggests the effect of other factors besides improved social conditions. Indeed, as the fall began during the 1930s depression and continued through the Second World War, improved social conditions may have been only a minor factor. Other improvements were as follows.

- Antibiotics: sulphonamides were introduced in 1937 and penicillin appeared during the Second World War. Death rates from puerperal sepsis quickly fell (Fig. 3.4).

- In 1936 the Midwives Act came into being, making it the responsibility of the local authorities to provide a salaried midwife who was responsible for attending births and thus limiting the previous role of unqualified birth attendants.
- Blood transfusion became safe during the 1940s.
- Ergometrine, for the treatment and prevention of postpartum haemorrhage, was introduced in the 1940s.
- Obstetrics became recognized as a specialty and the Royal College of Obstetricians and Gynaecologists was founded in 1929.
- Reduced parity: the average family size had already begun to fall before the oral contraceptive pill was introduced in 1961.
- Legalization of abortion in 1967 was followed by elimination of criminal abortion as a cause of maternal death.

Phase 3

Since 1985, there has been little change in the MMR in the UK, and although there are minor fluctuations, it is likely that we have now reached a steady state. This does not mean that the number of maternal deaths has reached an irreducible minimum, but any improvements will take much more effort. Also, whilst improvements can be made, the emphasis in maternity

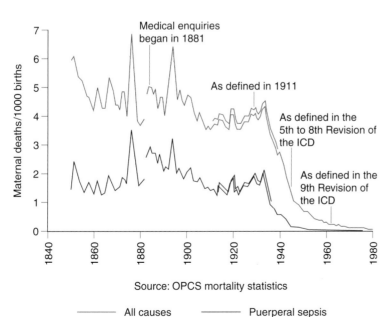

Figure 3.4 Maternal mortality rate in the UK, 1847–1980. (From *Report on Confidential Enquiries into Maternal Deaths in England and Wales 1982–84*).

Medical enquiries began in 1881

As defined in 1911

As defined in the 5th to 8th Revision of the ICD

As defined in the 9th Revision of the ICD

Maternal deaths/1000 births

Source: OPCS mortality statistics

——— All causes   ——— Puerperal sepsis

care has changed from a philosophy of achieving safety at all costs to one of trying to balance safety with the wishes of mothers to have choice in their care.

There are likely to be major changes in how maternity care is provided in the future. The establishment of neonatal networks will lead to scaling down of some maternity units, and the European Working Time Directive will lead to changes in trainees' experience. The role of the confidential enquiries will continue to be vital as a marker for changes in care for either the better or the worse.

Causes of maternal mortality

As noted above, the enquiries are conducted by clinicians: doctors including obstetricians, anaesthetists, pathologists and midwives.

Methods of enquiry

When a woman dies during or within a year following pregnancy, the Director of Public Health Medicine sends an enquiry form to the general practitioners, midwives, health visitors, obstetricians and any other staff involved in her care. The form requests full information about the case.

The completed form is then sent to regional assessors in obstetrics, midwifery, anaesthesia (if appropriate) and pathology. When they have added their comments, the form is sent to the Chief Medical Officer. It is made anonymous and then passed to central assessors of the same disciplines to assess the causes of death and decide whether any aspects of the care were substandard.

Every 3 years a national report is published, which collates all the cases, draws attention to areas of 'substandard care' and makes recommendations. The report excludes any details that might allow identification of individual cases.

This system originally applied to England, though arrangements were similar in the rest of the UK. The last four national reports have covered the whole of the UK, again making it difficult for individual cases to be identified (Fig. 3.5).

Causes of maternal mortality in the UK

In the triennium 1997–99 there were 378 maternal deaths, of which 242 were direct (106) or indirect (136) and the remainder were coincidental (29) or late (107) deaths. For the first time, the number of indirect deaths exceeded the number of direct deaths. The causes are shown in Table 3.1.

Direct deaths

Thromboembolism

During pregnancy, changes in the clotting factors occur and women enter a hypercoagulable state. Labour and the puerperium may cause venous stasis, particularly after Caesarean section. Death from thromboembolism can occur at any stage of pregnancy, even in the first trimester or after an ectopic pregnancy. The risk is

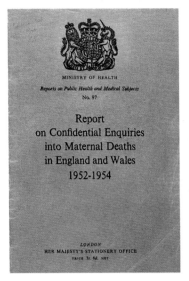

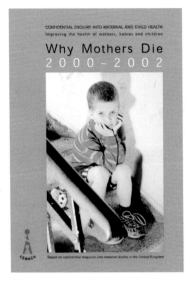

(a)   (b)

Figure 3.5 Maternal mortality reports. (Crown copyright material is reproduced with the permission of the Controller of Her Majesty's Stationery Office.)

Table 3.1 – Causes of direct and indirect maternal deaths, 1997–99

Cause of death	Number of deaths
Direct deaths	
Thrombosis and thromboembolism	35
Hypertensive disease	15
Haemorrhage	7
Sepsis	14
Amniotic fluid embolism	8
Ectopic pregnancy	13
Spontaneous miscarriage	2
Legal termination	2
Genital tract trauma	2
Anaesthetic	3
Fatty liver	4
Other direct causes	1
Indirect deaths	
Cardiac disease	35
Psychiatric disorder	15
Other indirect causes	75
Indirect malignancies	11

highest in the early puerperium and continues until about 6 weeks postnatally.

There has been a dramatic fall in deaths from thromboembolism after the previous enquiry recommended a schedule for thromboembolism prophylaxis after Caesarean section, from 2.1 to 1.45 deaths per 100 000 maternities. The rates had been gradually rising until this point.

Interestingly, the rates of death from pulmonary embolism after vaginal delivery have been rising. It is recognized that risk factors for thromboembolic disease include obesity and increasing age, both of which are becoming more common in the childbearing population.

More attention is now being focused on the recognition of higher risk amongst women delivering vaginally. In addition to the above factors, immobility and family history are also risk factors. Prophylaxis may include good hydration (many women become dehydrated during labour), thromboembolic deterrent stockings and intermittent subcutaneous heparin.

The most recent enquiry has published a guideline for thromboprophylaxis after vaginal delivery.

Hypertensive disorders
The number of deaths from hypertensive disease has been gradually declining since 1970. Better management of hypertension, the introduction of magnesium sulphate for the management of severe pre-eclampsia and eclampsia, and better anaesthetic care have all contributed to these improvements. The largest single cause of death due to hypertension amongst the 15 women who died was intracranial haemorrhage, accounting for seven deaths. This suggests that failure to control hypertension is now the major problem. Complications of hypertensive disease led to the deaths of four women. Interesting, only one woman had pulmonary complications (adult respiratory distress syndrome) and no women died from pulmonary oedema. This is a major improvement from previous enquiries and probably relates to much better understanding of fluid management in these women, leading to far less fluid overload.

The areas in which care was substandard continue to be:
• poor communication,
• late involvement of senior staff,
• delay in managing severe hypertension.

Haemorrhage
This is the leading cause of maternal death worldwide but in the UK it now only accounts for a few deaths each year. In the last report, seven direct deaths were investigated: three due to placenta praevia, three from abruption and one postpartum haemorrhage. The enquiry has noted repeatedly that deliveries where there is known to be a placenta praevia should be attended by a consultant obstetrician and anaesthetist. Life-saving decisions about proceeding to hysterectomy are made earlier by more senior doctors.

Genital tract sepsis
This, the other major cause of maternal death worldwide, accounted for 14 deaths in 1997–99 in the UK. The rate of death due to sepsis is rising (4 per million maternities in 1985–87 compared to 8.4 in the most recent report). In many cases, failure to recognize the severity of infection contributed to death. Group A *Streptococcus* continues to kill women in the UK, as it has done for many hundreds of years. We appear to have become more complacent with regard to infection than our forebears.

Amniotic fluid embolism

In this condition, amniotic fluid enters the maternal circulation and causes massive disseminated intravascular coagulopathy, activating the clotting cascade through a thromboplastin-mediated pathway. This leads to rapid consumption of clotting factors and platelets, with platelet–fibrin clumps being deposited in the lungs, kidneys and brain. Proof of the diagnosis is the finding of fetal squames in the maternal lungs at post mortem, though cases for which the index of suspicion is very high can now be reported. It causes sudden collapse, usually during labour, although cases have been reported after Caesarean section, and it carries a high mortality. It was formerly thought to be associated with high parity, but only one of the eight cases reported in 1997–99 was of high parity. Five out of the eight cases were associated with induction or augmentation of labour. The rates of death in this category have declined significantly (from 35 reported in 1994–96), although the reasons for this are not clear.

Early pregnancy deaths

Deaths occurring before 24 weeks' gestation are now included in this category (formerly the upper limit was 20 weeks). They include deaths due to ectopic pregnancy, spontaneous abortion and termination of pregnancy. Seventeen deaths due to early pregnancy were reported.

Ectopic pregnancy

The rate of death attributable to ectopic pregnancy has not fallen over the last four triennia, 13 women dying in 1997–99. However, it is known that the incidence of ectopic pregnancy across the UK has risen during the last decade to approximately 1 in every 150 pregnancies. The most commonly identified fault contributing to death was failure to consider ectopic pregnancy as a diagnosis. Many women presented with atypical urinary or gastrointestinal symptoms and without vaginal bleeding. If abdominal pain is associated with a positive pregnancy test, the woman should be referred to hospital. Clear guidelines for the management of suspected ectopic pregnancy should be followed, as it is sometimes a difficult diagnosis to make.

Miscarriage

Four deaths occurred from this cause in 1997–99, two of which were attributable to infection and were potentially avoidable.

Termination of pregnancy

It is now more than 15 years since the last maternal death from illegal abortion in Britain, but a small number of deaths from legal abortion continue to occur. In 1997–99, there were two deaths. One woman developed thrombotic thrombocytopenic purpura, and one woman appeared to have suffered an amniotic fluid embolism. It is unlikely that either of these deaths was avoidable.

Genital tract trauma

Only two deaths occurred as a result of genital tract trauma in 1997–99. One was associated with a ruptured uterus and the other was of a woman who delivered alone at home and sustained a vaginal wall tear.

Anaesthesia

Anaesthesia in obstetrics has undergone tremendous changes over the last 40 years. Regional techniques have taken over in the main from general anaesthesia, and epidural analgesia has become a safe technique for most women. The rates of death directly attributable to anaesthesia fell until 1996. In the last triennium, a small rise, to three cases, was seen. These were all difficult cases in which some substandard care contributed to the deaths. The recommendation that the dose of intravenous Syntocinon should be limited to 5 units has come about because of one of the deaths.

Indirect deaths

Cardiac disease

Heart disease is now the joint most common cause of maternal death, with 35 recorded deaths. Rheumatic heart disease is rarely encountered. The major groups comprise congenital heart disease, ischaemic heart disease and cardiomyopathy.

Pulmonary hypertension and Eisenmenger's syndrome carry maternal mortality rates of 30–50 per cent. Pulmonary vascular problems accounted for seven of the ten deaths due to congenital heart disease. Patients with known heart disease should be managed by a cardiologist in co-operation with an obstetrician. There may be some women for whom pregnancy should be avoided. However, care should be taken in counselling these women so that they do not feel unable to seek medical care if they do become pregnant.

Psychiatric deaths

In the 1994–96 report, deaths from psychiatric causes were discussed separately for the first time. Prior to this, they had been considered under the coincidental category. In the 1997–99 report, psychiatric disorder contributed to the deaths of 42 women, 28 due to suicide. As a single category, psychiatric disorder is the largest cause of death amongst women. The category covers a diverse range of problems, including suicide, illicit drug use, alcohol abuse and murder. The report once again recommends screening at booking for psychiatric disorder, substance abuse or severe social problems, and a liaison service provided for patients identified as at risk.

Other indirect deaths
Many diseases are exacerbated by pregnancy, but of the total of 75 deaths in 1997–99, epilepsy was a major contributor (as in the previous triennium), causing nine deaths. This is a large drop from the 19 reported in the previous report, after which recommendations were made to reduce the risk to mothers with epilepsy.

Multi-disciplinary care of women with medical disease is recommended to reduce the problems encountered in many cases.

Additional points in management

Improvements in case ascertainment in the last enquiry allow a complete picture of maternal mortality to develop. The clear relationship between maternal age and mortality continues to be seen. Deaths among the very young occur almost entirely in a group of women who are severely socially excluded, with physical and sexual abuse commonly encountered. Women undergoing fertility treatment are at particular risk: in-vitro fertilization (IVF) pregnancies have an estimated maternal mortality rate of 48.4 per 100 000.

Data relating to ethnicity are only estimated in the 1997–99 report, as the data collection method does not stratify by ethnic origin, only country of birth. Despite this, it is estimated that mortality rates are highest amongst women from a Pakistani/Indian or Bangladeshi background. Late booking and poor attendance were seen as major contributors in this group. Additionally, this group comprised the largest number of non-English speakers. The highest maternal mortality rates for ethnic groups occur amongst the travellers. These data are not reliably collected yet,

but ten deaths amongst travellers must be a disproportionately large number.

Social class data were analysed for the first time in the 1997–99 report and confirmed what had long been suspected, that women from the most deprived sectors of the community have a maternal mortality rate 20 times greater than women in the two highest social categories.

Recommendations have been made to encourage flexibility within the provision of antenatal care and to improve access to interpreters where language problems may occur.

The enquiries must not only gather accurate data, but must also interpret them intelligently. This involves regular reappraisal, particularly with a long-running enquiry. The recent realization that maternal suicide is now one of the major causes of mortality is an example of this, and highlights the need for better service provision.

'Near-miss' enquiries
As the number of maternal deaths has declined in Britain, there have been suggestions that instead of looking only at deaths, enquiries should be widened to include 'near misses' – incidents that might have resulted in a maternal death but for prompt and effective treatment. A 'near miss' is difficult to define, and national figures would probably be much less reliable than data on maternal deaths.

Nevertheless, 'near misses' have been examined on a local basis, using criteria such as admission to an intensive care unit. In a comprehensive survey in Pretoria, South Africa, a full list of criteria for 'near misses' has been developed. Life-threatening maternal haemorrhage affects 1 in 1000 pregnancies, most of which are well managed.

New developments

Low maternal mortality rates in developed countries are now taken for granted and there is a tendency for people to forget what risks there are when care is not available. The aim now is to remove unnecessary restrictions without compromising safety. It is unlikely that rates of maternal mortality will rise again while they are carefully monitored, but our aim should be to reduce them still further. This is quite a challenge, because as maternity care and maternal health improve, life-threatening events become even less common, and as a result staff are less practised in dealing with them.

Many units now practise emergency 'drills', along the same lines as cardiac arrest drills. These allow staff to develop team working and test systems in response to situations such as major haemorrhage, unexpected maternal collapse and eclamptic fits. Data that demonstrate the improvements in management with these are difficult to find, but many units can show an improvement in staff confidence in dealing with rare and life-threatening situations. Other professions that use similar training techniques have shown that local training is better than sending individuals away on courses, and that encouraging team working is the key to success.

Perinatal mortality

Perinatal death is about 100 times more common than maternal death. Perinatal mortality rates therefore often seem more relevant to day-to-day practice and, because of the larger numbers of cases, they perhaps give a clearer picture of the problems that may be encountered. However, analysis of individual cases at a national level is more difficult because of the large numbers.

As with maternal mortality data, the diagnosis of death is unequivocal. Comparison between countries is often difficult, as definitions of the dividing line between miscarriage and stillbirth vary.

Definitions

The definitions that follow are those used by CEMACH (Fig. 3.6), which is described below. Until 2003, the reports were written and published by the Confidential Enquiry into Stillbirths and Deaths in Infancy (CESDI). CEMACH has now taken over this role.

CESDI looked at all deaths from 20 weeks of pregnancy to the end of the first year of life, but only a proportion of these fulfil the definition of 'perinatal deaths'. For example, death between 20 and 24 weeks of pregnancy is not counted in the perinatal mortality statistics.

- Stillbirth: any fetus born with no signs of life after 24 weeks' gestation. (Note that the British definition of stillbirth was changed in October 1992. Before that time, only deaths after 28 weeks' gestation were included. The change in definition added nearly 30 per cent to the former official stillbirth rate.) Of particular importance in the definition is that it is *delivery* of the baby which

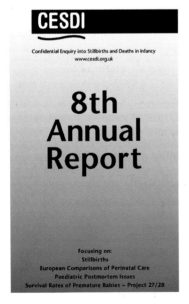

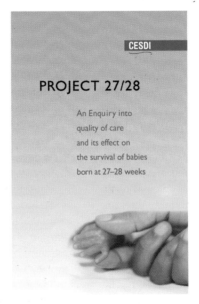

Figure 3.6 Confidential Enquiry into Stillbirths and Deaths in Infancy: (a) 8th Annual Report, (b) Project 27/28. Reproduced with permission.

(a)   (b)

dates the stillbirth and not the point in the pregnancy at which the baby was known to die. This is only usually of note where there has been a retained dead fetus for many weeks, such as may occur in multiple pregnancies.

- Early neonatal death: death in the first week after birth.
- Perinatal death: all stillbirths plus deaths in the first week after birth.
- Perinatal mortality rate (PMR): the number of stillbirths and early neonatal deaths per 1000 live births and stillbirths.
- Late fetal loss: deaths occurring between 20 + 0 weeks and 23 weeks + 6 days. If gestation is not sure, all births of at least 300 g are reported.

In addition to these cases, CEMACH gathers data on deaths beyond the first week after birth. These definitions are given below.

- Late neonatal death: death of a neonate from age 7 days to 27 completed days of life.
- Post-neonatal death: death of a baby at age 28 days and over, but under 1 year.
- Infant death: death at age under 1 year of a baby born alive.

Rates of neonatal and infant death are expressed as rates per 1000 live births (i.e. they do not include stillbirths and late fetal losses).

The worldwide picture

Across the world, there are wide differences in perinatal mortality rates. Overall, life expectancy in some countries is less than half that in others, and this is largely due to high death rates in small children.

Accurate figures for perinatal mortality worldwide are often lacking. The WHO estimates that there are between 7 and 8 million perinatal deaths annually: a global perinatal mortality rate of 50–60 compared to 7.9 in the UK.

Malnutrition, gastrointestinal disease, HIV infection and population dislocation due to war remain the commonest causes of child death.

Strategies aimed at improving the situation for the world's children include:

- promotion of breastfeeding,
- improving maternal education,
- encouraging contraceptive usage (especially barrier methods),
- settlement of Third World debt.

HIV poses a major problem in sub-Saharan Africa particularly. The risk of mother-to-child transfer of HIV is 25–35 per cent and 20 per cent of infected infants will develop AIDS or die within their first year. By 6 years of age, 23 per cent will have died and 30–40 per cent will have AIDS. The balance of risks still favours breastfeeding in areas of high prevalence, as the risk of death from gastroenteritis remains higher in this population.

Amongst developed countries, comparisons of PMRs can be misleading because different countries have minor variations in definitions.

History in the UK

Data on perinatal mortality have been collected in the UK for the last 60 years, during which time there has been a dramatic reduction in perinatal deaths. This has been mainly due to the improved health of the population, better nutrition and wider education, though the healthcare profession may also take some credit.

Since 1963, stillbirth and neonatal death rates in England and Wales have fallen steadily. In 1963, the stillbirth rate was over 17 per 1000 births and the neonatal death rate was over 14 per 1000 births. In 1999, these rates were respectively 5.0 and 3.9. The Eighth Annual Report published in 2002 gives the figures for 1999. There has been a fall in the perinatal mortality rate over a 6-year period, mainly due to a fall in stillbirths. This appears to be due to improvements in obstetric care.

Method of the confidential enquiry

CESDI was set up in 1992 to improve understanding of how the risks of death from 20 weeks of pregnancy to 1 year after birth might be reduced. In 2003, the roles of the two confidential enquiries were amalgamated into the single CEMACH. CEMACH attempts to identify risks that can be attributed to sub-optimal clinical care.

The enquiry covers England, Wales and Northern Ireland. A rapid reporting form is the notification system used. Its aims are:

- to obtain a data set within the CESDI range for all deaths between 20 weeks' gestation and 1 year of life,
- to provide information as soon as possible, to support the enquiry process.

All deaths are notified to the regional co-ordinator so that a full picture of the causes of death is obtained. In addition, a specialist panel within each region reviews a sub-set of anonymous cases. The regional data and enquiry findings are collated by a central secretariat to provide a national overview and are published in an annual report.

Each panel consists of experts from several disciplines, including, as a minimum, an obstetrician, paediatrician, midwife, specialist perinatal/paediatric pathologist, general practitioner and independent chairman. Others with appropriate expertise may also be involved. Panel members are sent anonymous case notes and they summarize their cases and meet for discussion. There is no feedback to individuals or units, but the findings are published as a report.

The panel comments on sub-optimal care, grading each case as follows.
- Grade 0: no sub-optimal care.
- Grade 1: sub-optimal care, but different management would have made no difference to the outcome.
- Grade 2: sub-optimal care, and different management might have made a difference to the outcome.
- Grade 3: sub-optimal care, and different management would reasonably have been expected to make a difference to the outcome.

The special programmes of CESDI

CESDI has also worked to look at individual topics as well as providing general statistics. These individual projects have been seminal in changing the care provided. The programme of special studies is shown below.

Enquiry topics
- Intrapartum-related deaths > 2.5 kg.
- Intrapartum-related deaths < 1.5 kg.
- 'Explained' sudden deaths in infancy.
- A 1 in 10 sample of all deaths > 1.0 kg.
- All deaths 4 kg and over.

Case control studies
- Sudden unexpected deaths in infancy.
- Antepartum stillbirths.
- Project 27/28 (deaths at these gestations).

Focus groups and review
- Shoulder dystocia.
- Ruptured uterus.

- Planned home delivery.
- Anaesthetic complications and delays.
- Breech presentation at the onset of labour.
- Stillbirths.

Audits and collaborative work
- Post-mortem reporting.
- Cardiotocography education.
- European comparisons of perinatal care.
- Use of electronic fetal monitoring.

Classification systems

CEMACH uses three systems of classification: the extended Wrigglesworth classification, the Obstetric (Aberdeen) classification and the Fetal and Neonatal Factor classification. There is wide overlap between these three systems.

Extended Wrigglesworth classification
- Category 1: congenital defect or malformation (lethal or severe).
- Category 2: unexplained antepartum fetal death.
- Category 3: death from intrapartum asphyxia, anoxia or trauma.
- Category 4: immaturity.
- Category 5: infection where there is clear microbiological support for the diagnosis.
- Category 6: other specific causes.
- Category 7: accident or non-intrapartum trauma.
- Category 8: sudden infant death, cause unknown.
- Category 9: unclassifiable (this category is used only as a last resort).

Obstetric (Aberdeen) classification
This classification includes 22 categories grouped under the following headings.
- Congenital anomaly.
- Iso-immunization.
- Pre-eclampsia.
- Antepartum haemorrhage.
- Mechanical (e.g. cord prolapse).
- Maternal medical disorder.
- Miscellaneous.
- Unexplained.

Fetal and Neonatal Factor classification
This system has 24 categories, grouped as follows.
- Congenital anomaly.
- Iso-immunization.
- Asphyxia before birth.

- Birth trauma.
- Severe pulmonary immaturity.
- Hyaline membrane disease.
- Intracranial haemorrhage.
- Infection.
- Miscellaneous.
- Unclassifiable/unknown.

In the Obstetric and Fetal and Neonatal Factor classifications, only one category can be ascribed. The highest on the list should be used, e.g. a baby born at 24 weeks may eventually die as a result of intracranial haemorrhage; however, this is due to severe pulmonary immaturity and is categorized under this heading.

The causes of death due to stillbirth, early or late neonatal death for 1999 are shown in Table 3.2.

Table 3.2 – Causes of death due to stillbirth, early or late neonatal death for 1999

	Number	Percentage
Antepartum fetal death	2472	41
Immaturity	1209	20
Congenital malformation	1063	18
Intrapartum anoxia	486	8
Others	798	13
Total	6028	

Source: CESDI Eighth Annual Report.

The potential for further reductions in perinatal mortality is considered under the four main categories of the extended Wrigglesworth classification.

Congenital malformation
Congenital abnormalities account for about 18 per cent of the perinatal deaths in the UK.

Cardiac anomalies form the major group. Although the ability of ultrasound to detect abnormalities is improving, cardiac lesions remain the most difficult to detect: subtle changes on ultrasound can represent lethal abnormalities in the fetus.

Neural tube defects (NTDs), spina bifida and anencephaly are now almost entirely detected by screening with serum alpha-fetoprotein (AFP), ultrasound or both. This has led to a reduction in these conditions as contributors to perinatal mortality. In addition, the government advice that all women should take periconceptual folic acid to reduce the incidence of NTDs has led to a significant decline in the numbers of fetuses with NTDs.

Biochemical screening for chromosomal abnormalities is now widely available through tests involving either serum or ultrasound screening or, in some areas, both combined. The most common chromosomal abnormality, Down's syndrome, does not usually cause neonatal death and therefore this screening programme has little effect on perinatal mortality.

Antepartum fetal death
Antepartum term stillbirth was the subject of a special study in the Fifth Annual CESDI Report. Cases were compared with controls and parents were interviewed in addition to the usual methods of gathering data. Of 86 cases studied, 27 were unexplained and 22 were associated with intrauterine growth restriction. Of the remainder, the two commonest conditions were placental abruption (nine cases) and abnormal glucose tolerance (nine cases). Many mothers had noted a change in fetal movements or abdominal pain before the death occurred. These symptoms are non-specific, but may point the way towards further research in the future.

The Eighth CESDI Report examined 422 stillbirths in 1996–97: 45 per cent of these were associated with sub-optimal care. The main areas of sub-optimal care were as follows.

- Failure to recognize a mother at risk, at booking.
- Inadequate monitoring of fetal growth, or failure to act once detected.
- Failure to realize the importance of diminished fetal movements, either by the mother or professional.
- Failure to act on:
  - high blood pressure or proteinuria,
  - suspicious cardiotocograph,
  - glucose intolerance.
- Poor communication.
- Mother unable or unwilling to stop smoking or to attend for antenatal care.
- Poor care after delivery (inadequate investigation, post-mortem or bereavement counselling).

Intrapartum asphyxia
The Fourth Annual CESDI Report examined 873 cases of intrapartum death from 1994 and 1995. The

risk of death in labour was 1 in 1561 births, and when the cases were looked at in detail, more than 78 per cent were criticized for sub-optimal care. Alternative management might (25 per cent) or 'would reasonably be expected to' (52 per cent) have made a difference to the outcome.

Although the risk of a baby dying in labour is less than 1 in 1000, it is very worrying that such a high proportion of cases had sub-optimal management. The main problem in antepartum care was failure to recognize risk factors, and the main problem in intrapartum care was inadequate assessment of the fetal condition by heart rate monitoring and fetal blood sampling. In 22 per cent of cases, there was also criticism of the resuscitation of the newborn.

Three recommendations are particularly important.
1. 'The training, assessment, supervision and practice of obstetricians and midwives of all grades need to be critically appraised by their parent bodies.'
2. Professional bodies should 'look again at how level of practical competence of professionals of all grades caring for women in labour and for babies following delivery is achieved and maintained'.
3. 'A multidisciplinary initiative at national level is needed to develop guidelines covering all aspects of fetal assessment before and especially during labour.'

The Royal Colleges of Midwives and of Obstetricians and Gynaecologists have responded to this recommendation by publishing guidelines for improved standards of care in labour, which recommend, among other things, more involvement of consultant obstetricians in the day-to-day running of delivery suites in Britain. In addition there are now national guidelines for electronic fetal monitoring in labour, published by NICE. The Eighth Annual CESDI Report has commented:

It is extremely encouraging to see that intrapartum related mortality has now decreased significantly from 0.95 (1994) to 0.62 (1999) per 1000 live births and stillbirths. Although it is not possible to predict if this is a continuing downward trend, it is hoped that by maintaining efforts to achieve the highest possible standard of intrapartum care this will prove to be the case.

Immaturity
Although only 8 per cent of babies are born prematurely, this group contains 50 per cent of neonatal deaths. The immediate causes of death amongst this group include respiratory distress syndrome, infection, neurological causes and gastrointestinal causes. Advances in neonatal care have improved the survival of many premature infants. The 27–28 weeks CESDI study showed that the overall survival for infants born at these gestations is 88 per cent. A reduction in the numbers of low-birth-weight babies born is a government target, but the reality is that this is a difficult area to impact upon, as the causes are varied and many are only amenable to improvements in social care.

The restriction on embryo replacement for IVF by the Human Fertility and Embryo Authority has had some small impact in areas where large fertility units are sited.

From an obstetric point of view, the single most significant contribution to improved survival in very small babies is the administration of antenatal corticosteroids. Steroids ideally need to be given at least 24 hours before delivery, though smaller effects are seen at shorter durations. The standard is that they should be administered where there is a real risk of premature delivery except where there are contraindications.

Clinical risk management

Every hospital providing obstetric care will have a system for clinical risk management. This can take many forms, but integral to this system is a reporting method that accurately collects data from cases where there has been a poor outcome and where a poor outcome was avoided but could have easily occurred (a near miss). These may take the form of:
• perinatal mortality meetings,
• perinatal morbidity forums,
• discussion of cases with low Apgar scores and pH measurements at birth or those that developed neonatal encephalopathy,
• discussion of cases of major haemorrhage or eclamptic fits,
• review of emergency Caesarean section cases.

The discussions must take place in an atmosphere of 'no blame' and encompass the views of staff from all areas and of all grades. Suggestions for improvements in care should be clearly recorded and, importantly, a strategy for leaning from mistakes and instituting change must be in place. All maternity units must become 'organizations with a memory' such that mistakes are not repeated.

🔑 Key Points

- Worldwide, the situation for childbearing women is only slowly improving.
- HIV is a continuing threat to the health of many mothers and babies.
- In the UK, the Confidential Enquiry into Maternal Deaths has shown significant improvements in the management of problems such as thromboembolism after Caesarean section and the management of severe hypertension.

- The rate of stillbirth appears to have declined. The reasons for this are unclear as yet.
- The rate of intrapartum fetal death has also declined recently. It is too early to know whether this fall will be sustained.
- There is always room for improvement, but this must be balanced against the wishes and needs of mothers.

Additional reading

Confidential Enquiry into Stillbirths and Deaths in Infancy. Eighth Annual Report. London: Maternal and Child Health Research Consortium, 2002.

Department of Health. *Report on Confidential Enquiries into Maternal Deaths in the UK 1997–1999.* London: RCOG Press, 2002.

Royal College of Obstetricians and Gynaecologists. *Report of the Working Party on Minimum Standards of Care in Labour.* London: RCOG Press, 1998.

Key document for reproductive health and maternal health, including benchmarks for maternal health care for coming years, are available on the website www.unfpa.org

Conception, implantation and embryology

OVERVIEW

Knowledge of the fundamental processes involved in conception, implantation and the early development of the human form will provide an understanding of many of the basic pathologies causing infertility, miscarriage, genetic disorders, abnormalities of fetal growth and placental function and even cardiovascular disease in later life.

Somatic and germ cells

The human body has two types of cells, somatic cells and highly specialized germ cells. Somatic cells are diploid. They contain 46 chromosomes, a pair of sex chromosomes, X and Y, and two copies of each of the autosomal chromosomes, one from the father and the other from the mother. Chromosomes are found in cells, for example, from the brain, liver or heart. These cells divide in a process known as mitosis, and prior to this each chromosome pair is duplicated. The two copies remain together as sister chromatids. During mitotic division, the sister chromatids are separated from each other and each of the two daughter cells inherits one copy of each pair (Fig. 4.1).

The mature germ cells (sperm or egg), unlike somatic cells, are haploid; they have only one copy of each chromosome, and either an X or a Y chromosome. Following fertilization, fusion of the male and female pronuclei re-establishes diploidy.

Mitosis and meiosis

Both mitosis and meiosis begin with diploid cells. However, whilst the product of mitosis is two diploid daughter cells, a meiotic division leads to four haploid daughter cells. Mitotic and meiotic divisions are compared in the diagram in Figure 4.1. Unlike mitosis, cell division occurs twice in meiosis. At the end of division one, two haploid daughter cells are produced. During the second division, no DNA replication occurs. Thus, 23 double-stranded chromosomes lined up in metaphase will separate as single-stranded chromosomes to form the nucleus of each daughter cell.

Pathophysiology: clinical importance

During the formation of haploid cells by meiotic division, chromosome maldistribution may occur. One of each pair of chromosomes should go to each

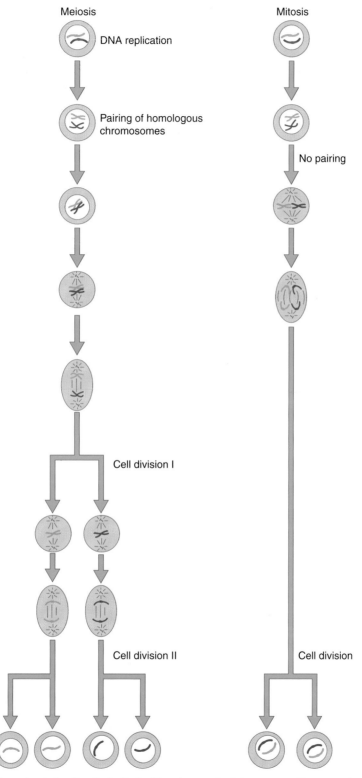

Figure 4.1 A comparison of meiosis with mitosis. To simplify, only one pair of chromosomes (known as a homologue) is shown. Note that pairing of homologues is unique to meiosis.

spermatozoon or mature egg. Fertilization leads to a chromosome complement of 46, 23 pairs. If an error occurs and both chromosomes in a pair pass to the same daughter cell, two abnormal cells are produced, one with a chromosome complement of 24 and the other with 22. Fertilization with a normal haploid cell (23 chromosomes) will then lead to cells with chromosome complements of either 47 or 45.

This error can occur with any chromosome pair. In the majority of cases pregnancy will fail at an early stage (and may not be recognized to have occurred). In recognized cases of spontaneous miscarriage, around 50 per cent can be demonstrated to have a chromosomal abnormality.

Continuing pregnancy is estimated to occur in 1:200 cases. An extra chromosome 21 produces Down's syndrome, the commonest survivable trisomy. Approximately 20 per cent of trisomy 21 cases survive to term if no therapeutic termination of pregnancy is performed. With trisomy 18, only 4 per cent survive to term. Monosomies are less common, with only 1:500 of Turner's cases (45XO, no second sex chromosome) surviving.

More rarely, there is chromosome breakage, with part of a chromosome being lost or attaching to another chromosome (translocation). If the transfer of material is between a single pair of chromosomes, both daughter cells will be abnormal: one will have too much material and the other too little. If the transfer is between unpaired chromosomes, it is possible for the correct complement to end up in the same haploid cell. If both affected chromosomes go to the same daughter cell, the total genetic complement will be present and this is known as a balanced translocation. Around 1:500 of normal people have a balanced translocation. Formation of their own haploid spermatozoa or eggs may lead to separation of the two balanced chromosomes. Subsequent fertilization leads to a lack or excess of genetic material in the embryo, which is an unbalanced translocation and usually causes miscarriage.

Single-gene mutations – base alterations at a single point in the DNA chain – occur during DNA replication. They are common and most will have no effect. Some are known to cause disease, for instance sickle-cell disease. These mutations will be inherited once they have occurred, although the phenotypic effect will depend upon dominance and penetrance. If an abnormal gene is dominant, only one copy is required to reveal the disease. If the normal gene is dominant, and so the abnormal gene is recessive,

both chromosomes need to have the mutation for the gene to be expressed. Achondroplasia is an example of a disease caused by a dominant mutation and cystic fibrosis a recessive. The mutant gene may be on the X chromosome, in which case it will be the only gene available in a male, but may act as a recessive in a female when a second normal X chromosome is present. Other genetic and environmental factors may affect the penetrance of a gene – that is, the actual effect it has on the individual's phenotype.

Conception, implantation and embryology

Conception

Conception is the consequence of several complex events that include the final maturation of the spermatozoa and oocyte, transport of the gametes in the female genital tract and, following the fusion of the male and female gametes, the assembly of a diploid number of chromosomes.

Spermatogenesis

Spermatogenesis is the production of mature sperm. It occurs in the seminiferous tubules of the testis. The primordial germ cells divide to produce spermatogonia, the precursors of mature sperm. The spermatogonia located at the basal lamina of the tubule begin to divide mitotically at the onset of puberty to produce primary spermatocytes. These undergo a first meiotic division to produce the secondary spermatocytes. The diploid secondary spermatocytes further divide (meiotic division II) to produce the haploid spermatids (Fig. 4.2a).

The differentiation of round spermatids to motile spermatozoa is called spermiogenesis. Round spermatids appear like any other somatic cells with a distinct nucleus. During differentiation, a series of changes occurs, which produces a motile sperm. The most visible change is the reduction in size and formation of a tail, which allows the sperm cells to swim. The chromosomes in the sperm cells are almost crystallized by a special set of sperm-specific proteins called protamines. In fact, this protamine-induced condensation of the sperm chromosomes is so extensive that the size of the sperm nucleus is about one-thirtieth the size of a mature human egg. This compact structure of the sperm is important for its motility. In the human it takes more than 3 weeks to complete meiosis and

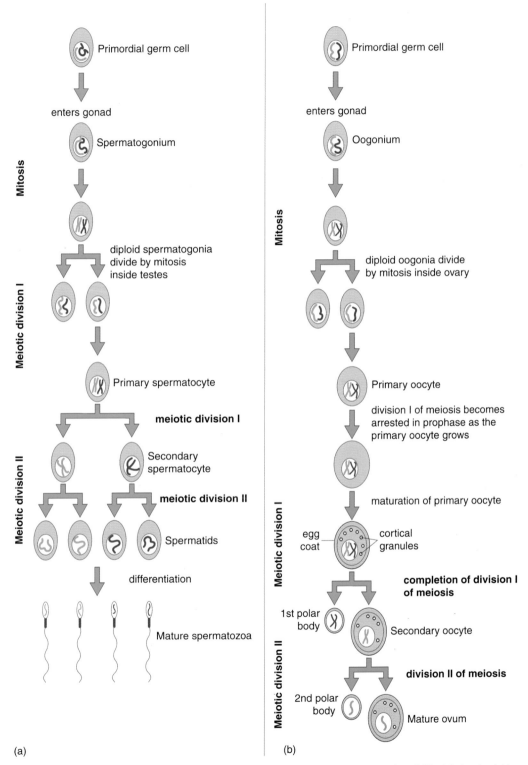

Figure 4.2 Various stages of spermatogenesis (a) and oogenesis (b). Note that one spermatogonium divides into four haploid mature spermatozoa, whereas one oogonium produces only one haploid mature ovum or egg.

more than 2 months for a spermatogonium to divide into four mature sperm.

Pathophysiology: clinical importance

Production of spermatozoa in the testes requires the presence of germ cells and their transformation and maturation under the control of hypothalamic and pituitary hormones and testicular androgens. In the survivable trisomy 47XXY (Klinefelter's syndrome), which occurs in approximately 1:500 male births, the germ cells are absent and azoospermia results. Deletions of parts of the Y chromosome will have a similar effect. Damage to the germinal epithelium and subsequent azoospermia or severe oligozoospermia may also be acquired following viral or, less commonly, bacterial infections.

Sperm development may be affected by infections or by impairment of hormonal control, for instance in the presence of cerebral or testicular tumours. Failure of descent of the testes into the scrotum (cryptorchidism) will also lead to poor sperm quality because of the resulting increase in testicular temperature.

Oogenesis and maturation of eggs

In principle, the development of a mature egg from a primordial germ cell producing oogonia in the ovary is very similar to the process of spermatogenesis in the testis. However, there are some distinct cellular and biochemical differences. Following the first meiotic division of primary to secondary oocytes, one of the two daughter cells, described as the first polar body, degenerates. Similarly, one of the two daughter cells produced after the second meiotic division, the second polar body, fails to survive. Therefore, one diploid oogonium after mitotic and meiotic divisions produces one haploid mature egg (Fig. 4.2b). In contrast, one diploid spermatogonium gives rise to four haploid mature spermatozoa.

⚲ Key Points

- In humans, most cells contain 46 chromosomes. These cells are in a diploid state.
- Meiosis generates mature (haploid) eggs or sperm containing 23 chromosomes.
- A diploid primary spermatocyte undergoes meiosis to produce four haploid mature sperm.
- A diploid primary oocyte undergoes meiosis. It produces only one haploid mature ovum (containing one polar body).

- During the second meiosis, the primary oocyte remains in meiotic arrest. Meiosis will resume once fertilization has occurred.
- All mature eggs (ova) contain 23 chromosomes.
- Mature sperm also contain 23 chromosomes.
- One of the 23 chromosomes in all ova and sperm is a sex chromosome.
- Unlike the female ovum, which contains only X chromosomes, the sperm contain either X or Y chromosomes.
- The resulting embryo contains 46 chromosomes, of which two will be sex chromosomes. Therefore a normal sex combination will be either XX (female) or XY (male).
- The sperm determines the sex of a child.
- Errors in meiotic divisions may lead to trisomies or monosomies or balanced or unbalanced translocation of genetic material.
- Many fetuses in spontaneous miscarriages have chromosomal defects.
- Point mutations may occur during DNA replication.

The sperm

Spermatozoa are produced at the onset of puberty in boys. Thereafter, the seminiferous tubules of the testis will go on producing sperm daily until 60 years of age and beyond.

Following spermatogenesis, the spermatozoa pass through the seminiferous tubules to the rete testis, on to the vasa deferentia, the head of the epididymis and thence, 12 days later, to the tail of the epididymis. Transport of the mature sperm is via muscular activity within the epididymis and vas. The seminal fluid is made up from the secretions of a number of glands, such as the bulbo-urethral, seminal vesicles and the prostate, to all of which must be added the half a millilitre or so of epididymal fluid. During this time, the sperm acquire motility and undergo the final biochemical changes that give them the ability to fertilize the ovum. The mature sperm containing a haploid number of chromosomes (22 + X or Y) is a few microns long. It travels a distance of 30–40 cm in the female genital tract to fertilize the oocyte. Spermatozoa have a complex structure that provides motility and propulsion (tail), an energy source (midpiece) and the acrosome for penetrating the oocyte (Fig. 4.3).

Seminal fluid containing sperm coagulates immediately following ejaculation. Under normal circumstances it liquefies within 20 minutes. The basic pH of the seminal fluid protects the spermatozoa from the acidity of the vagina. Within minutes after ejaculation, sperm may be found in the cervix and are released constantly over a period of up to 72 hours.

During this time the sperm will move with great speed towards the ampulla, where fertilization of the

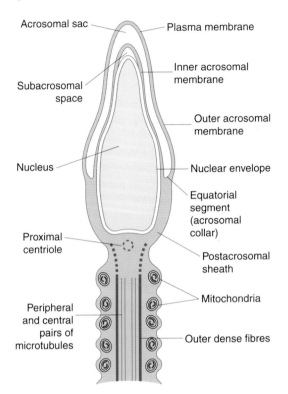

Figure 4.3 Outline of a spermatozoon.

mature, ovulated oocyte usually occurs. To achieve this, the sperm must undergo capacitation, which is oestrogen-dependent and calcium-dependent activation. During this process the inner membrane beneath the acrosome cap becomes primed for fusion with the inner membrane of the ovum.

The acrosome reaction exposes the inner membrane of sperm. This portion will fuse with the membrane of the ovum (Fig. 4.4).

Pathophysiology: clinical importance
Obstruction to sperm movement from the testis may be caused by congenital absence or blockage of the epididymis or vas deferens. Blockage may also be acquired following infection, for instance with *Neisseria gonorrhoeae*.

Movement of spermatozoa from the cervix to the ampulla of the Fallopian tube may be prevented by the consequences of disease in the female genital tract, or deliberately by mechanical methods of contraception. Cervicitis, the presence of pus and organisms in the cervix, may immobilize the sperm. Intratubal infection or scarring following infection may prevent passage of sperm through the tubes. Condoms, diaphragms and sterilization procedures effect artificial blockage.

The follicle
In the ovary, the primordial follicle is composed of primordial germ cells surrounded by mesenchymal cells derived from endodermal tissue. Having passed

Figure 4.4 Sperm undergoing acrosome reaction.

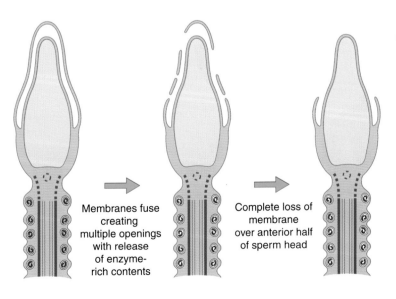

the first meiotic division at birth, the primary oocyte is arrested at metaphase of the second meiotic division until puberty. At the onset of puberty, a few follicles at a time recommence growth on a daily basis, the largest being 2–5 mm in the late luteal phase. It is from these follicles that the follicle destined for the next ovulation will be selected (Fig. 4.5). In each cycle, only one egg usually ovulates. Antral follicles are surrounded by inner granulosa cells and outer theca cell layers. These cell layers are derived from mesenchyme. The granulosa cells synthesize oestrogens, whereas the theca cells produce androgens (Fig. 4.6). Meiosis is not resumed until after the luteinizing hormone (LH) surge.

Complex mechanisms ensure that only one dominant follicle becomes pre-ovulatory and the other follicles undergo degeneration or atresia within the first week of the follicular growth phase prior to ovulation. The biochemical interactions between the oocyte and the surrounding granulosa and thecal cells within the

developing follicle are shown in Figure 4.6. The high oestrogen level in the follicle induces the pre-ovulatory surge of LH, which then initiates the resumption of meiosis. The completion of first meiotic division results in the extrusion and release of the first polar body. The oocyte, now described as an ovum, has acquired the competence to be fertilized (metaphase II of the meiotic cycle, Fig. 4.7).

Pathophysiology: clinical importance

The formation and release of a mature oocyte are dependent upon the hormones of the menstrual cycle, hypothalamic, pituitary and ovarian. Interference with the normal pattern of release of any one of these hormones is likely to lead to ovulation failure. This may occur naturally at extremes of reproductive age, in young women shortly after puberty and in women approaching the menopause. During lactation, prolactin production interferes with the hormonal cycle and causes anovulation. Anovulation can also be

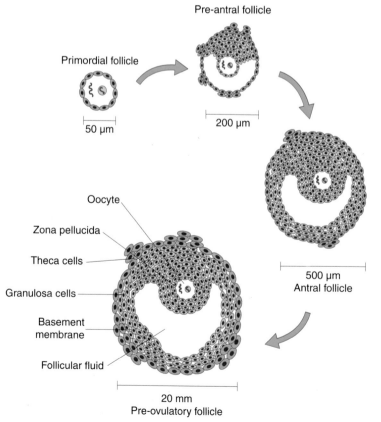

Pre-antral follicle

Primordial follicle

50 µm

200 µm

Figure 4.5 Development of a follicle.

500 µm
Antral follicle

Oocyte
Zona pellucida
Theca cells
Granulosa cells
Basement membrane
Follicular fluid

20 mm
Pre-ovulatory follicle

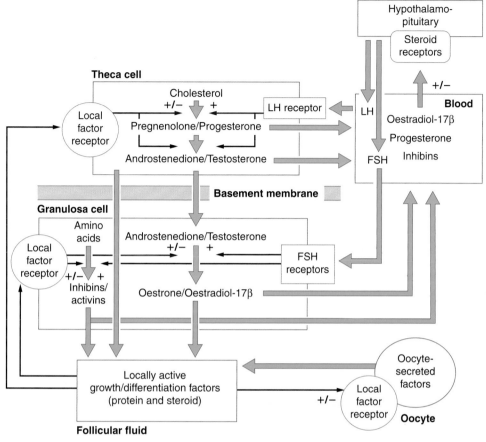

Figure 4.6 Biochemistry of hormone production in the ovary. (LH, luteinizing hormone; FSH, follicle-stimulating hormone.)

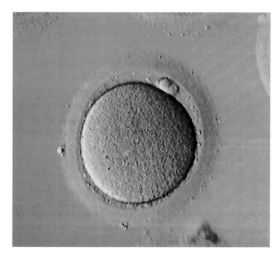

Figure 4.7 Mature ovum (metaphase II). The extruded polar body can be seen at 1 o'clock. (Kindly supplied by Dr Bruce Campbell.)

induced artificially by the hormones in combined oral contraceptive preparations. Endocrinological disease, for instance polycystic ovarian disease or thyrotoxicosis, may similarly interfere with the hormonal events, causing anovulation and subsequent infertility.

Fertilization

At ovulation, the ovum is surrounded by a jelly-like protective coating, which predominantly consists of cumulus cells. The ovulated egg is picked up by the fimbria of the Fallopian tube and then swept by ciliary action towards the ampulla, where fertilization occurs. The sperm penetrates the cumulus cell layer and subsequently interacts with egg-specific surface receptors in the zona pellucida, a thick glycoprotein sheet covering the cytoplasmic membrane of the egg. This interaction triggers the sperm acrosome reactions necessary for penetration of the sperm into the egg cytoplasm. At this point, a series of complex macromolecular events must occur within the sperm head to transform it into a male pronucleus (see Fig. 4.4). Similarly, the egg must complete its meiotic division II to form the haploid female pronucleus and a second polar body, which is extruded.

As described earlier, the sperm chromosomes are almost crystallized and are uniquely glued together by sperm-specific basic protamines. One of the earliest events in male pronuclear formation is the decondensation of sperm chromosomes by releasing the protamines. Once the protamines are stripped from the sperm chromosomes, a new set of egg-specific proteins bind the sperm chromosomes. This process is known as chromosome remodelling. Subsequently, new cytoplasmic organelles and a nuclear envelope assemble around the remodelled sperm chromosomes to produce the male pronucleus. Finally, the fertilization ends with successful fusion of the male and female pronuclei (Fig. 4.8), resulting in a single cell called a zygote. In humans, fertilization is completed within 20 hours, resulting in a return to a diploid genetic constitution of the embryo.

The coming together of the two haploid sets of chromosomes, called syngamy, is the final phase of fertilization. Soon after, anaphase and telophase are completed, and the one-cell zygote becomes a two-cell embryo.

Pathophysiology: clinical importance
In in-vitro fertilization (IVF) techniques the mature ovum is incubated with sperm on day zero. On day one, the ovum is inspected to ensure that two pronuclei are present, demonstrating that normal fertilization is underway. A four-cell embryo has formed by day two, and eight cells by day three. In cases where diagnosis of genetic disease is required, it is at this point that two cells can be removed for chromosome and DNA analysis.

Implantation

As soon as the zygote develops, it begins dividing very rapidly, and within 5 days a tiny mass of cells, the

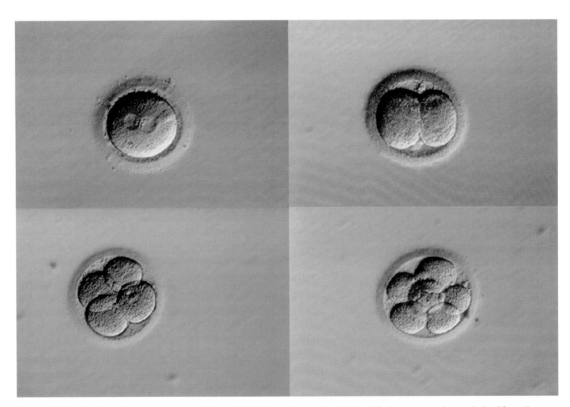

Figure 4.8 Fertilized egg showing two pronuclei: one derived from the egg (containing 23 chromosomes), one derived from the sperm (containing 23 chromosomes). The fertilized egg is diploid, containing 46 chromosomes in total. Subsequently, division into the two-cell, four-cell and eight-cell stages is shown. (Kindly supplied by Dr Bruce Campbell.)

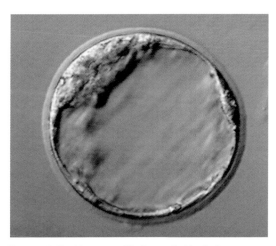

Figure 4.9 The blastocyst. (Kindly supplied by Dr Bruce Campbell.)

blastocyst, is formed (Fig. 4.9). For a pregnancy to be established, the embryo must hatch. This means that the embryo has to escape from the zona pellucida and the outer covering of the original egg and then begin to 'burrow' into the decidua. To prepare for this, the endometrium undergoes complex cyclical changes. In particular, extensive proliferation occurs under the influence of oestrogen released from the ovarian follicles during maturation of the eggs.

Following ovulation, the corpus luteum grows near the surface of the ovary as it produces oestrogen and progesterone. Under this hormonal influence, the endometrium and its glands undergo rapid morphological changes leading them to a secretory phase. Factors other than gonadal steroids influence uterine receptivity for implantation when appropriately conditioned by oestrogen and progesterone. Also assisting implantation are local peptides such as growth factors, including epidermal growth factor (EGF), insulin-like growth factor-I (IGF-I) and its binding protein (IGF-BP-1), prostaglandin (notably PGE2), plasminogen activators and possibly leukaemia inhibitory factor (LIF). Some of these have angiogenic properties.

The embryo remains in the Fallopian tube for 3–4 days until it reaches morula stage (8–32-cell stage). The embryo proceeds through the isthmus to the uterine cavity where it will float freely for up to 72 hours. By the sixth day, it orientates itself towards the decidua and begins to penetrate its epithelial surface by piercing its basement membrane. This is accomplished

by generating metalloproteinases. Once inside the decidua, it generates extracellular matrix (ECM) de novo, which is thought to enhance the chances of implantation. This process facilitates one of the earliest embryo–maternal interactions, the secretion of human chorionic gonadotrophin (hCG) by the trophoblastic cells, leading to the maternal recognition of pregnancy. There appear to be many changes that involve modulation of the immune responses within the uterus.

The early steps of implantation involve numerous cell–cell interactions, for example the binding to ECM (glycoproteins) with the basement membrane's (laminin and fibronectin) surface receptors. The embryo synthesizes integrins (cell adhesion molecules). There is activation of proteases and pericellular degradation of matrix components (matrix metalloproteinases). All these changes allow the invading cytotrophoblast easier access to the decidua for implantation. Indeed, de-novo expression of the gene for gelatinases A and B is activated, causing breakdown of the basement membrane, which facilitates contact of the cytotrophoblastic cells with the decidua's ECM through their fibronectin receptors (Fig. 4.10).

Endometrial cytokines modulate cytotrophoblastic proteolytic activity to control the depth of invasion. Twelve days after fertilization, the embryo is embedded within the decidual stroma, the trophoblast having already differentiated into cytotrophoblast and invasive syncytiotrophoblast. The developing embryo at 9 days is 500–600 mm in diameter, with predecidual cells surrounding the embryonic mass. Increased epithelial vasculature at the implantation site is observed due to oedema and localized hyperaemia. At 11–12 days, the implantation site can be seen as a 1 mm red spot on the mucosa due to maternal blood in lacunar spaces. By 14–21 days, the trophoblastic structure at the periphery of the embryo resembles the villi of the mature placenta as the inner cell mass has begun to undergo embryogenesis.

Pathophysiology: clinical importance
Human chorionic gonadotrophin is produced by the trophoblast. In the first week after implantation, serum hCG levels in the mother rise from 5 to 50 iu/L. By the time the mother has missed her first menstrual period, her hCG levels are around 100 iu/L. Commercial testing kits are available that are sensitive to 25 iu/L in urine. A quantitative serum hCG assay showing a level of >15 iu/L will usually denote a

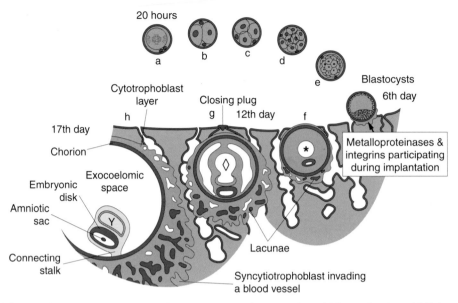

Figure 4.10 Sequential events post-fertilization. (a) Dividing zygote. (b) Two-cell embryo. (c) Four-cell embryo. (d) Eight-cell embryo. (e) Morula. (f) Implanting blastocyst: primary yolk sac (*star*). (g) Implanted blastocyst: developing secondary yolk sac: extra-embryonic mesoderm (*diamond*). (h) Gestational sac: the secondary yolk sac is broadly connected to the ventral aspect of the embryonic disk (Y). Note the expanded exocoelomic space and the small amniotic sac.

pregnancy. With a normal intrauterine pregnancy, the hCG level doubles approximately every 36–48 hours.

Delay or obstruction of the passage of the fertilized ovum down the Fallopian tube to the uterus may result in implantation in the Fallopian tube, or, more rarely, the ovary or peritoneal cavity. This is known as an ectopic pregnancy and although the pregnancy may continue to develop for some weeks, it will eventually fail. The increases in hCG are usually suboptimal. Some cases will cause rupture of the Fallopian tube and will present as an acute emergency.

Implantation is, as yet, a poorly understood phenomenon. Implantation failure may be due to deficiency in the embryo or in the maternal preparation for its reception in the uterus. Failure of implantation leads to early miscarriage. It is likely that in a majority of these cases the patient does not appreciate that she has been pregnant because the bleeding associated with a miscarriage is at or around the time when she would normally expect to have a menstrual period. More subtle deficiencies in implantation are likely to be part of the processes leading to obstetric diseases such as pre-eclampsia or to intrauterine growth restriction later in pregnancy. Inappropriate implantation may, more rarely, lead to morbid adherence of the placenta in conditions such as placenta accreta.

Embryology

In humans, following successful fertilization, the differentiation of cells into specialized tissues, to form inter-related organ systems, is known as the embryonic period. It starts with the generation of the embryonic disk during the second week post-fertilization (4 weeks after the last menstrual period) and, conventionally, ends on the last day of the eighth week (10 weeks after the last menstrual period). At this point, all organ systems are formed, but are not necessarily 'mature' or functioning.

Third week

On the dorsal aspect of the bilaminar germ disk, a faint groove, the primitive streak, appears on the midline near its caudal end (Fig. 4.11A). This is an important event during which a number of developmental landmarks are generated. For example, the primitive streak determines symmetry and defines the cephalic and caudal poles of the embryo. It follows that ventrality as well as laterality are generated at the same time. Definition of symmetry, polarity and laterality at the outset of organogenesis is fundamental for appropriate organ-system topology and a number of genes participate in this initial step.

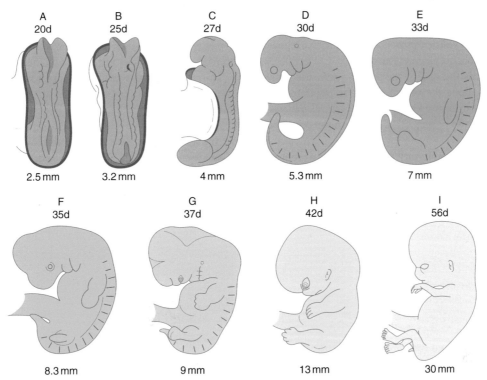

A	B	C	D	E
20d	25d	27d	30d	33d
2.5 mm	3.2 mm	4 mm	5.3 mm	7 mm

F	G	H	I
35d	37d	42d	56d
8.3 mm	9 mm	13 mm	30 mm

Figure 4.11 Sequential changes during the development of the external form in a normal human embryo from day 20 (A) through to the 56th day (I) post-fertilization (add 2 weeks to consider the gestational time from the last menstrual period). The crown–rump length is expressed in millimetres.

During the third week, two other structures become apparent on the embryonic disk: the neural plate and the somites, which appear as symmetrical eminences on either side of the midline.

Internally, the bilaminar embryo generates the mesodermal layer, which is made up of cells which, from the primitive node at the cephalic end of the primitive streak, migrate between the ectodermal and endodermal layers. The somites composed of paraxial mesodermal cells will appear on day 20, at a level corresponding to the future base of the skull.

Other structures intimately related to the embryonic disk develop during this time. The primary yolk sac grows rapidly into the expanding exocoelomic space. The yolk sac is an important organ for exchanging metabolites between the mother and the embryo at the time when there is no placenta but there are some chorionic villi undergoing vascularization. The life span of the yolk sac is limited: it attains full development by day 32 and its complex wall starts degenerating by the end of the sixth week. The amniotic membrane is another extra-embryonic element, which by day 17 is closely apposed to the embryonic disk.

There will be some time before the embryo is suspended in a well-expanded amniotic sac.

Fourth week

During this week the embryonic disk folds into an embryonic cylinder (Fig. 4.11B), within which is a cranio-caudal, blind-ending tube which has three segments, the foregut, the midgut opened to the developing yolk sac, and the hindgut. This stage marks the start of organogenesis.

The first organ to become apparent is the primitive heart in the shape of a forward-buckling loop (Fig. 4.11C). Cardiac activity is evident by day 22 post-fertilization.

Neurulation (the development of the nervous system) takes place at this stage of development. Briefly, the neural plate becomes a deep groove on the dorsal aspect of the embryo; it sinks deeper and the opposing crests fuse, generating the neural tube. As closure takes place, the cephalic neuropore closes during day 26 and the caudal neuropore at the end of the fourth week. A special population of cells detaches from the lips of the neural crest and migrates to several specific locations of the body. By the end of the fourth week, the central neural system has defined segments, the primary brain vesicles, prosencephalon, mesencephalon and rhombencephalon (Fig. 4.11D).

Towards the end of the fourth week, the foregut septates along the midline into the respiratory and digestive primitive elements. The ventral pancreatic bud migrates posteriorly to fuse with the dorsal pancreatic bud.

The lower respiratory system appears as septation of the foregut occurs. Two lung buds are evident at the end of the fourth week.

By day 26, the mesonephric duct and mesonephros differentiate. At 28 days, the ureteric buds and the metanephric blastema are defined structures.

In summary, it can be said that by the end of the fourth week almost all organ systems, albeit immature, can be readily identified.

Towards the end of the fourth week the body of the embryo is attached to the yolk sac by a broad vitelline duct and two connecting vitelline blood vessels. The yolk sac is placed within the exocoelomic space. The vitelline duct and the vitelline vessels are included within the umbilical cord just before the cord enters into the amniotic sac.

In the cephalic pole of the embryo, five pharyngeal arches appear in succession. Towards the end of the fourth week, the buccopharyngeal membrane perforates.

Changes in the external appearance

During the ensuing 3 weeks, the outer aspect of the human embryo changes dramatically. The head starts to grow faster than the rest of the body and is bent forward until the end of the seventh week (Fig. 4.11G and H). The face is formed by a series of transformations of the pharyngeal arches. The eyes are in a lateral position and after the 34th week they appear pigmented. As the embryo grows bigger, the eyes appear to 'migrate' towards the midline of the face. The eyelids develop after the sixth week and by the end of the eighth week the eyes are closed by the eyelids, which fuse with one another. The eyelids will separate after the 20th week of gestation.

The ears differentiate at either side of the neck early during the fifth week of gestation and appear to be displaced upwards as the body of the embryo gains length.

The nose is present early during the sixth week and the nostrils will be plugged with keratin until after the 20th week of gestation. The mouth can be recognized

after the sixth week of gestation. However, the palatal shelves will only fuse during the eighth week. The uvula remains bifid for a week or so, after which it assumes the shape observed later in gestation or after birth.

During the fourth week, the thorax is largely occupied by the heart. As embryonic growth proceeds, the lungs develop within the thorax.

The development of the upper limbs precedes that of the lower limbs. The upper limb buds appear at about the 27th day. The lower limb buds become evident a day later. Early during the sixth week, the hand plate presents lobulations which anticipate digit differentiation. The lower limbs lag behind. However, by the end of the eighth week, both the upper and lower limbs are fully differentiated, the head is slightly upright and the embryo has a distinct human appearance (Fig. 4.11I).

Clinical importance

Ultrasound examination is commonly used to detect early intrauterine pregnancies. Using transvaginal ultrasound, a gestation sac will be seen in the uterus between the fourth and the fifth week after the last menstrual period (2–3 weeks after fertilization). The fetal heart will be seen to be beating between 5 and 6 weeks after the last menstrual period. Abdominal ultrasound examination can be used to identify the gestation sac, but it will not be seen by this method until 6–7 weeks. Also, identification of the beating fetal heart is delayed by 1 week when compared with transvaginal ultrasound.

If the serum β-hCG level in the mother is >1500 iu/L, an intrauterine gestation sac should be seen using transvaginal ultrasound. If it is not with this level of hCG, it strongly suggests the possibility of an ectopic pregnancy.

New developments

The areas of conception, implantation and embryology are arguably the fastest moving in the whole of obstetrics and gynaecology. Many of the developments have been driven by the needs of IVF programmes:

- elucidation of the genetic basis of oocyte maturation,
- in-vitro growth of ovarian follicles,
- in-vitro maturation of oocytes,
- in-vitro blastocyst development,
- biopsy at eight-cell stage for pre-implantation genetic diagnosis,

- genetic basis of implantation,
- three-dimensional ultrasound and magnetic resonance imaging use in the evaluation of ovarian and uterine blood flow in the study of ovulation and implantation,
- development of inner cell mass cells to develop human embryonic stem-cell lines.

Key Points

- Embryos must synthesize integrins (cell adhesion molecules).
- The decidua must synthesize fibronectin and other ECM components.
- The above-mentioned activities are likely to be mediated by growth factors and cytokines. Both the decidua and the embryo are likely to make and release these factors.
- The embryo must produce cytotrophoblastic and syncytiotrophoblastic tissue in order to infiltrate the endometrial stroma successfully.
- It is now thought that cytokines are involved in initiating a localized immunosuppression, which would allow the developing embryo to avoid a rejection-like response from the womb.
- Leukocyte infiltration of the implantation site has been observed. Most of these seem to be T-suppressor cells.

Physiological changes in pregnancy

OVERVIEW

Textbooks of physiology conventionally present data obtained from young adult males. The norms for young adult females, particularly when pregnant, often differ significantly from these. Lack of appreciation of these differences may lead to inappropriate management of clinical problems in obstetrics.

This chapter outlines the major maternal physiological adaptations to pregnancy, indicating the potential for misinterpretation of clinical signs. Where possible, explanations for the changes are provided. Recent research is beginning to provide new insights into the mechanisms underlying the processes involved with physiological adaptation during normal and abnormal pregnancy.

Systemic changes

Volume homeostasis

One of the most fundamental systemic changes of normal pregnancy is fluid retention, which accounts for between 8 and 10 kg of the average maternal weight gain of 11–13 kg. There is some increase in intracellular water, but the most marked expansion occurs in extracellular fluid volume, especially circulating plasma volume (Fig. 5.1).

This change is pivotal to a series of other physiological adaptations, notably increases in cardiac output and in renal blood flow. It also has important consequences for the interpretation of haematological indices in normal pregnancy (Fig. 5.2). Relatively larger increases in plasma volume have been reported in women taking regular exercise during pregnancy and relatively smaller increases occur in the pregnancy

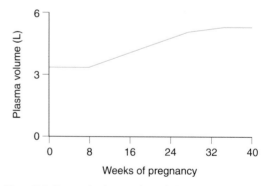

Figure 5.1 Changes in plasma volume during normal human pregnancy. There is an increase in mean values from 3 L in the non-pregnant state to between 4 and 4.5 L during late pregnancy.

complications of intrauterine growth restriction (IUGR) and pre-eclampsia.

The precise mechanisms responsible for this important adaptation remain uncertain. In the non-pregnant situation, sodium is the most important determinant

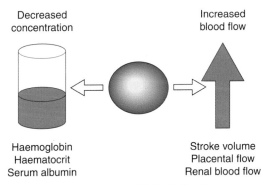

Decreased concentration

Increased blood flow

Haemoglobin
Haematocrit
Serum albumin

Stroke volume
Placental flow
Renal blood flow

Figure 5.2 The consequences of fluid retention during pregnancy. The concentrations of certain substances in the circulation decrease, whereas there are marked increases in haemodynamics.

of extracellular fluid volume. There is a net retention of sodium during normal pregnancy, amounting to a total of 900 mmol (or 3–4 mmol per day). In keeping with this finding are the very marked increases in the concentration of the anti-natriuretic hormones aldosterone and deoxycorticosterone observed during pregnancy. However, natriuretic factors, such as atrial natriuretic peptide and progesterone, also increase during pregnancy. Furthermore, a substantial proportion of the retained sodium must be sequestered within fetal tissues (including placenta, membranes and amniotic fluid). Maternal plasma sodium concentration actually decreases slightly during pregnancy and it is therefore possible that other factors, such as alterations in intracellular metabolism, may also contribute to the fluid retention.

One noteworthy feature of this change in fluid homeostasis is that plasma osmolality decreases by about 10 mosmol/kg. In the non-pregnant state such a marked decrease would be associated with a rapid diuresis in order to maintain volume homeostasis. However, the pregnant woman appears to accept this new level of osmolality, as evidenced by infusion experiments in which urinary concentration is regulated in order to maintain the new equilibrium. Interestingly, there is also evidence of a decrease in the thirst threshold so that pregnant women feel the urge to drink at a lower level of plasma osmolality than they do in the non-pregnant state.

Not only does plasma osmotic pressure decrease during pregnancy, but oncotic pressure (colloid osmotic pressure) is also markedly reduced. Plasma oncotic pressure is predominantly determined by the concentration of albumin, and this decreases by about

20 per cent during normal pregnancy to levels (28–37 g/L) that would be considered pathological in a non-pregnant woman. The significance of this change is that plasma oncotic pressure is a major contributor to the Starling equilibrium, which determines the degree to which fluid passes into and out of capillaries (including glomerular capillaries). Thus the decrease in plasma oncotic pressure is one of the factors responsible for the marked increase that occurs in glomerular filtration rate during normal pregnancy (see p. 55). It is also likely to contribute to the development of peripheral oedema, a feature of normal, uncomplicated pregnancy.

The factors contributing to fluid retention are:
- sodium retention
- resetting of osmostat
- decrease in thirst threshold
- decrease in plasma oncotic pressure.

The consequences of fluid retention are:
- haemoglobin concentration falls
- haematocrit falls
- serum albumin concentration falls
- stroke volume increases
- renal blood flow increases.

Blood

The marked increase in plasma volume associated with normal pregnancy causes dilution of many circulating factors. Of particular note is the haemodilution of red blood cells. Although pregnancy is associated with an increase in the production of erythrocytes, this increase is outstripped by the relative increase in plasma volume. Thus haematological indices, which depend upon the proportion of plasma in a measured blood sample, tend to decrease. Such indices include red cell count, haematocrit and haemoglobin concentration.

The mean haemoglobin concentration falls from 13.3 g/dL in the non-pregnant state to 10.9 g/dL at the 36th week of normal pregnancy. This physiological change may be mistaken for the development of pathological anaemia most commonly due to iron deficiency. Pregnant women require increased amounts of iron, and absorption of dietary iron from the gut is increased. Despite this adaptation, women who do not take supplementary iron during pregnancy show a reduction in stainable iron in the bone marrow as well as a progressive reduction in mean cell volume and serum ferritin. Therefore pregnant women are often given 'prophylactic' haematinics, notably oral iron. This drug can cause unpleasant side effects, including nausea and constipation. Pregnant women are already predisposed to these symptoms, making compliance with oral iron therapy a well-recognized problem. The use of supplementary oral iron in pregnancy is controversial. Most would agree that it is indicated if the haemoglobin concentration is less than 10 g/dL, although others have higher cut-offs. Iron stores are most reliably assessed using serum ferritin measurements. Iron deficiency is endemic in certain parts of the world and there are many women who, for personal or cultural reasons, take a diet that is relatively deficient in iron. Furthermore, certain pregnant women, such as those with multiple gestations, have a greater than normal dietary iron requirement. Iron supplementation should not be unreasonably withheld in such cases.

Folic acid supplementation is also widely advocated to prevent macrocytic anaemia. Renal clearance of folic acid increases substantially during normal pregnancy and plasma folate concentrations fall. However, red cell folate concentrations do not decrease to the same extent. Routine folate supplementation for haematinic purposes in women eating an adequate diet and carrying a single fetus is not indicated. However, there is clear evidence that supplementation with folic acid over the time of conception and during the first trimester of pregnancy can reduce the frequency of neural tube defects, and women in the UK are advised to take 0.4 mg folic acid from the cessation of contraception until 12 weeks of pregnancy.

Unlike red blood cells, white cell concentrations do not show a dilutional decrease during normal pregnancy. Conversely, the total white cell count increases, and the average value during the third trimester is 9×10^9/L. This is predominantly because of a substantial increase in the numbers of polymorphonuclear leukocytes. This is especially marked during the immediate puerperium, when values of $>20 \times 10^9$/L have been found in healthy women. Alterations in the concentrations of other circulating white cells, including both T and B lymphocytes, are relatively slight in comparison with these changes in neutrophils. There is, however, a slight reduction in the platelet count, with an increased proportion of larger, younger platelets.

There are also substantial changes in coagulation during normal human pregnancy, producing a hypercoagulable state. There are significant increases in the production of several procoagulant factors and a reduction in plasma fibrinolytic activity. There is a marked increase in plasma fibrinogen concentration.

This is thought to be responsible for the substantial augmentation of erythrocyte sedimentation rate that occurs during pregnancy, since it enhances rouleaux formation. The need for relative hypercoagulability is particularly apparent at the time of placental separation. At term, about 500 mL of blood flows through the placental bed per minute. Without effective and rapid haemostasis, a woman could die from exsanguination within a few minutes. Myometrial contraction is the first line of defence, compressing the blood vessels supplying the placental bed (see Fig. 5.5, p. 53). Almost immediately, fibrin begins to be deposited over the placental site and ultimately between 5 and 10 per cent of all of the fibrinogen in the circulation is used up for this purpose. Factors that impede this haemostatic process, such as inadequate uterine contraction or incomplete placental separation, can therefore rapidly lead to depletion of fibrinogen reserve.

The disadvantage of the potentially life-saving physiological adjustment of hypercoagulation is the substantially increased risk of thromboembolism. Venous thromboembolism remains the largest cause of direct maternal death in the UK.

🔑 Key Points

Haematological changes

Decreases in:
- red cell count
- haemoglobin concentration
- haematocrit
- plasma folate concentration.

Increases in:
- white cell count
- erythrocyte sedimentation rate
- fibrinogen concentration.

Cardiovascular system

Early pregnancy is characterized by peripheral vasodilatation. The precise order of events causing this phenomenon is speculative, but there is evidence to implicate vasoactive factors derived from the endothelium, such as nitric oxide. Initially, the vasodilatation appears to be perceived centrally as circulatory under-fill, similar to that which might occur following haemorrhage. A significant increase in heart rate can be demonstrated as early as the fifth week of pregnancy (3 weeks after conception) and this contributes to an increase in cardiac output detectable at this time (cardiac output = stroke volume × heart rate). However, the increase in stroke volume cannot be detected until several weeks later. This presumably occurs when plasma volume expands, following fluid retention by the mechanisms described above.

Further changes in the factors regulating cardiac output continue as pregnancy advances (Table 5.1; Fig. 5.3). A progressive increase in heart rate continues until the third trimester of pregnancy, when rates are typically 10–15 beats per minute greater than those

Table 5.1 – Changes in cardiac output with labour

	Increase in cardiac output (%)
Latent phase (cervix <3 cm dilated)	17
Active labour	23
Late 1st stage/2nd stage	34

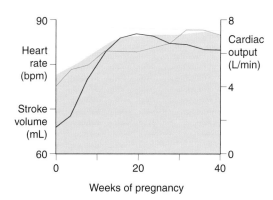

Figure 5.3 There is a marked increase in maternal cardiac output during pregnancy. Increases in both heart rate and stroke volume contribute, but changes in these components are not synchronous.

found in the non-pregnant state. There is also a progressive augmentation of stroke volume (10–20 mL) during the first half of pregnancy, probably related to the incremental changes in plasma volume at this time. As a consequence of these changes, cardiac output increases from an average of less than 5 L/min before pregnancy to approximately 7 L/min at the 20th week of pregnancy. Thereafter, changes are less dramatic. During the third trimester the gravid uterus impairs venous return to the heart in the supine position.

A proportion of women will, in consequence, develop significant supine hypotension, and loss of consciousness is possible. By rolling over on to the left side, cardiac output is almost instantly restored.

Key Points

Cardiovascular changes
- Heart rate increases (10–20 per cent).
- Stroke volume increases (10 per cent).
- Cardiac output increases (30–50 per cent).
- Mean arterial pressure decreases (10 per cent).
- Peripheral resistance decreases (35 per cent).

Normal changes in heart sounds during pregnancy

- Increased loudness of both s1 and s2.
- Increased splitting of mitral and tricuspid components of s1.
- No constant changes in s2.
- Loud s3 by 20 weeks' gestation.
- <5 per cent develop s4.
- >95 per cent develop a systolic murmur that disappears after delivery.
- 20 per cent have a transient diastolic murmur.
- 10 per cent develop continuous murmurs due to increased mammary blood flow.

Despite the marked increases in circulating plasma volume and in cardiac output described above, the greater part of normal pregnancy is characterized by a reduction in arterial blood pressure (Fig. 5.4). This implies that there must be very substantial decreases in total peripheral vascular resistance during pregnancy, but the mechanisms responsible for this dramatic alteration are not fully elucidated. Peripheral arterial tone is the result of a balance of opposing vasoconstrictor and vasodilator influences and, since substantial alterations have been reported in the production of both types of agents, it is unlikely that a single simple unifying hypothesis will be sufficient to explain this remarkable physiological phenomenon.

High blood pressure is a major contributor to maternal and perinatal disease and death. The accurate measurement of maternal blood pressure is therefore of critical importance in the assessment of pregnancy. The decrease in diastolic blood pressure is

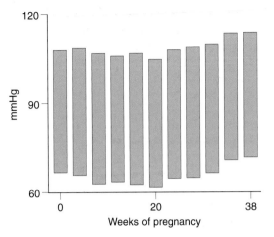

Figure 5.4 Arterial blood pressure decreases during the first half of pregnancy but gradually increases during the third trimester. This has major implications for the management of hypertensive disorders during pregnancy.

increases significantly to levels that are at least equivalent to those found in the non-pregnant state. The precise determination of diastolic pressure is therefore critically important. Recent studies have demonstrated that more reproducible and accurate measurements are obtained when the fifth Korotkoff sound (disappearance of sounds) is used rather than the fourth (muffling). This should be standard practice in pregnancy.

Reproductive organs

The uterus

Changes in circulating hormone concentrations markedly affect the tissues of the genital tract. The uterus is formed from fusion of the two Mullerian ducts in the midline, which gives rise to the adult structure of the uterus comprising three layers. These are a thin, inner layer of circular muscle fibres; a thin, outer layer consisting predominantly of longitudinal muscle fibres; and a thicker, central layer of interlocking fibres. In addition, the ratio of muscle to connective tissue

more marked during the antenatal period than the decrease in systolic pressure (Fig. 5.4). Thus early pregnancy is associated with a relative increase in pulse pressure. Later, however, diastolic blood pressure

CASE HISTORY

A 21-year-old Bangladeshi woman presents to the accident and emergency department. She arrived in the UK 4 months earlier. She is so short of breath that she is unable to give a history, but her partner tells you that she is 2 months' pregnant and was well until 3 days ago. On examination, you find that her pulse is 100 bpm, her blood pressure is 90/60 mmHg and she has a respiratory rate of 36. Examination of her chest reveals signs of pulmonary oedema.

What is the diagnosis?

Sudden onset of breathlessness could be due to chest infection, pulmonary embolism or pulmonary oedema. This patient had no temperature, and a careful cardiovascular examination revealed a facial rash, a tapping, undisplaced apex beat, atrial fibrillation and a low-pitched, mid-diastolic murmur, consistent with the diagnosis of mitral stenosis.

Why has the woman presented at this time?

Early pregnancy is associated with hormonal changes resulting in fluid retention and expansion of the plasma volume. This, with increased heart rate and stroke volume (Starling's law of the heart), causes an increase in cardiac

output early in the first trimester of pregnancy. With stenosis of the mitral valve, the increased blood flow through the heart cannot be accommodated; there is a rise in pulmonary venous pressure and pulmonary oedema results. Thus a person who normally has few symptoms unless very active can become very unwell as she does not cope with the physiological changes of pregnancy.

What is the treatment?

The pulmonary oedema should be treated with oxygen and diuretics. In extreme cases, venesection is sometimes necessary to rapidly reduce the circulating volume, and therefore the pulmonary venous pressure. As left ventricular filling is limited by the stenosis, beta-blockers will reduce the cardiac rate and allow more time for filling to occur. Balloon valvotomy or closed mitral valvotomy has good results in pregnancy and there is an increasing literature on full cardiopulmonary bypass in pregnancy. For many couples, termination of pregnancy, reversing the physiological changes that have precipitated the acute problem, will be an option, allowing definitive treatment (valve replacement) to occur before a subsequent pregnancy is planned.

increases from the lower part of the uterus towards the fundus. High levels of maternal oestradiol and progesterone stimulate both hyperplasia and hypertrophy of the myometrial cells, increasing the weight of the uterus from 50–60 g prior to pregnancy to 1000 g by term. In early pregnancy, uterine growth is independent of the growing fetus, and occurs equally rapidly with an ectopic pregnancy. As gestation increases, myometrial cell division is less important and hypertrophy of individual cells accounts for most of the increase in uterine size. The growing size of the uterine contents is an important stimulus at this stage, with individual muscle fibres increasing in length by up to fifteen-fold. In the second half of pregnancy, a growth-restricted fetus (see Chapter 13) may be detected on abdominal palpation, by finding a uterine size smaller than expected for gestational age. The uterine arteries also undergo hypertrophy in the first half of pregnancy, although in the second half of gestation the increasing uterine distension is matched by arterial stretching.

As well as changes in the size and number of myometrial cells, specialized cellular connections also develop with increasing gestation. These intercellular gap junctions allow changes in membrane potential to spread rapidly from one cell to another, facilitating the spread of membrane depolarization, and subsequent myometrial contraction. As these junctions mature, uterine contractions become more frequent. These are apparent initially as Braxton–Hicks, painless contractions that are increasingly apparent to the woman in the second half of pregnancy. Subsequently, these allow the pacemaker activity of the uterine fundus to promote the co-ordinated, fundal-dominant contractions necessary for labour.

Conventionally, the uterus is divided into the lower and upper segments. The lower segment is the part of the uterus and upper cervix which lies between the attachment of the peritoneum of the uterovesical pouch superiorly and the level of the internal cervical os inferiorly. This part of the uterus contains less muscle and fewer blood vessels, is thinner, and is the site of incision for the majority of Caesarean sections.

Immediately after the placenta has separated from the wall of the uterus, the interlocking muscle fibres of the uterus contract (Fig. 5.5). This occludes the blood vessels that were supplying the placenta and reduces blood loss. If the placenta has been attached to the lower uterine segment, the relative lack of muscle in this part of the uterus makes the haemostatic mechanism less efficient, and postpartum haemorrhage can occur.

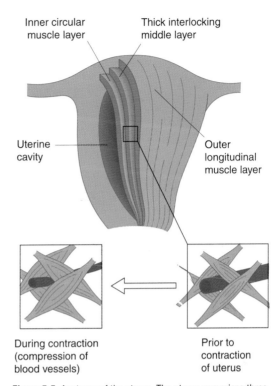

Figure 5.5 Anatomy of the uterus. The uterus comprises three muscle layers, derived from the layers of the Mullerian ducts. The muscle fibres in the inner layer are arranged in a predominantly circular pattern. The thicker intermediate layer comprises interlocked muscle fibres. The outer layer of muscle fibres runs longitudinally, over the fundus.

The cervix

Under the influence of oestradiol and progesterone, the cervix becomes swollen and softer during pregnancy (Fig. 5.6). Oestradiol stimulates growth of the columnar epithelium of the cervical canal that becomes visible on the ectocervix, and is called an ectropion. This is of significance as it is a less robust epithelium and is prone to contact bleeding. The cervix is often described as looking 'bluer' during pregnancy. This is a function of increased vascularity. In addition to these changes, the mucous glands of the cervix become distended and increase in complexity. Prostaglandins induce a remodelling of cervical collagen, particularly towards the end of gestation, whilst collagenase released from leukocytes also aids in softening the cervix.

Under the influence of oestrogens, the vaginal epithelium becomes thicker during pregnancy, and there is an increased rate of desquamation resulting

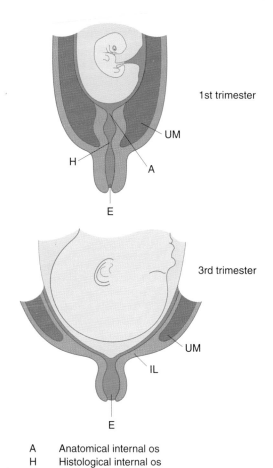

1st trimester

UM

H

A

E

3rd trimester

UM

IL

E

A   Anatomical internal os
H   Histological internal os
E   External os
UM Uterine muscle
IL Intermediate layer

Figure 5.6 Formation of the lower uterine segment. With increasing gestation, uterine stretch occurs. This has the effect of drawing the anatomical internal cervical os (A) further from the histological internal cervical os (H). The retraction of the thick intermediate layer (IL) of muscle with increasing gestation thins the lower segment.

in increased vaginal discharge during pregnancy. This discharge has a more acid pH than non-pregnant vaginal secretions (4.5–5.0) and may protect against ascending infection. The vagina also becomes more vascular with increasing gestation.

Breasts and lactation

Cyclical changes are seen in breast tissue in response to the menstrual cycle, and during pregnancy these changes are amplified. There is considerable deposition

of fat around the glandular tissue. The number of glandular ducts is increased by oestrogen, whilst progesterone – and human placental lactogen (hPL) – increases the number of gland alveoli. The hPL may also stimulate alveolar casein, lactoglobulin and lactalbumin synthesis.

Although the serum prolactin concentration increases throughout pregnancy, it does not result in lactation, as its effect is antagonized at an alveolar receptor level by oestrogen. It is the rapid fall in oestrogen concentration over the first 48 hours after birth that removes this inhibition and allows lactation to begin. Towards the end of pregnancy, and in the early puerperium, the breasts produce colostrum, a thick yellow secretion rich in immunoglobulins.

Lactation is promoted by early, frequent suckling, which stimulates both the anterior and posterior pituitary to release prolactin and oxytocin respectively. Stress and fear reduce the synthesis and release of prolactin through increased dopamine (prolactin inhibitory factor) synthesis. During the first 2 or 3 days of the puerperium, prolactin promotes breast engorgement, as the alveoli become distended with milk. Oxytocin released from the posterior pituitary causes contraction in myoepithelial cells surrounding the alveoli and small ducts. This squeezes milk into the larger ducts and subareolar reservoirs. In addition, oxytocin may inhibit dopamine release, further promoting successful lactation (Fig. 5.7).

The urinary tract and renal function

Vasodilatation, such as occurs in pregnancy, results from the relaxation of vascular smooth muscle. Other organs that have a significant component of smooth muscle also exhibit a change in function during pregnancy. Thus, in the alimentary tract there is delay in gastric emptying (important in the management of women requiring general anaesthesia) and reduced colonic motility (contributing to constipation). Similarly, the urinary tract becomes dilated during pregnancy. By the third trimester, about 97 per cent of women have been shown to have some evidence of stasis or hydronephrosis. This physical change, together with certain alterations in the composition of the urine itself (see later), predisposes pregnant women to ascending urinary tract infection, a common and important complication of pregnancy.

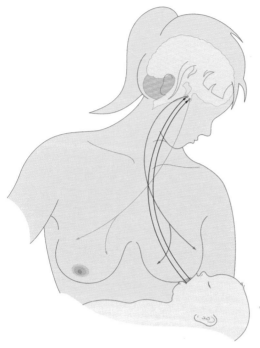

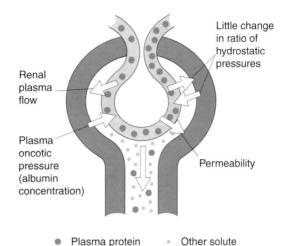

Figure 5.8 Factors contributing to enhanced glomerular filtration during pregnancy. The marked increase in renal blood flow is the major factor but there are significant contributions from the decrease in plasma oncotic pressure and enhanced permeability. Although systemic arterial pressure decreases during pregnancy, there is little difference in the relative pressures at either end of the glomerular capillary loop and in intra-renal pressure.

Suckling causes:
Afferent signals to posterior pituitary increasing oxytocin release, inducing myoepithelial cells to contract and express milk.
Afferent signals to anterior pituitary increasing prolactin release, thus increasing milk synthesis.

Figure 5.7 Schematic representation of lactation. Suckling induces afferent signals to the anterior and posterior pituitary. This results in the release of prolactin and oxytocin. Prolactin induces milk production by the glandular tissue of the breast. Oxytocin causes contraction of the myoepithelial cells surrounding the glandular ducts, squeezing milk towards the nipple.

One consequence of vasodilatation, reduction in blood pressure, has already been discussed. Another important consequence is increase in blood flow. There is evidence that in pregnant women blood flow to many organs is increased, notably the uterus, breasts and skin (hence the glow of health with pregnancy). There is also a marked (60–75 per cent) increase in renal blood flow. This leads to a substantial augmentation of glomerular filtration rate by about 50 per cent (Fig. 5.8). Filtration of the plasma is of critical importance in the maintenance of fluid balance, the excretion of waste products and the regulation of essential nutrients.

The increase in glomerular filtration rate is responsible for an increase in the clearance of a number of substances from the bloodstream. Thus the plasma concentrations of urea and creatinine, used as markers for the severity of renal disease, are reduced during normal pregnancy. It is important to use appropriate pregnancy-specific normal ranges when managing both normal pregnancies and those in women with renal diseases. There is also an increase in total protein excretion (particularly microalbuminuria) during pregnancy. The upper limit of urinary protein excretion in pregnancy increases to 0.3 g per day.

Glycosuria, which is rare in the absence of diabetes in the non-pregnant state, is very common during pregnancy. Glycosuria varies during any given pregnancy and does not relate reliably to disorders of carbohydrate metabolism. It is not a reliable screen for gestational diabetes. The increase in glomerular filtration rate may be partially responsible for this glycosuria, and a reabsorptive mechanism in the proximal renal tubule may become saturated so that the 'renal threshold' is exceeded, explaining the increased amount of this solute in the urine. Glucose reabsorption occurs secondarily to the absorption of sodium and therefore other factors contributing to volume homeostasis and sodium retention may be involved in the physiological glycosuria of pregnancy.

Key Points

Renal changes
- Blood flow increases (60–75 per cent).
- Glomerular filtration increases (50 per cent).
- Clearance of most substances is enhanced.
- Plasma creatinine, urea and urate are reduced.
- Glycosuria is normal.

Respiratory tract

Increases in cardiac output affect both sides of the heart. Therefore pregnancy is associated with very substantial increases in pulmonary blood flow. There is also a significant increase in tidal volume (see below) and the lungs are therefore able to function more efficiently, facilitating gas transfer. In consequence, there is a marked decrease (15–20 per cent) in the partial pressure of carbon dioxide (P_{CO_2}). Furthermore, there is a slight increase in the partial pressure of oxygen (P_{O_2}). These changes facilitate gas transfer to and from the fetus (Fig. 5.9).

During pregnancy there is an increase in 2,3-diphosphoglycerate (2,3-DPG) concentration within

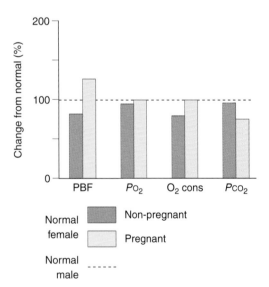

Figure 5.9 Human pregnancy is associated with marked changes in respiratory physiology. This diagram illustrates the percentage changes in normal values found in non-pregnant and pregnant women in comparison with typical male values for pulmonary blood flow (PBF), partial pressure of oxygen (P_{O_2}), oxygen consumption (O_2 cons), and partial pressure of carbon dioxide (P_{CO_2}).

maternal erythrocytes. This anion, which binds preferentially to deoxygenated haemoglobin, promotes the release of oxygen from the red cell at relatively lower levels of haemoglobin saturation (i.e. shifting the oxygen–haemoglobin dissociation curve to the right). This increases the availability of oxygen within the tissues. Furthermore, the fetus is also adapted to take maximum advantage of this alteration in maternal physiology. Fetal haemoglobin differs from adult haemoglobin in that the two beta-chains are replaced by gamma-chains. Binding of 2,3-DPG to haemoglobin occurs preferentially to beta-chains, with the result that in the fetus the oxygen–haemoglobin dissociation curve is shifted to the left relative to the maternal state. Thus oxygen transfer from mother to fetus is facilitated.

The reduction in P_{CO_2} also has implications for maternal homeostasis. Since carbon dioxide forms carbonic acid in the presence of water, it is a major factor in acid–base balance. There is an elaborate system of buffering which compensates for fluctuations in acid production. Reductions in P_{CO_2} activate these mechanisms so that potentially hazardous alkalosis is prevented. Compensation for such a respiratory-induced alkalosis classically involves the activity (predominantly within the erythrocytes) of the enzyme carbonic anhydrase, which converts carbonic acid to bicarbonate, thus releasing hydrogen ions to restore pH. The bicarbonate formed is excreted by the kidney. In human pregnancy there is evidence of such compensation: renal excretion of bicarbonate increases significantly and maternal arterial pH changes very little. Furthermore, there is evidence of an increase in the concentration of carbonic anhydrase within maternal erythrocytes, but whether this is a primary event (contributing directly to the reduction in P_{CO_2}) or a secondary adaptation is uncertain.

There are significant changes in the mechanical aspects of ventilation during pregnancy. These are of particular importance in the management of women with chronic respiratory diseases. Dyspnoea is a common symptom during normal pregnancy. Even in dyspnoeic women, the enhanced ventilation of pregnancy appears to result from increased tidal volume rather than from an increase in respiratory rate. The changes in lung volumes are demonstrated graphically in Figure 5.10. The enhanced tidal volume contributes to an increase in inspiratory capacity and there is a slight increase in vital capacity, which represents the total functional capacity of the lungs.

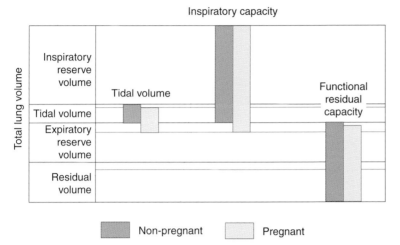

As a result, there is a relative decrease in the non-inspiratory fraction of vital capacity – the expiratory reserve. There is also a reduction in the non-ventilated part of the lung volume – the residual volume – so that there is a fairly substantial reduction in the sum of these two volumes, known as functional residual capacity. The main reason for this reduction is thought to be an alteration in thoracic anatomy during pregnancy when the ribcage is displaced upwards and increases in transverse diameter. Such changes improve airflow along the bronchial tree. Women with respiratory problems tend to deteriorate less during pregnancy than those with other chronic disorders, such as cardiac failure. The physiological changes do not affect the interpretation tests of ventilation such as forced expiratory volume in 1 second (FEV_1) and peak expiratory flow rate. Therefore these tests may be used in the management of pregnant asthmatics and women with other obstructive pulmonary disorders.

🔑 Key Points

Blood gas and acid–base changes
- P_{CO_2} decreases (15–20 per cent).
- P_{O_2} increases (slight).
- Oxygen availability to tissues and placenta improves.
- pH alters little.
- Bicarbonate excretion increases.

🔑 Key Points

Ventilatory changes
- Thoracic anatomy changes.
- Tidal volume increases.
- Vital capacity decreases.
- Functional residual capacity decreases.

Endocrinological changes

Complex endocrinological changes occur in pregnancy. Many of the peptide and steroid hormones produced by the endocrine glands in the non-pregnant state are produced by intrauterine tissues during pregnancy (Table 5.2). The precise contributions of these alternative sources to circulating concentrations of hormones, as well as their possible feedback activities, are not fully understood. Many hormones exert their actions indirectly, by interacting with cytokines and chemokines. The production and activity of many of these substances are also significantly altered during human pregnancy.

Many pregnancy-specific peptides are produced within the uterus, but not all have been shown to have definite endocrine roles. Of those that have, the best known is human chorionic gonadotrophin (hCG). This hormone is composed of α and β subunits and the β subunit is pregnancy specific,

---

Table 5.2 – Hormones produced within the
pregnant uterus

Pregnancy specific
Human chorionic gonadotrophin (hCG)
Human placental lactogen (hPL)

Hypothalamus related
Gonadotrophin-releasing hormone (GnRH)
Corticotrophin-releasing factor (CRF)

Pituitary related
Prolactin
Human growth hormone (hGH)
Adrenocorticotrophic hormone (ACTH)

Other peptides
Insulin-like growth factor I and II (IGF)
1,25-Dihydroxycholecalciferol
Parathyroid hormone-related peptide
Renin
Angiotensin II

Steroids
Oestradiol
Progesterone

Note that this list is not exhaustive.

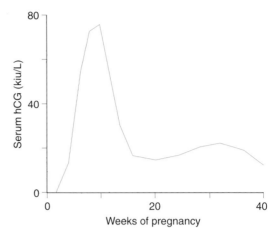

Figure 5.11 Serial changes in the plasma concentration of human chorionic gonadotrophin (hCG) during pregnancy. Note the marked increment during the first trimester.

being widely used in modern practice as a sensitive pregnancy test. The hormone is produced by trophoblast cells and is detectable within the maternal circulation in small quantities within days of implantation.

Production of hCG is influenced both by the cytokine leukaemia inhibitory factor (LIF) and by an isoform of gonadotrophin-releasing hormone (GnRH), which is also produced within the placenta. Human chorionic gonadotrophin has a major role during early pregnancy in maintaining the function of the corpus luteum. When the importance of this ovarian source of maternal progesterone diminishes (as the placental production of progesterone becomes dominant during the later weeks of the first trimester), concentrations of circulating hCG decrease from peak values around the 10th week of pregnancy to plateau after the 12th week (Fig. 5.11).

The α subunit of hCG differs only slightly from the α subunits of luteinizing hormone (LH), follicle-stimulating hormone (FSH) and thyroid-stimulating hormone (TSH) and can interact with receptors for at least some of these hormones. For example, hCG is widely used clinically in assisted reproduction to mimic the physiological LH surge in order to induce ovulation from stimulated ovarian follicles. During normal pregnancy, hCG suppresses the secretion of FSH and LH by the gonadotrophs of the anterior pituitary gland, perhaps by similar hormone/receptor interaction at the hypothalamic level.

Human placental lactogen, another peptide produced from the placenta, has partial homology with both prolactin and human growth hormone (hGH). It has major effects upon maternal production of these hormones (see later).

Sex steroid hormones are produced in large quantities by the placenta and fetus. Concentrations of oestrogens, including the active hormone oestradiol, and progesterone increase substantially from the earliest weeks of pregnancy, then plateau for the remainder of the pregnancy. These hormones were previously used to assess fetal well-being, but this practice has been superseded by more specific biophysical methods. Both oestrogen and progesterone have effects upon the myometrium (oestrogen encourages cellular hypertrophy, whereas progesterone discourages contraction) and, together with prolactin, the tissues of the breast (see p. 54). It is likely that they exert effects on many other target tissues during pregnancy, such as the smooth muscle of the vascular tree and of the urinary and gastrointestinal tracts.

Concentrations of prolactin reach levels during pregnancy that would be considered pathological in a non-pregnant woman. Oestrogen may have a stimulatory role in this process and hPL may be inhibitory. The endocrinological mechanisms that regulate prolactin production in the non-pregnant state, such as sleep (which increases prolactin concentrations) and dopamine agonists (which reduce them), remain effective during pregnancy. Therefore prolactin production by the lactotrophs of the anterior pituitary gland probably continues despite intrauterine production, especially from cells within the decidua. Receptors for prolactin are present on trophoblast cells and within the amniotic fluid. The increased prolactin production is essential for lactation (see p. 54).

In contrast to prolactin, there is evidence that hGH production by the anterior pituitary gland is suppressed during pregnancy. A reduction has been reported in the number of pituitary somatotrophs, and responses to conventional provocation tests are blunted. Circulating concentrations of hGH are also reduced during pregnancy. It is likely that hPL suppresses hGH release by the maternal pituitary: in women who have a pregnancy in which hPL is deficient (for example in trophoblastic disease), it appears that pituitary growth hormone production is not suppressed.

Fetal growth is not regulated primarily by hGH. Insulin and the insulin-like growth factors (IGFs) appear to be more important. There are two major types of these somatomedins and the relative concentrations of each vary from site to site and from time to time during pregnancy. IGF-II predominates in the fetal circulation throughout pregnancy. Both IGF-I and IGF-II are produced by fetal cells (in the liver) and by maternal cells (in the uterus). The relative proportions of maternal IGFs and of the specific binding proteins that regulate their activity vary during the menstrual cycle and during the early part of pregnancy. Fetal growth is now known to be of major importance in determining an individual's susceptibility to several disorders later in life. Control of fetal growth is therefore currently the subject of intensive research.

Factors controlling carbohydrate metabolism

During the first half of pregnancy, fasting plasma glucose concentrations are reduced but there is relatively little change in plasma insulin levels. A standard oral glucose tolerance test at this time shows an enhanced response compared to the non-pregnant state, with a normal pattern of insulin release but reduced blood glucose values. This pattern changes during the second half of pregnancy, at least in women who eat a Western-style diet. There is a delay in reaching peak glucose values and an increase in these values throughout the test despite significant increases in plasma insulin concentrations, a pattern suggestive of relative insulin resistance. This change may involve hPL or other growth-related hormones, which reduce peripheral insulin sensitivity. Pregnancy is also associated with alterations in the characteristics of insulin binding to its receptor, similar to those described in non-pregnant women who are obese or have non-insulin-dependent diabetes mellitus. If such women become pregnant, they are liable to have babies of higher mean birth weight than normal women. Whether this phenomenon results from increased transplacental transfer of glucose or from the growth-promoting characteristics of insulin and somatomedins (see above) is unclear.

Thyroid function

Human chorionic gonadotrophin has thyrotrophic activity (perhaps as a result of α subunit homology with TSH), and maternal TSH production may be suppressed during the first trimester of pregnancy, when hCG levels are maximal. The TSH response to injection of thyrotrophin-releasing hormone (TRH) is blunted during the first trimester but later returns to normal.

Some have suggested a role for hCG or TSH in the nausea and vomiting often experienced by normal pregnant women, which usually improves after the first trimester. Hyperemesis gravidarum, an extreme and pathological form of nausea and vomiting, may be associated with a biochemical hyperthyroidism with high levels of free thyroxine (T4) and a suppressed TSH. In general, however, thyroid function is considered to remain normal throughout the remainder of pregnancy.

Some workers have reported a physiological increase in the size of the thyroid gland in pregnancy, but such observations have been in populations of women who were relatively iodine deficient. These increases have not been confirmed in women from Iceland and the Netherlands, where iodine intake is greater. Maternal iodine requirements increase because of active transport to the feto-placental unit and because iodine excretion in the urine is increased. Because the plasma level falls, the thyroid gland increases iodine uptake from the blood. If there is already dietary insufficiency of iodine, the thyroid gland hypertrophies in order to trap sufficient iodine.

Pregnancy is associated with a marked increase in thyroid-binding globulin and also in the bound forms of T4 and tri-iodothyronine (T3). The circulating concentrations of unbound/free (and therefore active) forms of these hormones are altered less, although they do fall a little in the second and third trimesters.

Factors controlling calcium metabolism

In the circulation, about 40 per cent of calcium is bound to albumin. Since plasma albumin concentrations decrease markedly during pregnancy (see above), total plasma calcium concentrations also decrease. There is little change in the circulating concentration of unbound, ionized calcium. There is a substantial fetal demand for calcium, and transplacental flux rates of about 6.5 mmol per day have been calculated. Such a quantity would represent about 80 per cent of the net amount absorbed from the upper gastro-intestinal tract in a non-pregnant woman. However, the pregnant woman increases absorption and slightly decreases excretion, thereby coping with little net change in transfer rates into and out of bone stores. This new equilibrium is finely poised: women who are unable to sustain this level of fetal transfer from dietary sources alone may develop osteopenia during and after pregnancy.

The marked increase in calcium absorption is a direct result of increased production of one metabolite of vitamin D3, 1,25-dihydroxycholecalciferol (1,25-$[OH]_2$D3). Production of 1,25-$(OH)_2$D3 is under the influence of parathyroid hormone (PTH), which increases by about one-third during human pregnancy. No consistent changes have been reported in circulating concentrations of other agents with roles in calcium metabolism, notably calcitonin and other metabolites of vitamin D3. The fetus has higher plasma concentrations of calcium than the mother, and hormones such as PTH and calcitonin appear to be independently regulated by mother and fetus and are not thought to cross the placenta. Placental sources of 1,25-$(OH)_2$D3 and of a PTH-related peptide have been identified.

Placental corticotrophin-releasing factor and the onset of human labour: the placental clock theory

From mid-pregnancy onwards, the trophoblast is able to synthesize corticotrophin-releasing factor (CRF). CRF stimulates the fetal pituitary to increase fetal adrenocorticotrophic hormone (ACTH), and thereby fetal dihydroepiandrosterone (DHEA) production by the fetal adrenal is increased. DHEA is the main precursor for placental oestrogen secretion. The high levels of oestrogens towards the end of pregnancy increase gap junction synthesis between uterine myometrial cells, aiding conduction and therefore regular uterine contractions. CRF synthesis is regulated in a positive feedback loop by oestrogens.

The placental regulation of its own metabolism via effects on the fetus, with subsequent effects on maternal uterine physiology, and possibly the onset of labour, has been christened the placental clock theory.

Corticosteroids and the renin–angiotensin system

Trophoblast cells produce both CRF and ACTH. These placental hormones have roles in regulating the activity of the fetal adrenal glands and the myometrium and possibly the mother's adrenal glands. There is a progressive increase in maternal circulating concentrations of cortisol throughout pregnancy, despite a relative decrease in the concentration of ACTH during the later weeks. Much of the cortisol is bound to cortisol-binding globulin (CBG), which doubles in concentration during pregnancy, but there is also a slight increase in unbound cortisol. The lack of diurnal fluctuation of cortisol and the attenuated response to dexamethasone suppression suggest that placental ACTH may have a role in regulating maternal cortisol levels.

Circulating concentrations of the anti-natriuretic hormones aldosterone and deoxycorticosterone increase up to ten-fold in pregnancy. Progesterone has natriuretic properties, and other factors that may influence aldosterone production, notably atrial natriuretic peptide and angiotensins, are produced in increased amounts during pregnancy. The increased production of angiotensins, including the vasoactive angiotensin II, is the result of an augmented production of the enzyme renin and its substrate angiotensinogen. Intrauterine tissues, both maternal and fetal in origin, also produce the elements of this system.

Mechanisms of change

Maternal homeostasis

Pregnancy results in marked changes in homeostatic equilibria. Many of these changes occur early in pregnancy and are underpinned by alterations in gene expression. For example, the gene for LIF, which is known to be involved in implantation of the blastocyst in mice, is expressed in human endometrial tissue and decidua at the appropriate stage of human pregnancy. LIF is thought to stimulate the production of hCG by trophoblast cells, and a receptor for LIF is expressed by trophoblast cells early in pregnancy.

🔑 Key Points

Endocrine changes
- Prolactin concentration increases markedly.
- Human growth hormone is suppressed.
- Insulin resistance develops.
- Thyroid function changes little.
- Transplacental calcium transport is enhanced.
- Corticosteroid concentrations increase.

CASE HISTORY

A 34-year-old woman had an uncomplicated first pregnancy. She was admitted to the delivery suite at term and had a slow labour, with a first stage lasting 16 hours and a 3-hour second stage, prior to assisted vaginal delivery with forceps. She subsequently had hypotension and a significant postpartum haemorrhage, losing 1500 mL of blood. After resuscitation, she went to the postnatal ward and, despite a desire to breastfeed her son, this proved unsuccessful. When seen by her GP at 8 weeks after the delivery, she felt tired and lethargic. The GP initially ascribed these symptoms to the new arrival; however, when they persisted 2 months later, and she had still not had a period, he referred the patient back to the obstetrician.

What investigations will help with the diagnosis?

Whilst it is not unreasonable to blame postpartum tiredness on the arrival of a new baby, the inability to establish lactation in a well-motivated mother, and the lack of menstruation after a postpartum haemorrhage, require that pituitary infarction (Sheehan's syndrome) is excluded. The anterior pituitary increases markedly in size during pregnancy and is particularly vulnerable to hypotension. The diagnosis of hypopituitarism is made by finding reduced plasma concentrations of T4, TSH (which may be inappropriately normal in the context of a low serum T4), cortisol, ACTH, FSH, LH and hGH. The secretion of ACTH, hGH and prolactin in response to hypoglycaemia (an insulin stress test) is reduced. The differential diagnosis of hypopituitarism includes lymphocytic hypophysitis and tumour. Computerized tomography (CT) or magnetic resonance imaging (MRI) of the pituitary fossa is therefore mandatory.

What is the management?

Cases of Sheehan's syndrome have resolved spontaneously. This patient did not present acutely, suggesting some pituitary function was retained. In general, patients will require thyroid and glucocorticoid hormone replacement. A lack of FSH and ovulation will require oestrogen replacement therapy to prevent osteoporosis. As the woman still has a uterus, progestogen therapy to induce a withdrawal bleed will also be required.

How will Sheehan's syndrome affect future pregnancies?

Spontaneous pregnancies have been reported after a confirmed diagnosis of Sheehan's syndrome. However, for most women it is likely that ovulation induction with exogenous gonadotrophins would be required to induce ovulation. If hormone replacement is inadequate, an increased risk of miscarriage, stillbirth and maternal morbidity (hypotension and hypoglycaemia) has been reported. Where hormone replacement is adequate prior to and during pregnancy, outcome is normal.

Uterine activity

The mechanisms by which the myometrium remains quiescent for most of pregnancy but is able to function in a co-ordinated manner to enable normal parturition to take place are not fully understood. Variations in gene expression, probably modulated by hormones and cytokines, are of fundamental importance in permitting the expression of anti-contractile factors early in pregnancy and of factors encouraging contraction and intercellular communication later.

Most of the maternal physiological changes described in this chapter result from similar changes in gene expression.

Additional reading

De Swiet M. *Medical disorders in obstetric practice*, 4th edn. Oxford: Blackwell Science, 2002.

Dunlop W. Normal pregnancy: physiology and endocrinology. In: Edmonds DK (ed.), *Dewhurst's textbook of obstetrics and gynaecology for postgraduates*, 6th edn. Oxford: Blackwell Science, 1999.

Chamberlain G, Broughton Pipkin F. *Clinical physiology in obstetrics*, 3rd edn. Oxford: Blackwell Science, 1991.

Nelson-Piercy C. *Handbook of obstetric medicine*, 2nd edn. London: Martin Dunitz, 2002.

Normal fetal development and growth

OVERVIEW

An appreciation of normal development, growth and maturation is important for understanding the complications that may arise in pregnancy and for the neonate.

At the end of embryogenesis, organogenesis is complete and the fetus is completely formed. The ensuing 6 months in utero will be devoted to maturation and growth.

Fetal growth and maturation

Determinants of birth weight are multi-factorial, and reflect the influence of the natural growth potential of the fetus and the intrauterine environment. The latter is controlled by both maternal and placental factors.

Fetal growth is dependent on adequate transfer of nutrients and oxygen across the placenta. This in itself is dependent on appropriate maternal nutrition and placental perfusion. Factors affecting these are discussed in Chapter 13. Other factors are important in determining fetal growth, for example fetal hormones. They affect the metabolic rate, growth of tissues and maturation of individual organs. In particular, insulin-like growth factors (IGFs) co-ordinate a precise and orderly increase in growth throughout late gestation. Insulin and thyroxine (T4) are required through late gestation to ensure appropriate growth in normal and adverse nutritional circumstances. Fetal hyperinsulinaemia,

which occurs in association with maternal diabetes mellitus when maternal glycaemic control is sub-optimal, results in fetal macrosomia with, in particular, excessive fat deposition.

Conversely, in growth-restricted fetuses, fetal insulin levels are low, thus further reducing fetal tissue accretion. Lack of thyroid hormone produces deficiency in skeletal and cerebral maturation, characteristic of cretinism, and surfactant production is delayed. Cortisol has a limited role in stimulating growth, but is essential for the structural and functional development of a wide variety of individual fetal tissues. In the lung, it increases compliance and surfactant release, which ensures that spontaneous breathing can occur at birth. In the fetal liver, cortisol induces beta-receptors and glycogen deposition to maintain a glucose supply to the neonate immediately after birth. In the gut, cortisol is responsible for villus proliferation and induction of digestive enzymes, which enable the neonate to switch to enteral feeding at birth.

In developed countries, the average birth weight is about 3.5 kg at the end of a normal pregnancy lasting an average of 40 weeks. About one-third of the eventual birth weight is reached by 28 weeks, half by 31 weeks, and two-thirds by 34 weeks. The average fetus gains approximately 25 g per day between 32 weeks' gestation and term.

Each baby has its own optimal growth potential, which is, to a degree, predictable from physiological characteristics known at the beginning of pregnancy. The principal known factors are maternal weight and height, parity, race or ethnic group, and the baby's sex. Maternal age is also a factor, but the variation is mostly accounted for by parity. Of paternal characteristics, height is associated with birth weight, but to a lesser extent than any of the maternal variables. The main coefficients are listed in Table 6.1.

Table 6.1 – Physiological variables affecting normal fetal growth

---

Pre-pregnancy weight and maternal booking weight
Maternal height
Maternal age and parity
Ethnic group
Fetal sex
Paternal height

The physiological variation in normal birth weight in any heterogeneous maternity population can be considerable. For example, a mother from India who weighs 5 kg less and is 5 cm shorter than the population average would be expected to have a baby that weighs [185 g (ethnic group) + 45 g (weight) + 40 g (height)] 270 g less than the average birth weight at 40 weeks. However, a European mother of average size but in her third pregnancy would have a baby that is approximately 150 g heavier than a mother with the same characteristics but in her first pregnancy (Table 6.2). Such differences become magnified if it is attempted, on the basis of birth weight alone, to determine what is an abnormally small baby. In an average birth-weight distribution, a 150 g adjustment at the tenth centile cut-off for small for gestational age (SGA) is enough for reclassification of up to 50 per cent of babies. It is important to note that not all

SGA fetuses are growth restricted; some of these babies are constitutionally small and have reached their full growth potential. In addition, not all growth-restricted fetuses are SGA.

Table 6.2 – Optimal birth weight

Maternal weight	9 g/kg
Maternal height	8 g/cm
Parity	
Para 1	+110 g
Para 2+	+150 g
Ethnic group	
South Asian (India, Pakistan)	−185 g
Afro-Caribbean	−130 g
Baby's gender	
Male > female	±60 g

Approximate coefficients used for individually adjusting the predicted birth weight at the end of a normal pregnancy, i.e. pathology-free birth weight. The baseline birth weight for a baby of a non-smoking Anglo-European mother in her first pregnancy, of average height (163 cm) and booking weight (64 kg), is about 3480 g at 40.0 weeks.

It is important to exclude the known pathological influences on birth weight when calculating the optimal weight that a baby can reach. Most of the factors listed in Chapter 13 are too rare and/or too heterogeneous in their effect to result in a statistically significant value in multivariate analysis of birth weight in a maternity population. However, smoking has an all too high prevalence in an average National Health Service (NHS) population: about 25 per cent of mothers admit to being smokers at the time of the booking visit, and most of them continue to smoke throughout pregnancy. The effect of smoking on birth weight is significant, consistent and dose dependent (Fig. 6.1).

Growth-restricted fetuses who have failed to achieve their growth potential have significantly higher perinatal mortality and morbidity rates than normally grown babies of a similar gestation. They are more likely to suffer intrauterine hypoxia/asphyxia and, as a consequence, be stillborn or demonstrate signs and symptoms of hypoxic–ischaemic encephalopathy (HIE), including seizures and multi-organ damage or failure

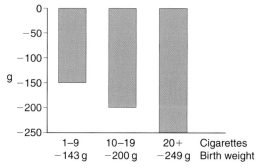

Figure 6.1 Deficit in birth weight due to smoking as recorded in early pregnancy (adjusted for other variables listed in Table 6.2).

in the neonatal period. Other complications to which these growth-restricted babies are more prone include neonatal hypothermia, hypoglycaemia, infection and necrotizing enterocolitis. In the medium term, cerebral palsy is more prevalent and in adulthood they are at greater risk of cardiovascular complications such as hypertension and ischaemic heart disease and of metabolic disorders such as non-insulin-dependent diabetes.

Cardiovascular system

The fetal circulation is quite different from that of the adult (Fig. 6.2). Its distinctive features are as follows.
- Oxygenation occurs in the placenta not the lungs.
- The right and left ventricles work in parallel rather than in series.
- The heart, brain and upper body receive blood from the left ventricle, while the placenta and lower body receive blood from both right and left ventricles.

Three modifications in fetal vascularity ensure that the best, oxygenated blood from the placenta is delivered to the fetal brain. These are:
1. the ductus venosus, which shunts blood away from the liver;
2. the foramen ovale, which shunts blood from the right to left atrium;
3. the ductus arteriosus, which shunts blood from the pulmonary artery to the aorta.

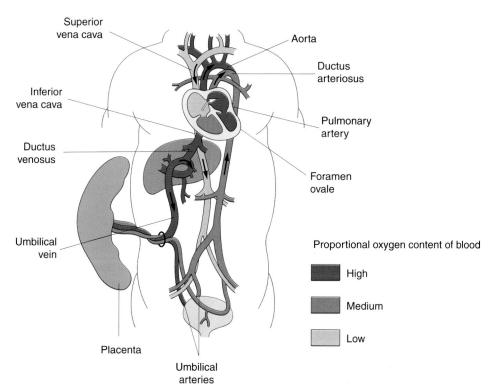

Figure 6.2 Diagrammatic representation of fetal circulation. (Reproduced from *A Colour Atlas of Doppler Ultrasonography in Obstetrics*, by K. Harrington and S. Campbell. London: Arnold, 1995.)

Oxygenated blood from the placenta returns to the fetus through the umbilical vein. This vein divides into two main branches, one that supplies the portal vein in the liver, and another narrow vessel called the ductus venosus, which joins the inferior vena cava as it enters the right atrium. Fifty per cent of the blood will pass to the portal system and 50 per cent to the ductus venosus. The ductus is a narrow vessel and high blood velocities are generated within it. This streaming of the ductus venosus blood, together with a membranous valve in the right atrium (the crista dividens), prevents mixing of the well-oxygenated blood from the ductus venosus with the desaturated blood of the inferior vena cava. The ductus venosus stream passes across the right atrium through a physiological defect in the atrial septum called the foramen ovale to the left atrium; from here, blood passes through the mitral valve to the left ventricle and hence to the aorta. About 50 per cent goes to the head and upper extremities; the remainder passes down the aorta to mix with blood of reduced oxygen saturation from the right ventricle.

Blood from the inferior vena cava and the superior vena cava is directed across the tricuspid valve to the right ventricle. Only a small portion of blood from the right ventricle passes to the lungs, as they are not functional. Most of the blood is directed through a narrow vessel called the ductus arteriosus into the descending aorta below the origin of the head and neck vessels from the aortic arch. By this means, the desaturated blood from the right ventricle passes down the aorta to enter the umbilical arterial circulation and thence to the placenta.

Prior to birth, the ductus remains patent due to the production of prostaglandin E2 and prostacyclin, which act as local vasodilators. Premature closure of the ductus has been reported with the administration of cyclo-oxygenase inhibitors.

At birth, the cessation of umbilical blood flow causes cessation of flow in the ductus venosus, a fall in pressure in the right atrium and closure of the foramen ovale. Ventilation of the lungs opens the pulmonary circulation, with a rapid fall in pulmonary vascular resistance. The ductus arteriosus closes functionally within a few days of birth.

Occasionally, this transition from fetal to adult circulation is delayed, usually because the pulmonary vascular resistance fails to fall despite adequate breathing. This delay, termed persistent fetal circulation, results in left-to-right shunting of blood from the aorta through the ductus arteriosus to the lungs. The baby remains cyanosed and can suffer from life-threatening hypoxia.

This delay in closure of the ductus arteriosus is most commonly seen in premature infants. It results in congestion in the pulmonary circulation and a reduction in blood flow to the gastrointestinal tract and brain, and is implicated in the pathogenesis of necrotizing enterocolitis and intraventricular haemorrhage.

Respiratory system: lung

Full differentiation of capillary and canalicular elements of the fetal lung is apparent by 20 weeks' gestation. Alveoli develop after 24 weeks. Numerous, but intermittent, fetal breathing movements occur in utero, especially during rapid eye movement (REM) sleep, and along with an adequate amniotic fluid volume appear to be necessary for lung maturation. Fetal breathing occurs for 15 per cent of the observation time in the second trimester, rising to 30 per cent in the third trimester. The fetal lung is filled with fluid, the production of which starts in early gestation and ends in the early stages of labour. At birth, the production of this fluid must cease and the fluid present is absorbed. Adrenaline, to which the pulmonary epithelium becomes increasingly sensitive towards term, appears to play a major role in this process.

Lung alveoli are lined by a group of phospholipids known collectively as surfactant. Surfactant prevents the collapse of small alveoli during expiration by lowering surface tension. The surfactant is continually replaced by synthesis from type 2 alveolar cells, with maximal production after 28 weeks. These cells make up 10 per cent of the lung parenchyma. The predominant phospholipid (80 per cent of the total) is phosphatidylcholine (lecithin). The production of lecithin is enhanced by cortisol, growth restriction and prolonged rupture of the membranes, and is delayed in diabetes. Other phospholipids may be more potent in reducing surface tension. For example, levels of phosphatidylglycerol in the amniotic fluid are more predictive of respiratory distress syndrome, especially in pregnancies complicated by diabetes.

Normal lung development requires an adequate amniotic fluid volume and fetal breathing movements. Oligohydramnios (reduced amniotic fluid volume), decreased intrathoracic space (e.g. diaphragmatic hernia), or chest wall deformities can result in pulmonary hypoplasia, which leads to progressive respiratory failure from birth.

Respiratory distress syndrome (RDS) is specific to babies born prematurely and is associated with surfactant deficiency. It typically presents within the first few hours of life with signs of respiratory distress, including tachypnoea and cyanosis. It occurs in more than 80 per cent of infants born between 23 and 27 weeks, falling to 10 per cent of infants born between 34 and 36 weeks. Acute complications include hypoxia and asphyxia, intraventricular haemorrhage and necrotizing enterocolitis. The incidence and severity of RDS can be reduced by administering steroids antenatally to mothers at risk of preterm delivery.

Fetal blood

The first fetal blood cells are formed on the surface of the yolk sac from 14 to 19 days after conception. Haemopoiesis continues from this site until the third post-conceptual month. During the fifth week of embryonic life, extramedullary haemopoiesis begins in the liver and to a lesser extent in the spleen. The bone marrow starts to produce red cells at 7–8 weeks and is the predominant source of red cells from 26 weeks' gestation.

Most haemoglobin in the fetus is fetal haemoglobin (HbF), which has two gamma-chains (alpha-2, gamma-2). This differs from the adult haemoglobins HbA and HbA2, which have two beta-chains (alpha-2, beta-2) and two delta-chains (alpha-2, delta-2) respectively. Ninety per cent of fetal haemoglobin is HbF between 10 and 28 weeks' gestation. From 28 to 34 weeks, a switch to HbA occurs, and at term the ratio of HbF to HbA is 80:20; by 6 months of age, only 1 per cent of haemoglobin is HbF. A key feature of HbF is a higher affinity for oxygen than HbA. This, in association with a higher haemoglobin concentration (at birth, the mean capillary haemoglobin is 18 g/dL), enhances transfer of oxygen across the placenta.

Abnormal haemoglobin production results in thalassaemia. The thalassaemias are a group of genetic haematological disorders characterized by reduced or absent production of one or more of the globin chains of haemoglobin. Beta-thalassaemia results from reduced or absent production of the beta-globin chains. As the switch from HbF to HbA described above occurs, the absent or insufficient beta-globin chains shorten red cell survival, with destruction of these cells within the bone marrow and spleen. Beta-thalassaemia major results from the inheritance of two abnormal beta genes; without treatment, this leads to severe anaemia, fetal growth restriction, poor musculoskeletal development and skin pigmentation due to increased iron absorption. In the severest form of alpha-thalassaemia, in which no alpha-globulin chains are produced, severe fetal anaemia occurs with cardiac failure, hepatosplenomegaly and generalized oedema. The infants are stillborn or die shortly after birth.

Immune system

The fetus requires an effective immune system to resist intrauterine and perinatal infections. Lymphocytes appear from 8 weeks, and by the middle of the second trimester all phagocytic cells, T and B cells and complement are available to mount a response. Early infection with any of the TORCH organisms (toxoplasmosis, rubella, cytomegalovirus, herpes) will affect a number of systems, including the immune defences themselves. Immunoglobulin G (IgG) originates mostly from the maternal circulation and crosses the placenta to provide passive immunity.

The fetus normally produces only small amounts of IgM and IgA, which do not cross the placenta. Detection of IgM/IgA in the newborn, without IgG, is indicative of fetal infection.

General immunological defences include the amniotic fluid (lysosymes, IgG), the placenta (lymphoid cells, phagocytes, barrier), granulocytes from liver and bone marrow and interferon from lymphocytes.

Skin and homeostasis

Fetal skin protects and facilitates homeostasis. The thickness of the skin increases progressively from the first month of gestation until birth. A stratum corneum forms in the fifth month and after approximately 23 weeks the appearance of the skin approaches that of the adult epidermis. During the last weeks, skin is covered by vernix, which consists of desquamated skin cells, cholesterol and glycogen. Preterm babies have no vernix and thin skin; this allows a proportionately large amount of insensible water loss.

Thermal control in cool, ambient temperatures is limited by a large surface-to-body-weight ratio and poor thermal insulation. Heat may be conserved by peripheral vasoconstriction and can be generated by brown fat catabolism, but this is deficient in preterm or growth-restricted babies because of the small amount of subcutaneous fat and immaturity of vascular tone regulation in the former. The response to warm ambient temperatures is also poor, because the poor responses of the eccrine glands will preserve heat and can result in overheating of the infant.

Alimentary system and energy stores

The primitive foregut and hindgut are present by the end of the fourth week and at this stage the intestine is almost a straight tube, suspended by the mesentery from the dorsal body wall. The abdominal cavity is too small to accommodate the enlarging liver and intestine and as a consequence the midgut herniates into the base of the umbilical cord during the sixth week. While herniated, the gut undergoes rotation prior to re-entering the abdominal cavity by 12 weeks. Failure of the gut to re-enter the abdominal cavity results in the development of an omphalocele.

From the time that the gastrointestinal tract is fully formed, the lumen is patent. The swallowing reflex develops and matures gradually. The fetus continually and increasingly swallows amniotic fluid, up to approximately 20 mL/h at term. A failure in this swallowing mechanism, as a consequence of either a neurological abnormality, e.g. anencephaly, or an obstruction in the gut, e.g. atresia of the oesophagus, will result in an increase in fluid within the amniotic cavity (polyhydramnios).

Peristalsis in the intestine occurs from the second trimester. The large bowel is filled with meconium at term. Defecation in utero, and hence meconium in the amniotic fluid, is associated with post-term pregnancies and fetal hypoxia. Aspiration of meconium-stained liquor by the fetus at birth can result in meconium aspiration syndrome and respiratory distress.

While body water content gradually diminishes, glycogen and fat stores increase about five-fold in the last trimester. Preterm infants have virtually no fat, and a severely reduced ability to withstand starvation. This is aggravated by an incompletely developed alimentary system, and may manifest in a poor and unsustained suck, uncoordinated swallowing mechanism, delayed gastric emptying, and poor absorption of carbohydrates, fat and other nutrients. Growth-restricted fetuses also have reduced glycogen stores and are therefore more prone to hypoglycaemia within the early neonatal period.

Liver and gallbladder

The primitive liver appears at about the 18th day of embryonic life as a diverticulum arising from the duodenum. By the 25th day, it has developed into a T-shaped outgrowth which is invaded by blood vessels. The larger portion of this diverticulum gives rise to the parenchymal cells and the hepatic ducts, while the smaller portion gives rise to the gallbladder. In utero, the normal metabolic functions of the liver are performed by the placenta. For example, unconjugated bilirubin from haemoglobin breakdown is actively transported from the fetus to the mother, with only a small proportion being conjugated in the liver and secreted in the bile (the mechanism after birth). The fetal liver also differs from the adult organ in many processes, for example the fetal liver has a reduced ability to conjugate bilirubin because of relative deficiencies in the necessary enzymes such as glucuronyl transferase. The loss of the placental route of excretion of unconjugated bilirubin, in the presence of reduced conjugation, particularly in the premature infant, may result in transient unconjugated hyperbilirubinaemia or physiological jaundice of the newborn. The fetal liver plays an important role in haemopoiesis, which starts at 6 weeks, peaks at 12–16 weeks and continues until approximately 36 weeks. Glycogen is stored within the liver in small quantities from the first trimester, but storage is maximal in the third trimester, with abundant stores being present at term. Growth-restricted and premature infants have deficient glycogen stores; this renders them prone to neonatal hypoglycaemia.

Kidney and urinary tract

After regression of the mesonephros or Wolffian duct, the metanephros forms the renal collecting system (ureter, pelvis, calyces and collecting ducts) and induces the formation of the renal secretory system (glomeruli, convoluted tubes, loops of Henle) from the mesenchyme of the nephrogenic cord. Nephrogenesis is complete by 36 weeks, but the maturation of the excretory and concentrating ability of the fetal kidneys is gradual. It is immature in the preterm infant, and this may lead to abnormal water, glucose, sodium or acid–base homeostasis.

Fetal urine forms much of the amniotic fluid, which is a protein-free and sugar-free hypotonic ultra-filtrate of fetal plasma. Fetal urine production rises gradually with fetal maturity, from about 12 mL/h at 32 weeks to 38 mL/h at 40 weeks. Renal agenesis will therefore result in severe reduction or absence of amniotic fluid (oligohydramnios).

Fetal behaviour

Fetal movement can be first perceived by the mother by about 18 weeks in primiparae and several weeks earlier in multiparae ('quickening'). Self-monitoring or formal counting of fetal movements is an important method of monitoring fetal well-being. A sensation of diminished fetal activity may be associated with chronic hypoxia and growth failure, and may be a precursor of fetal death. Reduced fetal movements are an important screening tool for further investigation.

With maturation of the central nervous system, the fetus develops more complex patterns and well-defined behavioural states that have been named 1F to 4F. State 1F is similar to quiet (non-REM) sleep, with an absence of eye and body movements. In state 2F, periodic eye and body movements are present (REM sleep). State 3F has eye movements but no body movements (i.e. is equivalent to quiet wakefulness), and 4F is an active phase with ongoing eye movements and fetal activity. For most of the time (>80 per cent), the fetus alternates between the sleep cycles 1F and 2F. This is particularly relevant when interpreting tests of fetal well-being, e.g. cardiotocography (CTG) and the biophysical profile. An unreactive CTG may reflect the fact that the fetus is in a sleep pattern (1F; 2F) and not compromised.

In this situation, providing there are not other indicators of potential compromise, the trace should be repeated after a reasonable time interval when the fetus is in a more active behavioural state (4F).

Amniotic fluid

By 12 weeks' gestation, the amnion comes into contact with the inner surface of the chorion and obliterates the extra-embryonic coelom. The two membranes become adherent, but never intimately fuse. Neither the amnion nor the chorion contains vessels or nerves, but both do contain a significant quantity of phospholipids as well as enzymes involved in phospholipid hydrolysis. Choriodecidual function is thought to play a pivotal role in the initiation of labour through the production of prostaglandins E2 and F2a.

The amniotic fluid is initially secreted by the amnion, but by the 10th week it is mainly a transudate of the fetal serum via the skin and umbilical cord. From 16 weeks' gestation, the fetal skin becomes impermeable to water and the net increase in amniotic fluid is through a small imbalance between the contributions of fluid through the kidneys and lung fluids and removal by fetal swallowing. Amniotic fluid volume increases progressively (10 weeks: 30 mL; 20 weeks: 300 mL; 30 weeks: 600 mL; 38 weeks: 1000 mL), but from term there is a rapid fall in volume (40 weeks: 800 mL; 42 weeks: 350 mL). The reason for the late reduction has not been explained.

The function of the amniotic fluid is to:
- protect the fetus from mechanical injury,
- permit movement of the fetus while preventing limb contracture,
- prevent adhesions between fetus and amnion,
- permit fetal lung development in which there is two-way movement of fluid into the fetal bronchioles; absence of amniotic fluid in the second trimester is associated with pulmonary hypoplasia.

Major alterations in amniotic fluid volume occur when there is reduced contribution of fluid into the amniotic sac in conditions such as renal agenesis, cystic kidneys or intrauterine growth restriction; oligohydramnios results. Reduced removal of fluid in conditions such as anencephaly and oesophageal/duodenal atresia is associated with polyhydramnios (see Chapter 11).

CASE HISTORY

A 26-year-old is admitted to the labour ward at 32 weeks' gestation. She gives a history suggestive of preterm rupture of membranes and is experiencing uterine contractions. On vaginal examination, the cervix is found to be 8 cm dilated and she rapidly goes on to deliver a male infant weighing 1650 g. At birth he is intubated because of poor respiratory effort and transferred to the neonatal intensive care unit.

As a premature infant, which complications is he particularly at risk of?

Fetal growth
Deficient glycogen stores in the liver increase the risk of *hypoglycaemia*. This is compounded by the increased glucose requirements of premature infants.

Cardiovascular system
Patent ductus arteriosus may result in pulmonary congestion, worsening lung disease and decreased blood flow to the gastrointestinal tract and brain. The duct can be closed by administering prostaglandin synthetase inhibitors, e.g. indomethacin, or by surgical ligation.

Respiratory system
Respiratory distress syndrome and *apnoea of prematurity* may lead to hypoxia. The administration of antenatal steroids to the mother reduces the risk and severity of respiratory distress syndrome. For benefit to be gained, steroids need to be administered at least 24 hours before delivery. In this case, delivery occurred too rapidly for steroids to be administered. The severity of respiratory distress syndrome can also be reduced by giving surfactant via the endotracheal tube used to ventilate the baby.

Fetal blood
Anaemia of prematurity is common because of low iron stores and red cell mass at birth, reduced erythropoiesis and decreased survival of red blood cells. Treatment is by blood transfusion, iron supplementation or, in some cases, the use of erythropoietin.

Immune system
Preterm babies have an increased susceptibility to *infection* due to impaired cell-mediated immunity and reduced levels of immunoglobulin. Suspected infection should be treated early with antibiotics because deterioration in these premature small infants can be rapid.

Skin and homeostasis
Hypothermia is common in preterm infants secondary to a relatively large body surface area, thin skin, lack of subcutaneous fat and lack of a keratinized epidermal layer of skin. High insensible water losses due to skin immaturity may aggravate dehydration and electrolyte problems secondary to immaturity in renal function (see below). The environment can be controlled by nursing this type of infant in an incubator.

Alimentary system
Necrotizing enterocolitis is an inflammatory condition of the bowel leading to necrosis, and is thought to be secondary to alterations in gut blood flow, hypotension, hypoxia, infection and feeding practices. *Feeding problems* are common in preterm infants because they have immature suck and swallowing reflexes and gut motility. Parenteral nutrition is usually required in these very premature infants, with gradually increasing volumes of milk given by nasogastric tube.

Liver and gallbladder
Jaundice (hyperbilirubinaemia) secondary to liver immaturity and a shorter half-life of red blood cells is common in premature infants. Treatment with phototherapy is required because premature infants are at greater risk of bilirubin encephalopathy.

Kidney and urinary tract
Immaturity of the kidneys can lead to a poor ability to concentrate or dilute urine. This can result in *dehydration and electrolyte disturbances*: hypernatraemia and hyponatraemia, hyperkalaemia and metabolic acidosis.

Neurological
Periventricular and intraventricular haemorrhages result from bleeding from the immature rich capillary bed of the germinal matrix lining the ventricles. Such haemorrhages are more likely in the presence of hypoxia. Major degrees of haemorrhage can result in hydrocephalus and neurological abnormalities such as cerebral palsy. *Periventricular leukomalacia* is ischaemic necrosis in the white matter surrounding the lateral ventricles, and commonly leads to cerebral palsy.

CASE HISTORY

A 16-year-old is admitted to the labour ward at 38 weeks' gestation. She gives a history suggestive of rupture of membranes and is experiencing uterine contractions. She was seen at 10 weeks' gestation for consideration of termination of pregnancy and had a scan at that time which confirmed her gestational age. She opted to continue with the pregnancy but did not attended for antenatal care. She admitted to smoking 20 cigarettes per day. Vaginal examination confirms that the cervix is 8 cm dilated. A CTG demonstrates a baseline fetal heart rate of 165 bpm with variable decelerations, and fetal scalp pH is 7.14 with a base deficit of 12 mmol/L. A Caesarean section is performed and a male infant weighing 1900 g is delivered. Apgar scores are 3 at 1 minute and 8 at 5 minutes.

Which complications are such severely growth-restricted infants particularly at risk of?

Reduced oxygen supply in utero can result in the fetus being *stillborn* or suffering damage from acute *asphyxia*. In the latter case, the neonate may demonstrate features of *HIE*, which may lead to death from multi-organ failure. If the infant survives, neurological damage and *cerebral palsy* may result. Chronic hypoxia in utero can also result in neurological damage without the acute manifestations of HIE. Other consequences of reduced oxygen supply in utero include increased *haemopoiesis* and *cardiac failure*. Increased haemopoiesis can in turn result in coagulopathy, polycythaemia and jaundice in the newborn.

Neonatal *hypothermia* and *hypoglycaemia* are also more common in this type of infant and result from reduced body fat and glycogen stores. Both of these conditions, if untreated, can lead to increased mortality and neurological damage.

Reduced supply of amino acids in utero can impair immune function, increasing the risk of *infection* in the newborn.

Growth-restricted babies are also at increased risk of *chronic diseases* such as coronary heart disease, stroke, hypertension and non-insulin-dependent diabetes in adulthood. This is thought to be because the fetal adaptation to under-nutrition in utero results in the permanent resetting of homeostatic mechanisms, and this leads to later disease.

Key Points

Determinants of birth weight are multi-factorial, and reflect the influence of the natural growth potential of the fetus and the intrauterine environment.

- The fetal circulation is quite different from that of the adult. Its distinctive features are:
  - oxygenation occurs in the placenta, not the lungs,
  - the right and left ventricles work in parallel rather than in series,
  - the heart, brain and upper body receive blood from the left ventricle, while the placenta and lower body receive blood from both right and left ventricles.
- Surfactant prevents collapse of small alveoli in the lung during expiration by lowering surface tension. Its production is maximal after 28 weeks. Respiratory distress syndrome is specific to babies born prematurely and is associated with surfactant deficiency.
- The fetus requires an effective immune system to resist intrauterine and perinatal infections. Lymphocytes appear from 8 weeks and, by the middle of the second trimester, all phagocytic cells, T and B cells and complement are available to mount a response.

- Fetal skin protects and facilitates homeostasis.
- In utero, the normal metabolic functions of the liver are performed by the placenta. The loss of the placental route of excretion of unconjugated bilirubin, in face of conjugating enzyme deficiencies, particularly in the premature infant, may result in transient unconjugated hyperbilirubinaemia or physiological jaundice of the newborn.
- Growth-restricted and premature infants have deficient glycogen stores; this renders them prone to neonatal hypoglycaemia.
- The function of the amniotic fluid is to:
  - protect the fetus from mechanical injury,
  - permit movement of the fetus while preventing limb contracture,
  - prevent adhesions between fetus and amnion,
  - permit fetal lung development in which there is two-way movement of fluid into the fetal bronchioles; absence of amniotic fluid in the second trimester is associated with pulmonary hypoplasia.

Antenatal care

OVERVIEW

The overall purpose of antenatal care is to optimize the outcome of pregnancy for the mother, her child and the rest of her family.

History taking, examination and the use of investigations are tailored to each individual pregnancy to assess risk and to screen for potential physical, psychological and social problems.

If a potential problem is identified, appropriate action can be taken to minimize the impact it has on the pregnancy. This may involve recruiting help from other professionals.

Aims of antenatal care

The aims of antenatal care are:
- to prevent, detect and manage those factors that adversely affect the health of mother and baby;
- to provide advice, reassurance, education and support for the woman and her family;
- to deal with the 'minor ailments' of pregnancy;
- to provide general health screening.

The original model of antenatal care established in the 1930s involved as many as 15 visits to a doctor or a midwife. This scheme was not evidence based, but persisted for many years because of fears that reducing the number of visits would lead to an increase in maternal and perinatal morbidity and mortality. Newer models of antenatal care have questioned the need for so many reviews and in *problem-free low-risk* pregnancies there is no evidence that fewer visits has compromised outcomes. However, the initial risk assessment of the pregnancy is vital if more intensive levels of care are to be appropriately targeted to women at higher risk of complications. Risk assessment should be viewed as an ongoing exercise throughout the pregnancy so that the type of care offered to a woman can change if her level of risk changes. If a pregnancy is deemed to be 'low risk', a minimum standard of care is still to be expected. This chapter focuses on this minimum standard of antenatal care and describes how the process of risk assessment is carried out.

Classification of antenatal care

Shared care

This is the term given to antenatal care that is provided jointly by a hospital maternity team, a general practitioner (GP) and community midwives. Women receiving this form of care are 'booked' under a named hospital consultant and are seen in hospital for the booking visit by a member of this consultant's team.

Some hospital consultants still see all their antenatal patients again routinely at 28–32 weeks; however, there is no evidence that this improves outcomes for low-risk women and it certainly makes the hospital antenatal clinics extremely busy.

Mostly, 'low-risk' women are not reviewed again by the hospital team until they have gone past their expected delivery date. All other routine check-ups are carried out by the community team. If potential problems are detected, an appointment in the consultant antenatal clinic is organized. Women with risk factors identified at booking may have extra hospital appointments organized from the outset, making this form of care ideal for those women whose pregnancies are not entirely straightforward.

Community-based care

The booking appointment is carried out by a community midwife. Routine scans and investigations are also requested by the community midwife, performed in the hospital and interpreted by the community team. GPs have a variable involvement in the provision of community-based antenatal care and ideally only 'low-risk' women are offered this option. If potential problems arise, a referral to a hospital consultant team may become necessary. Community-based care is often accompanied by intrapartum care provided by the same team of community midwives. Women often appreciate the continuity that this provides and see this form of care as less interventional due to minimal medical involvement.

Hospital-based care

This is really an extension of shared care. Ultimately, even the women who are at highest risk are likely to benefit from some community midwifery input. However, this form of care involves a structured programme of visits to a hospital antenatal clinic which may well be highly specialized (e.g. an antenatal clinic for women with diabetes).

Whichever form of care is chosen, a pregnant woman will receive a set of *patient-held records* in which all healthcare professionals will write each time she is seen. The booking proforma (Fig. 7.1) is found within these notes, as are the results of investigations and plans for the delivery. This improves communication and allows access for all healthcare staff to the same information.

Most maternity units now also provide *day-care facilities*. Hospital-booked or community-booked patients can be referred to these units for assessment or review of a wide variety of antenatal problems, including hypertension in pregnancy and reduced fetal movements. The units are staffed by experienced midwives, many of whom are trained in ultrasonography. Day-care units help to reduce admissions to antenatal wards which can cause enormous social and domestic disruption.

Advice, reassurance and education

Pregnancy is a time of great uncertainty, and the physical changes experienced by the woman during her pregnancy add to this. She may need explanation and reassurance to help her cope with a wide variety of symptoms, including nausea, heartburn, constipation, shortness of breath, dizziness, swelling, backache, abdominal discomfort and headaches. Mostly, these represent the physiological adaptation of her body to the pregnancy and are often called the 'minor complaints' of pregnancy. Although usually of minimal harm, they can be extremely distressing and cause significant anxiety. Occasionally they will be the first presentation of a more serious problem. A skilled community midwife will differentiate those women who need referral to hospital from those who can be reassured and managed with simple advice.

Information regarding smoking, alcohol consumption and the use of drugs during pregnancy (both legal and illegal) is extremely important. In some populations almost a third of women smoke during pregnancy despite its association with fetal growth restriction, preterm labour, abruption and intrauterine fetal death. A major role of antenatal care is to help women limit these harmful behaviours during pregnancy, for example by inclusion in smoking cessation programmes. Alcohol or illegal substance misuse may require more specialized skills from a psychiatric service. Women also need advice on work, exercise, sexual intercourse and maternity benefits.

Parentcraft is the term used to describe formal group education of issues relating to pregnancy, labour and delivery and care of the newborn. These sessions offer an opportunity for couples to meet others in the same

NAME/ADDRESS/POSTCODE: Parvinder Singh 7, Birchwood Avenue Newtown	AFFIX PATIENT IDENTIFICATION LABEL HERE IF AVAILABLE ALTERNATIVELY WRITE INFORMATION IN BOX PROVIDED	D.O.B: 31-01-63	DATE OF BOOKING	05-02-02	
		Religion:	Marital Status:	Married	
			Previous Name/s:	/	
			Country of Origin:	Pakistan	
			ETHNIC GROUP	Patient	Partner
			White		

Telephone Home:	Telephone Work:	Black Caribbean		
HOSPITAL No.	OCCUPATION: Housewife	Black African		
CONSULTANT: Mr. Jackson	PARTNER'S OCCUPATION: Plumber	Black Other		
PLACE OF DELIVERY: Newtown maternity unit	NHS No:	Indian		
LMP: 12/11/01 EDD: 19/08/02	Silver Stat Card Y/N	Pakistani	✓	✓
FAMILY DOCTOR: Address: Telephone No: Name: Dr. P. Smith Newtown M/C		Bangladeshi		
		Chinese		
HUSBAND/PARTNER Address: Telephone No: Name: Davinder Singh - as above		Any other group		
		Not Given		

NEXT OF KIN: Address: Telephone No:

Relationship: Husband – as above

Computer information explained Y/N	Signature of Midwife	Printed Name:
Social Worker	Telephone:	Referral Date:

MEDICAL AND SURGICAL HISTORY						ANTENATAL INVESTIGATION			
	YES	NO		YES	NO	BOOKING	DATE	RESULT	
1. Cardiac/Hypertension	✓		14. Special Diet		✓	B.T.S. Number			
2. Thromboembolism	✓		15. Vegetarian		✓	ABO Group		B Pos	
3. Respiratory		✓	16. Drug Misuse*		✓	Antibodies		Neg	
4. Renal		✓	17. Bacterial Infections		✓	H.I.V.		Neg	
5. Alimentary		✓	18. Viral Infections		✓	VDRL		Neg	
6. Liver		✓	19. Chickenpox		✓	Hepatitis	A	Neg	
7. Endocrinological	✓		20. Genetic		✓		B	Neg	
8. Neurological		✓	21. Previous Surgery	✓			C		
9. Haematological	✓		22. Previous Infertility		✓	Electrophoresis			
10. Blood Transfusion	✓		23. Other		✓	Rubella Titre		Immune	
11. Contraception		✓	24. Mental Health		✓	AFP			
12. Drugs in Pregnancy		✓	25. Alcohol (units per week)		✓	MSU			
13. Allergies		✓	26. Smoking		✓	Cytology			

COMMENTS:

1. Previous pre-eclampsia
   Essential hypertension also
2. Previous deep vein thrombosis (left)
7. Hypothyroidism: on thyroxine
9. Anaemia in previous pregnancy
10. and 21. Previous transfusion after C/S.

Amniocentesis
CVS
Down's Screening
Other
PREVIOUS ANTI-D GIVEN   YES/NO
DATES GIVEN

Figure 7.1 A typical booking proforma contained in patient-held records.

Name: *Parvinder Singh*　　　　Hospital No. ....

PREVIOUS ANAESTHETIC PROBLEMS
(see anaesthetic referral guide lines)

Booking:- Weight

　　Height

	YES	NO
BM Index 42		
REFERRAL		

FAMILY HISTORY

	YES	NO		YES	NO		YES	NO
1. Multiple Birth		✓	4. Diabetes	✓		6. Congenital Abnormalities		✓
2. Hypertension	✓		5. Tuberculosis		✓	7. Deafness (Congenital)		✓
3. Thromboembolism	✓		Other					

Comments:

2. Essential hypertension – both Parvinder's parents.
3. Parvinder's mother and sister have both had pulmonary emboli
4. Parvinder's mother has non-insulin dependent diabetes mellitus

OBSTETRIC HISTORY

Menstrual Cycle: $\frac{5}{28}$　　　GRAVIDA: 6　　PARTIY: 4 + 1

LMP: 12/11/01　　EDD: 19/08/02　NORMAL YES/NO　　BLEEDING SINCE LMP YES/NO

DATE	PLACE	DURATION OF PREGNANCY	METHOD OF DELIVERY	SEX	WT.	CONDITION AT BIRTH	NAME OF CHILD
1985	NMU	38 wks	NVD	♂	2.7 kg	A + W	
			(Induced for PET)				
1987	NMU	39 wks	NVD	♀	2.65 kg	A + W	
1990	NMU	39 wks	NVD	♀	2.8 kg	A + W	
1992	NMU	8/40	Miscarriage				
1993	NMU	40 wks	Elective Caesarean section. Transverse lie. PPH. Transfusion	♂	3.0 kg	A + W	

INFORMATION GIVEN

HEA. Pregnancy Booklet　Yes/No　　Screening Tests　Yes/No　　FW8 Form　Yes/No

Figure 7.1 *(continued)*.

situation and help to establish a network of social contacts that may be useful after the delivery. They usually include a tour of the maternity department, the aim of which is to lessen anxiety and increase the sense of maternal control surrounding delivery.

The booking visit

The degree of risk in a pregnancy is determined by the use of repeated history taking, physical examination and investigations. The *first* risk assessment is usually made at the booking visit, which can be carried out in hospital or in the community. If risk factors are identified at this visit, the woman is likely to be referred directly for hospital-based or shared care. Issues raised at the booking visit may need to be pursued in some depth.

Before the risk assessment begins, the pregnancy should be confirmed and the expected date of delivery (EDD) should be calculated.

Confirmation of the pregnancy

The symptoms of pregnancy (breast tenderness, nausea, amenorrhoea, urinary frequency) combined with a positive urinary or serum pregnancy test are usually sufficient confirmation of a pregnancy, and an internal examination to assess uterine size is not often necessary. In many regions, all pregnant women are referred for a 'dating scan' (see below), which both confirms the pregnancy and accurately dates it. It may be possible to hear the fetal heart with the Doppler ultrasound from approximately 12 weeks onwards.

Dating the pregnancy

Setting a reliable EDD is an important function of the booking visit. Precise dating of a pregnancy becomes extremely important both at preterm gestations, when it may influence the timing of the delivery if there are fetal or maternal problems, and when the pregnancy is prolonged. A number of different screening tests also rely on an accurate gestation if their interpretation is to be meaningful (see serum screening for neural tube defects and Down's syndrome, Chapter 9). A pregnancy can be dated either by using the date of the first day of the last menstrual period (LMP) or by ultrasound scan.

Menstrual EDD

Naegele's rule states that the EDD is calculated by adding 7 days to the first day of the LMP and taking away 3 months. For example, if the LMP was 2 December 2003, the EDD by this rule would be 9 September 2004. This can be more easily determined by using an obstetric 'wheel'. This rule assumes a 28-day menstrual cycle, ovulation on day 14 of this cycle, and an accurate recollection by the woman of her LMP. In reality, the timing of ovulation is variable within a cycle and most women do not have a period every 28 days. Furthermore, many studies have shown poor recollection of the LMP.

Dating by ultrasound

For these reasons, dating by an ultrasound scan in the first or early second trimester is generally considered to be more accurate, especially if there is menstrual irregularity or uncertainty regarding the LMP. Many regions offer all women a dating scan.

Benefits of a dating scan

- Accurate dating in women with irregular menstrual cycles or poor recollection of LMP.
- Reduced incidence of induction of labour for 'prolonged pregnancy' (see Chapter 17).
- Maximizing the potential for serum screening to detect fetal abnormalities (see Chapter 9).
- Early detection of multiple pregnancies.
- Detection of otherwise asymptomatic failed intrauterine pregnancies.

Before 15–16 weeks' gestation there is minimal variation in fetal size between individual pregnancies, so measurements of the crown–rump length (CRL), biparietal diameter (BPD) and femur length (FL) can be plotted on standard fetal biometry charts and the gestation calculated (Fig. 7.2). If the EDD predicted by the dating scan differs by more than 7 days from the menstrual EDD, the scan EDD is usually chosen as the final EDD.

Beyond 20 weeks' gestation, the effects of genes and environmental factors will cause significant variability in fetal size. Dating a pregnancy by ultrasound

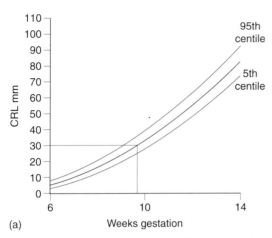

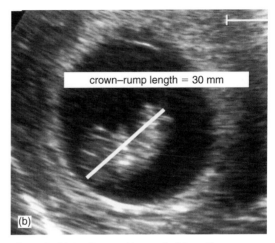

Figure 7.2 (a) Typical crown–rump length (CRL) chart showing normal growth. (b) An ultrasound image of a fetus with crown–rump length measurement.

CASE HISTORY

Mrs A attends an antenatal booking clinic on 26th June 2003. She has an irregular menstrual cycle and has a poor memory regarding her LMP; she thinks it was 3rd April 2003. From this LMP, her EDD should be 10th January 2004 and at this booking visit she should be 12 weeks' gestation. An ultrasound is requested to date the pregnancy and the result is shown in Figure 7.2. The CRL of the fetus is 30 mm. This is plotted to the 50th centile on the CRL chart and found to correspond to 9 weeks and 4 days. This differs by more than 7 days from her menstrual EDD and a new EDD, based on the scan of 25th January, is established.

scan therefore becomes progressively less accurate as the gestation advances.

The booking history

Past medical, obstetric and gynaecological histories are explored in depth, as these may have a major impact on the pregnancy risk assessment. Family history and social factors may have an even greater impact on the pregnancy than clinical factors. Age and racial origin must be noted at booking. Women at the extremes of reproductive ages are at greater risk of certain pregnancy complications (e.g. fetal chromosomal abnormalities in older women) and specific racial groups carry higher risks of medical conditions, both genetic (e.g. sickle-cell disease and thalassaemias) and otherwise (fibroids, for example in Africans). Women from ethnic minorities may find it more difficult to access medical care and there may be a need to arrange interpreters for those with language difficulties.

A detailed guide to obstetric history taking is given in Chapter 1. A few examples are discussed in the paragraphs below to emphasize how important this initial assessment really is.

Past medical history

The interaction between pregnancy and medical, surgical and psychiatric conditions has given rise to a clinical specialty called maternal medicine. The disease in question, and its treatments, may adversely affect the pregnancy and fetus in a number of different ways. Medications may be teratogenic or may alter fetal physiology. There may be an associated increased risk of placental dysfunction leading to fetal growth restriction, pregnancy-induced hypertension and/or preterm labour. The pregnancy itself may cause an improvement or deterioration in the co-existing medical condition. Pregnant women with other health problems are often managed jointly by obstetricians and physicians in 'high-risk' clinics. The details are discussed elsewhere, but the example booking pro-forma sheet (see Fig. 7.1) illustrates how the history is used to screen for these potential complications.

Past obstetric history

Pregnancy complications of most kinds carry a recurrence risk. The knowledge of previous complicating factors may influence the management of subsequent pregnancies. Details of previous labours and deliveries may also determine choices in the future. For example, careful discussion is needed with a woman who delivered her previous baby by Caesarean section (see Chapter 17).

Previous gynaecological history

A previous history of infertility or recurrent miscarriage may be extremely relevant to an ongoing pregnancy, not least in that it is likely to have a significant psychological impact on the woman and how she perceives the current pregnancy. Even with an ongoing pregnancy, a history of recurrent miscarriage may be a marker for other pregnancy complications such as fetal growth restriction, pre-eclampsia and fetal chromosomal abnormality. A history of gynaecological surgery may also be important. A cone biopsy, for example, may cause cervical incompetence or stenosis and myomectomy may weaken the uterus and increase the risks of uterine rupture during labour (see Chapter 19).

Family history

A number of medical conditions with familial tendencies may complicate the pregnancy. Gestational diabetes is more common in women with a family history of type II diabetes, and thromboembolic disease within the family may point to a higher risk of deep vein thrombosis and pulmonary emboli for the woman herself during her pregnancy. A wide variety of single-gene disorders can be tested for antenatally, but only if a recognized family history exists. General terms such as 'cerebral palsy' or 'mental handicap' are often used by women to describe the problems suffered by their relatives. These terms are not diagnostic and include a wide range of aetiologies, some of which are environmental and do not increase the recurrence risks within a family overall, and some of which are genetic, and do. Fragile X syndrome is a common inheritable cause of severe learning difficulty caused by a mutation on the X chromosome. It mostly affects boys, and female family members may be asymptomatic carriers. Failure to explore problems within a family may therefore mean the opportunity is missed for prenatal diagnosis in the index pregnancy.

Social history

The impact of smoking and alcohol misuse on pregnancy is discussed in other chapters. Direct questioning at booking is essential if women are to be offered appropriate support in reducing or stopping harmful activities during pregnancy. This also applies to the use of illegal substances such as cocaine, heroin and amphetamines.

Social deprivation is associated with poorer obstetric outcomes and its importance as a marker for pregnancy complications should be recognized. Domestic violence and child neglect raise serious concerns for the welfare of the woman and her unborn child.

CASE HISTORY

Mrs Singh is 12 weeks' gestation and attends a booking visit with her community midwife, who fills out her patient-held records. The history page is shown in Figure 7.1. A number of issues have been raised which must be addressed when planning her antenatal care.

Mrs Singh is originally from Pakistan, although she has been a UK citizen for many years. This makes a language problem less likely. However, there is no record of a thalassaemia screen having been performed. This is important, as thalassaemia trait might contribute to maternal anaemia. Also, if Mrs Singh's husband is a carrier as well, her offspring would have a 1 in 4 chance of being fully affected. It is reassuring that all the children are fit and well.

Of greater importance is Mrs Singh's age (39). This slightly increases the risks of dysfunctional labour and pre-eclampsia, but more significantly is associated with an increase in the risk of certain fetal chromosomal abnormalities, namely Down's syndrome. The decision to undergo screening and invasive testing is a personal one, often affected by cultural and religious beliefs, but the offer of testing should be made to all women. Women booking over the age of 37 are often offered an amniocentesis and may choose to bypass screening tests such as nuchal translucency scanning and serum biochemistry.

Mrs Singh has essential hypertension (probably related to her body weight) but is not treated with medication. This, her previous history of pre-eclampsia (in her first pregnancy), and her age all increase the risk of pre-eclampsia occurring in this pregnancy. Regular antenatal checks will be needed to detect a recurrence. There is a worrying personal history of deep vein thrombosis and a close family history of pulmonary emboli. It is highly likely that this family has an inherited thrombophilia (increased blood-clotting tendency) such as protein C or S deficiency or anti-thrombin III deficiency. Confirming or excluding this possibility is important because thrombophilias are associated with a high thrombotic risk in pregnancy (especially the puerperium) and an increase in the risk of fetal growth restriction, placental abruption and pre-eclampsia. Many of these complications can be prevented by the use of antenatal and postnatal low-dose aspirin or heparin injections.

Mrs Singh's children have all been of low birth weight. It is difficult to determine whether they were constitutionally small but healthy or whether they were pathologically small (i.e. growth restricted). It would be important to organize serial growth scans during this pregnancy as surveillance for fetal growth restriction.

Hypothyroidism corrected by thyroxine supplements rarely causes complications during pregnancy. Anaemia is common and usually responds to oral iron supplements. Dietary advice may be necessary and other causes of anaemia must always be considered. The blood transfusion after her last delivery has been noted. No red cell antibodies have occurred as a result, but these will need to be checked for again later in the pregnancy.

Mrs Singh has a raised body mass index (BMI) and this increases her risks of anaesthetic complications (such as failure to intubate or successfully site a spinal anaesthetic) and also her risks of developing gestational diabetes. An oral glucose tolerance test will be recommended at 28 weeks' gestation to screen for this.

Finally, the previous Caesarean section is a risk factor which will require discussion. The transverse lie was probably secondary to uterine laxity, but this would need to be confirmed by reading the old notes. It may occur again, but even if it does not, the risks of a trial of labour (in the presence of a previous Caesarean section scar) or a repeat elective Caesarean section will need to be discussed.

Clearly Mrs Singh is not a low-risk case. The booking history has produced a number of issues that increase her risk of complications during her pregnancy. Shared care under a hospital consultant would be the appropriate form of antenatal care.

The booking examination

Historically, a full physical examination was carried out at the booking visit. This included cardiovascular and respiratory systems as well as an abdominal, full pelvic and breast examination. The value of this has been questioned, as the detection of significant pathology in the absence of focal symptoms is uncommon. Loud heart sounds and flow murmurs can be heard in most pregnant women and usually result from the hyperdynamic circulation rather than from pathology. Speculum examination in the absence of bleeding or discharge is likely to be unhelpful, uncomfortable and embarrassing for the woman, and breast examination has a higher false-positive rate due to pregnancy-related physiological changes in breast tissue.

Furthermore, excessive anxiety can be caused by the subsequent referrals that are made to appropriate specialists when these 'signs' are found.

Most of these 'rituals' have been dispensed with in low-risk women, but thorough examination must be carried out if there are symptoms of concern.

For most healthy women without complicating medical problems, the booking examination will include the following.

- Accurate measurement of blood pressure.
- Abdominal examination to record the size of the uterus.
- Recognition of any abdominal scars indicative of previous surgery.
- Measurement of height and weight for calculation of the BMI. Women with a low BMI are at greater

risk of fetal growth restriction and obese women are at significantly greater risk of most obstetric complications, including gestational diabetes, pre-eclampsia, need for emergency Caesarean section and anaesthetic difficulties.

- Urine examination: asymptomatic bacteriuria is more likely to ascend and cause pyelonephritis in pregnancy. This causes significant maternal morbidity, but also predisposes to pregnancy loss and preterm labour. All women at booking should either have a midstream urine sent for culture or be tested with a dipstick which recognizes nitrates, the presence of which sensitively predicts the presence of significant bacteria.

Booking investigations

All pregnant women are encouraged to undergo screening for a number of health issues which may have an impact on the pregnancy or the fetus. Tests above and beyond these may be requested at booking if the history or examination demands it.

The following blood tests are usually performed.

Full blood count

This screens for anaemia and thrombocytopenia (low platelet count), both of which may require further investigation. Anaemia in pregnancy is most frequently caused by iron deficiency; however, a wide variety of other causes must be considered, especially if the haemoglobin value is <9.0 g/dL.

Blood group and red cell antibodies

Recording the blood group at this point will help with cross-matching blood at a later date if an emergency arises. Red cell antibodies most commonly arise from previous blood transfusions and may cause problems with rapid cross-matching and/or haemolytic disease of the newborn (HDN, see Chapter 11). Women found to be rhesus negative will be offered prophylactic anti-D administration at 28 and 34 weeks' gestation to prevent rhesus iso-immunization and future HDN. Other possible iso-immunizing events, such as threatened miscarriage after 12 weeks' gestation, antepartum haemorrhage and delivery of the baby, may require additional anti-D prophylaxis in rhesus-negative women.

Rubella

Vertical transmission of rubella from a mother to her fetus carries a high risk of causing serious congenital abnormalities, especially in the first trimester. Women who are found to be rubella non-immune should be strongly advised to avoid infectious contacts and should undergo rubella immunization after the current pregnancy to protect themselves for the future. The theoretical risk of viral reactivation from the vaccine means it should not be given during pregnancy, and pregnancy should be avoided for the 3 months following immunization. A history of previous immunization is not a guarantee of permanent immunity.

Hepatitis B

The presence of antibodies to the surface antigen represents immunity resulting either from previous infection or from immunization and should not cause concern. The presence of the surface antigen itself, or the 'e' antigen, represents either a recent infection or carrier status. Vertical transmission to the fetus may occur, mostly during labour, and horizontal transmission to staff or the newborn infant can follow contact with body fluids. A baby born to a hepatitis B carrier should be actively and passively immunized at delivery.

Human immunodeficiency virus

Without screening, less than half of all pregnant women infected with human immunodeficiency virus (HIV) are aware of their status. In known HIV-positive mothers, the use of antiretroviral agents, elective Caesarean section and avoidance of breastfeeding reduces vertical transmission rates from approximately 30 per cent to less than 5 per cent. Knowledge of HIV infection is therefore vital if the offspring are to be protected. Screening only those women at high risk of HIV infection (e.g. intravenous drug abusers, recent immigrants from central Africa) misses a significant number of cases. The Department of Health guidelines now recommend that all pregnant women should be offered an HIV test at booking.

Syphilis

Although only 200–300 new cases of syphilis are reported each year, it can be vertically transmitted to the fetus, with serious consequences. This transmission can be prevented simply by treatment of the mother with antibiotics. Because of this, and because the incidence is rising, testing for syphilis in pregnancy continues.

Haemoglobin studies

Tests for thalassaemia and sickle-cell disease are usually reserved for women who have an ethnic background from outside Northern Europe (especially Eastern Mediterranean, Indian, West Indian, South-East Asian and those from the Middle East). If a woman is found to be a carrier for any of the haemoglobinopathies, the father of the fetus should also be offered testing, as there is a 1 in 4 chance that their offspring will have the full clinical condition if he too is a carrier. Formal prenatal testing is offered to couples when both are carriers.

Gestational diabetes

Policies for screening for gestational diabetes mellitus (GDM) vary widely within regions and across the country. No universally accepted screening or diagnostic criteria exist for this condition, making it a very complex and confusing aspect of routine antenatal care (see Chapter 15). The policy of screening pregnant women only if they have one of a number of risk factors will inevitably miss a proportion of women with GDM. The alternative is to screen all pregnant women, a policy adopted in some centres. Screening may occur at booking but is more usefully performed at 28 weeks, when the metabolic changes of GDM have usually progressed to a level detectable with current screening tests. The screening tests themselves also vary. A random blood sugar, a fasting blood sugar or a formal oral glucose tolerance test may be employed and many different screening schedules exist, as do the criteria for diagnosis of GDM.

Other routine investigations

Cervical smears and vaginal swabs are not routinely taken at the booking visit. However, smears should be performed during pregnancy on women with an abnormal cervix on examination or those who are unlikely to attend postnatally and who are overdue for a smear. The request form should state clearly that the woman is pregnant, as this will affect interpretation of the cytology.

There is no evidence that a 'routine' fetal growth scan in the third trimester is of any value in low-risk women.

Screening for fetal abnormalities

This is a routine aspect of antenatal care, offered to all women in some form or another. Initial discussion of these screening tests usually occurs at the booking visit to establish the wishes of the couple. The tests themselves are carried out between 11 and 22 weeks' gestation and include:

- nuchal translucency scanning (11–13 weeks) or serum screening (15–19 weeks) for Down's syndrome,
- maternal serum alpha-fetoprotein (15–19 weeks) for neural tube defects, e.g. spina bifida, anencephaly,
- the 'detailed' or 'anomaly' ultrasound scan (19–22 weeks) for structural congenital abnormalities.

These tests are discussed in detail in Chapter 9. However, it is important to note that these screening tests, as with the blood tests mentioned earlier, are optional and should only be performed with the verbal consent of the woman after careful discussion regarding the relative pros and cons of the testing process.

Follow-up visits

Pattern of follow-up visits

A similar schedule of antenatal visits is offered regardless of the choice of shared or community-based care. The precise number of visits is a contentious point and should be tailored to the individual. Four-weekly appointments from 20 weeks until 32 weeks, followed by fortnightly visits from 32 weeks to 36 weeks and weekly visits thereafter, was a common pattern of antenatal care previously adopted for women in their first pregnancy. Pre-eclampsia is a common complication of first pregnancies, particularly in the late third trimester (see Chapter 13). It can develop quickly, over a period of a few days, and for this reason weekly visits after 36 weeks are still recommended by some authorities. Women with a normal past obstetric history are much less likely to have complications such as pre-eclampsia and therefore are often reviewed less frequently. The minimum number of 'visits' recommended by the Royal College of Obstetricians and Gynaecologists is five, occurring at 12, 20, 28–32, 36 and 40–41 weeks.

The content of follow-up visits

Each follow-up antenatal appointment should be viewed as an opportunity for screening and education. At every visit, the following should be carried out:

- General questions regarding maternal well-being.
- Enquiry regarding fetal movements (from 24 weeks).
- Measurement of blood pressure (a screen for pregnancy-related hypertensive disorders).
- Urinalysis, particularly for protein, blood and glucose: this is used to help detect infection, pre-eclampsia and gestational diabetes.
- Examination for oedema: oedema is common in pregnancy and is mostly an insensitive marker of pre-eclampsia. Oedema of the hands and face is somewhat more important as a warning feature of pre-eclampsia.
- Abdominal palpation for fundal height: if repeated symphysis–fundal height measurements are made throughout a pregnancy, the detection of fetal growth problems and abnormalities of liquor volume is increased.
- Auscultation of the fetal heart: there is no evidence that this practice is of any benefit in a woman confident in the movements of her baby; however, it provides considerable reassurance and will occasionally detect an otherwise unrecognized intrauterine fetal death.
  The following are carried out in addition to the above.
- A full blood count and red cell antibody screen is repeated at 28 and 36 weeks.
- Depending on the screening policy of the particular unit, women at 28 weeks may be tested for gestational diabetes.
- From 36 weeks, the lie of the fetus (longitudinal, transverse or oblique), its presentation (cephalic or breech) and the degree of engagement of the presenting part should be assessed and recorded. It is often at this appointment that a decision is made regarding the mode of delivery (i.e. vaginal delivery or planned Caesarean section).
- At 41 weeks' gestation, a discussion regarding the merits of induction of labour for prolonged pregnancy should occur. An association between prolonged pregnancy and increased perinatal morbidity and mortality means that women are usually advised that delivery of the baby should occur by 42 completed weeks' gestation. This will usually mean organizing a date for induction of labour at approximately 12 days past the EDD.

Common problems detected in routine antenatal care are hypertensive disorders of pregnancy, anaemia, abnormalities of uterine size ('small-for-dates' and 'large-for-dates') and abnormal fetal presentations. Further investigation in hospital will be necessary.

The routine use of iron supplements is debated. Pregnancy is undoubtedly a major drain on total body iron stores, and iron-deficiency anaemia is common in pregnancy. A haemoglobin value of <10.6 g/dL is often used as a threshold for commencing iron supplements, but more precise measures of iron deficiency such as serum ferritin and zinc protoporphyrin levels may help target treatment more sensibly. Women at high risk of anaemia (e.g. those with multiple pregnancies) or at higher risk of haemorrhage (e.g. women with placenta praevia) should be advised to take iron throughout their pregnancy. Oral iron supplements commonly cause nausea and gastrointestinal upset and compliance can be poor. Iron syrups may be better tolerated than tablets, but ultimately intramuscular injections of iron may be necessary for the most severe cases if the oral route fails.

Rhesus-negative women should be offered and advised to have prophylactic anti-D administration at 28 and 34 weeks. Although this practice is recommended for all rhesus-negative women, there exists geographical variation in its provision.

Each follow-up visit should be seen as an opportunity for women to express their anxieties and to educate them in the details of delivery, infant feeding and parenting skills.

Customized antenatal care

Through the process of booking and routine antenatal follow-up, it may become apparent that a woman and her pregnancy have risk factors or special needs not met by standard care. Referrals to other hospital consultants, psychiatric services, social services and physiotherapists are common in pregnancy. Indeed, 'high-risk' antenatal clinics staffed by interested obstetricians and doctors from other specialties can usually be found in tertiary centres.

Antenatal complications dealt with in customized antenatal clinics

- Endocrine (diabetes, thyroid, prolactin and other endocrinopathies)
- Miscellaneous medical disorders (e.g. secondary hypertension, autoimmune disease)
- Haematology (thrombophilias, bleeding disorders)
- Substance misuse
- Preterm labour
- Multiple gestation
- Teenage pregnancies

Furthermore, a number of regions are fortunate in having dedicated 'mother-and-baby' teams to care for pregnant women with psychiatric problems. Included in the team are psychiatrists, counsellors, community psychiatric nurses and social workers who have a special interest in pregnancy and its interaction with psychiatric and psychological problems (see Chapter 21).

Key Points

- Antenatal care improves pregnancy outcomes and a variety of models exist.
- There are key visits during the pregnancy when essential investigations or decisions are taken regarding antenatal care and delivery.
- Antenatal care should be seen as an opportunity for education, reassurance and screening for potential problems.
- Continued efforts should be made to improve access of disadvantaged groups to antenatal care.

Chapter 8

Antenatal imaging and assessment of fetal well-being

OVERVIEW

There is one principal imaging modality in obstetrics, namely diagnostic ultrasound, which is employed in many clinical situations and indeed is used routinely to screen all pregnancies in most developed countries. Ultrasound is used to date and chart antenatal growth of the fetus and to identify congenital abnormalities. Colour and spectral Doppler can identify placental and fetal blood vessels and provide information on placental function and the fetal circulatory response to hypoxia. The new development of three-dimensional ultrasound can provide further information when a fetal abnormality is suspected.

Antenatal tests of fetal well-being are now principally based on ultrasound techniques and are designed to identify the fetuses that are in the early or late stages of fetal hypoxia. Continuous wave (CW) Doppler ultrasound is employed to provide continuous tracings of the fetal heart rate, the patterns of which alter when the fetus is hypoxic.

Magnetic resonance imaging (MRI) is only occasionally used to provide further information when a fetal structural abnormality is suspected.

Diagnostic ultrasound

This technique employs high-frequency (3–7.5 MHz), low-intensity sound waves, which are transmitted through the abdomen or pelvis by an ultrasound transducer. The transducer consists of piezoelectric crystals, usually mounted in a curved array. Small groups of crystals are triggered in sequence and each emits a focused ultrasound beam in a series of pulses and then receives the reflected signals from within the uterus between the pulses. These returning signals generate small electric charges (piezoelectricity), which are transformed into visual signals on a cathode ray tube or video screen. This means that a two-dimensional map of the contents of the uterus is provided in thin slices. Because the complete array is triggered 20 or

more times per second, the image is constantly updated in real time and fetal, cardiac and other movements can be studied. Also, as the operator can move the transducer easily across the abdomen, the two-dimensional slices can be built into a three-dimensional mental image of the uterine contents. For imaging in the first trimester, a small array is mounted on a long probe and placed in the vagina (Fig. 8.1a). Transvaginal sonography is also useful for examining the cervix later in pregnancy and for identifying the lower edge of the placenta. In general, however, after 12 weeks an abdominal transducer, which is a flat probe with a much wider array, is used (Fig. 8.1b).

Before the applications of diagnostic ultrasound are discussed, certain aspects of ultrasound imaging should be stressed at this stage. The obtaining of good images is very dependent on the skill of the operator.

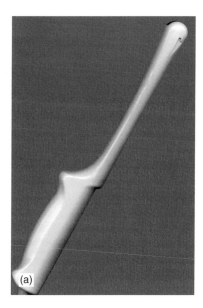

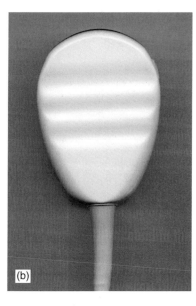

Figure 8.1 (a) Transvaginal ultrasound transducer. (b) Transabdominal ultrasound transducer.

The manipulation of the probe and transducer is a key factor in obtaining good diagnostic sections of the fetus and uterine contents.

There is good reason to suppose that ultrasound scanning is safe for both mother and fetus, which is why routine scanning is recommended by many governments and by the Royal College of Obstetricians and Gynaecologists. The safety of ultrasound has been studied epidemiologically by analysing the incidence of childhood cancer, dyslexia, speech development and other variables in women exposed to routine antenatal ultrasound examination, compared to those who had an ultrasound examination on indication. These studies have been reassuring, and no woman or baby has ever been shown to have been damaged directly by the use of diagnostic ultrasound in pregnancy. This is all the more striking when one considers that routine ultrasound scanning has been used in most developed countries for many years and many millions of women have been exposed prenatally. However, it is not true to say that ultrasound is a non-invasive method of investigation. Ultrasound can cause bio-effects on cells by inducing heating and other effects. Some of the newer ultrasound equipment uses more focused beams, which result in higher focal intensity than has been hitherto used. Furthermore, the development of spectral Doppler and transvaginal scanning may expose the fetus to higher intensities than those used in the older machines, which were shown to be safe. While there are no restrictions on the use of ultrasound in pregnancy, care should be taken to avoid unnecessarily prolonged exposure or the use of ultrasound for frivolous indications.

Clinical applications of ultrasound

Ultrasound in the first trimester

Early pregnancy problems
Transvaginal ultrasound plays a pivotal role in the diagnosis of disorders of early pregnancy, such as incomplete or missed miscarriage and ectopic pregnancy. In a missed miscarriage, for example, the fetus can be identified, but with an absent fetal heart and in a blighted ovum, the absence of fetal development results in the presence of a gestational sac which does not contain a fetus. An ectopic pregnancy is suspected if, in the presence of a positive pregnancy test, an ultrasound scan does not identify a gestation sac within the uterus, there is an adnexal mass with or without a fetal pole, or there is fluid in the pouch of Douglas.

The early pregnancy scan (11–14 weeks)
An increasing number of hospitals are routinely offering an early scan at about 11–14 weeks' gestation. This scan is normally performed transabdominally,

but in some countries the transvaginal route is preferred.

The principal aims of this scan are:
- to confirm fetal viability,
- to provide an accurate estimation of gestational age,
- to diagnose multiple gestation, and in particular to determine chorionicity,
- to identify markers which would indicate an increased risk of fetal chromosome abnormality such as Down's syndrome,
- to identify fetuses with gross structural abnormalities.

Estimation of gestational age

Fetal age can be assessed accurately before 12 weeks by measuring the crown–rump length (CRL: Fig. 8.2) and from 12 to 20 weeks the biparietal diameter (BPD),

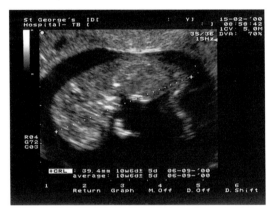

Figure 8.2 Crown–rump length measurement taken at 12 weeks' gestation. This view is also used for measurement of the nuchal translucency.

head circumference (HC) or femur length (FL) (Fig. 8.3). At this stage in pregnancy, the range of values around the mean is narrow. In clinical practice, the CRL and BPD are the most often used, because they are the most reproducible measurements. Essentially, the earlier the measurement is made, the better the prediction, and measurements made from an early CRL (accuracy of prediction ±5 days) will be preferred to a biparietal diameter at 20 weeks (accuracy of prediction ±7 days).

Predictions of gestational age by ultrasound before 20 weeks have been shown to be more accurate than predictions from the last menstrual period (LMP), even if the woman is certain of her dates. This has led

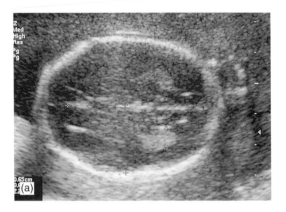

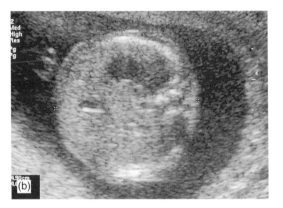

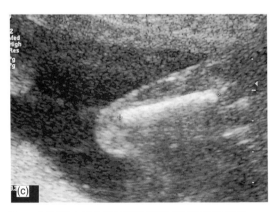

Figure 8.3 Measurements of (a) biparietal diameter, head circumference, (b) abdominal circumference, (c) femur length taken at 24 weeks' gestation.

to calls for the ultrasound prediction to be accepted for all pregnancies, but conventionally the ultrasound date is only taken if the discrepancy in the estimated date of delivery (EDD) calculated from ultrasound and the date of the LMP is >10 days.

Multiple pregnancy and chorionicity

Monochorionic twin pregnancies are associated with an increased risk of pregnancy complications and a higher perinatal mortality rate than dichorionic twin pregnancies. It is therefore clinically useful to be able to determine chorionicity early in pregnancy (see Chapter 12).

The dividing membrane in monochorionic twins is formed by two layers of amnion and in dichorionic twins by two layers of chorion and two of amnion. Dichorionic twins therefore have thicker membranes than monochorionic twins and this can be perceived qualitatively on ultrasound. Ultrasonically, dichorionic twin pregnancies in the first trimester of pregnancy have a thick inter-twin separating membrane (septum) flanked on either side by a very thin amnion. This is in contrast to a monochorionic twin pregnancy, which, on two-dimensional ultrasound, have a very thin inter-twin septum.

Another method of determining chorionicity in the first trimester uses the appearance of the septum at its origin from the placenta. On ultrasound, a tongue of placental tissue is seen within the base of dichorionic membranes and has been termed the 'twin peak' or 'lambda' sign. The optimal gestation at which to perform such ultrasonic chorionicity determination is 9–10 weeks.

Dichorionicity will also be confirmed by the identification of two placental masses and later in pregnancy by the presence of different-sex fetuses.

Nuchal thickness measurement and chromosomal abnormalities

In normal pregnancy during the first trimester, a fluid-filled area may be seen on the posterior surface of the fetal neck. This can be measured, and an association is now recognized between this nuchal translucency (NT) measurement and chromosomal and cardiac defects. At any given maternal age, the measurement of NT can be used to modify the underlying age-related risk of a fetal trisomy (see Chapter 9).

Ultrasound in the second trimester

The mid-pregnancy scan (18–22 weeks)

A routine scan is performed between 16 and 22 weeks in many hospitals in Europe. There is now a tendency to delay this to between 20 and 22 weeks, as this improves the opportunity to diagnose cardiac and late-developing abnormalities such as microcephaly. Furthermore, performing the mid-pregnancy scan slightly later will provide improved opportunities to identify women at increased risk of pre-eclampsia and preterm labour by assessment of the uterine artery flow velocity waveforms and measurement of the cervical length to assess the risk of premature delivery.

This scan has the following aims.

- To provide an accurate estimation of gestational age if an early scan has not been performed, through measurement of the BPD, HC and FL.
- To carry out a detailed fetal anatomical survey to detect any fetal structural abnormalities or markers for chromosome abnormality. At the present time, this is probably the principal reason for the mid-pregnancy scan. The vast majority of fetal abnormalities will not be anticipated and, therefore, would not be detected without this routine scan.
- To establish the presence of multiple gestation if an early scan has not been performed and to determine the chorionicity.
- To locate the placenta and identify the 5 per cent of women who have a low-lying placenta. A small percentage of such women will eventually be shown to have a placenta praevia.
- To estimate the amniotic fluid volume.
  Also, in some centres:
- to perform Doppler ultrasound examination of maternal uterine arteries to screen for adverse pregnancy outcome,
- to measure cervical length to assess the risk of preterm delivery.

Fetal anatomy

In 3 per cent of all pregnancies, there will be a serious structural abnormality of the fetus, the most common being central nervous system abnormalities and cardiac defects. The detection of these defects is discussed in Chapter 9. The most detailed survey of fetal anatomy is carried out at the mid-pregnancy scan at 20–22 weeks' gestation, but a screen of fetal anatomy will be carried out at any stage if there are risk factors for congenital abnormality. The fetal measurements and anatomical features that should be visualized are summarized in Table 8.1. The overall detection rate for abnormalities varies from centre to centre, but most studies report a 70–80 per cent detection rate for disabling or lethal conditions.

Table 8.1 – Fetal measurements and anatomical features visualized on the routine scan between 18 and 22 weeks' gestation

Standard fetal measurements Biparietal diameter Head circumference Abdominal circumference Femoral length	*Chest* Heart: four-chamber view, aortic root and arch, pulmonary artery and ductus Lungs

Fetal anatomical features and measurements
Brain
Ventricular section: anterior and posterior horns of
  the cerebral ventricles
measurement: anterior and posterior ventricle:
  hemisphere ratio
Posterior fossa section: cerebellum, vermis, cisterna
  magna, and nuchal skinfold
measurement: transcerebellar diameter and nuchal
  skinfold thickness
	Abdomen
	Diaphragm
	Cord insertion
	Liver, stomach, and intestines
	Both kidneys for parenchyma and renal
	  pelvis size
	Bladder
	Genitalia

Skull
Shape, e.g. lemon-shaped as in spina bifida
	Limbs
	Femur, tibia, fibula, foot and toes
	  (both limbs)
	Humerus, radius, ulna, hand and fingers
	  (both limbs)

Face Orbits (and both lenses) measurement: interorbital, external orbital diameters Nose, lips, palate and mandible	*Placenta* Morphology and site

Spine
'Anterior' view of spinous processes down to tip
  of sacrum; clear view of skin margin throughout
  length of spine
	Cord
	Number of vessels
	
	Amniotic fluid
	Volume assessment

Fortunately, the false-positive rate is low and termination of a normal fetus because of a mistaken diagnosis is a rare event. However, anxiety is engendered in some parents when waiting for a second opinion on a suspected abnormality. Once a serious abnormality is detected, evidence shows that parents will elect to terminate the pregnancy in 80–90 per cent of cases.

Placental location

Placenta praevia is a cause of life-threatening haemorrhage in pregnancy. Before any major antepartum haemorrhage occurs, there is usually a warning haemorrhage, and any woman with a bloodstained vaginal loss should immediately have a scan to determine placental location. If the lower edge of the placenta

appears to lie close to the cervix, a gentle transvaginal scan should be performed to determine whether the placenta covers the internal os, indicating a major placenta praevia (Fig. 8.4). In the third trimester, if the lower edge of the placenta lies within 3 cm of the internal os, the provisional diagnosis would be type I (minor) placenta praevia. At the mid-pregnancy scan, it is customary to identify women who have a low-lying placenta. At this stage, the lower uterine segment has not yet formed and most low-lying placentas will appear to 'migrate' upwards as the lower segment stretches in the late second and third trimesters. About 5 per cent of women have a low-lying placenta at 20 weeks, and only 5 per cent of this group will eventually be shown to have a placenta

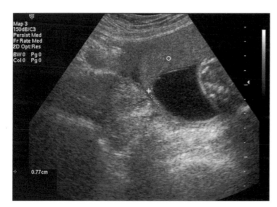

Figure 8.4 Transvaginal scan showing cervix and placenta covering internal os. o = placenta; + = placenta covering the internal os.

praevia. Recent studies have shown that a transvaginal scan performed in women with a low-lying placenta will identify cases of true placenta praevia with more precision.

Amniotic fluid volume
The fetus has a role in the control of the volume of amniotic fluid. It swallows amniotic fluid, absorbs it in the gut and later excretes urine into the amniotic sac. Congenital abnormalities that impair the fetus's ability to swallow, e.g. anencephaly or oesophageal atresia, will result in an increase in amniotic fluid. Congenital abnormalities that result in a failure of urine production or passage, e.g. renal agenesis and posterior urethral valves, will result in reduced or absent amniotic fluid. Variation from the normal range of amniotic fluid volume calls for a further detailed ultrasound assessment of possible causes.

Umbilical cord
Some abnormalities of the umbilical cord can be identified by ultrasound during the antenatal period, and visualization is improved with the use of colour Doppler. A single umbilical artery is associated with congenital abnormalities of the fetus and intrauterine growth restriction and is looked for at the time of the mid-pregnancy scan.

Doppler ultrasound and the prediction of adverse pregnancy outcome
The ability to identify blood vessels in the uterus, placenta and fetus and to measure aspects of blood velocity has led to major advances in the management of pregnancy. Doppler ultrasound makes use of the phenomenon of the Doppler frequency shift, where the reflected wave will be at a different frequency from the transmitted one if it interacts with moving structures, such as red blood cells flowing along a blood vessel. If the red blood cells are moving towards the beam, the reflected signal will be at a higher frequency than the transmitted one; the reflected beam will be at a lower signal if the flow is away from the beam. The original equipment displayed spectral signals with inexpensive continuous wave (CW) Doppler equipment. As the vessels are not visualized, this equipment is only suitable for detailing signals from the umbilical artery, which is easy to isolate from surrounding vessels. In modern equipment, the same transducer has the ability to perform conventional imaging and display Doppler frequency shifts. The Doppler shifted signals can be displayed as a colour map of blood vessels superimposed on top of the grey scale image. This is called colour Doppler imaging (or just colour Doppler). Blood flowing towards the transducer is shown in shades of red, the brighter shades indicating high velocity. Flow away from the transducer is shown in shades of blue. By this means, nearly all the major blood vessels in the placenta and fetus can be displayed (Fig. 8.5). Quantitative information about

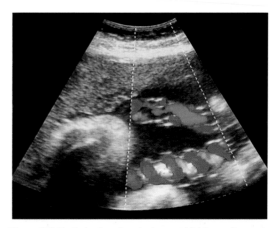

Figure 8.5 Typical colour Doppler image of fetal vessels.

the velocity or resistance to flow in any of these vessels can be obtained by means of pulsed or spectral Doppler. In this modality, signals from a particular vessel can be isolated (gated) and displayed in graphic form, with the velocity plotted against time. Arterial flow is pulsatile; venous flow is usually constant, but is pulsatile in veins that are close to the heart (central veins). In general, most studies have been carried out on arterial flow, although recently there has been an increasing interest in central veins.

The pulsatile arterial flow velocity waveform has a systolic and a diastolic component. If the angle of the ultrasound beam to the long axis of the vessel is known, the absolute blood velocity in centimetres per second can be determined. However, velocity has not been used much in obstetrics, except in assessing the rhesus-affected fetus when high blood velocities are associated with fetal anaemia. Most studies have looked at resistance to flow, which is reflected in the diastolic component. A small amount of diastolic flow implies high resistance downstream to the vessel being studied and implies low perfusion. A high diastolic component indicates low downstream resistance and implies high perfusion (Fig. 8.6). A measure of the amount of diastolic flow relative to systolic is provided by several indices, such as the pulsatility index or resistance index, which essentially compare the amount of diastolic flow to systolic flow. When these indices are high, this indicates high resistance to flow; when the indices are low, resistance to flow is low. Another feature of the waveform is a 'notch' in the waveform in early diastole. This is particularly important in the uterine artery because it indicates that the spiral arteries, which are downstream from the uterine artery, are muscular and compliant and, therefore, that trophoblast invasion of these arteries is incomplete or inadequate.

The proposed pathogenic model of pre-eclampsia is one of incomplete physiological invasion of the spiral arteries by the trophoblast, with a resultant increase in uteroplacental vascular resistance; this is reflected in the Doppler waveforms obtained from the maternal uterine circulation. Doppler ultrasound studies of the uterine arteries by means of the identification of a uterine arterial notch (Fig. 8.7), considered to result from increased vascular resistance in the uteroplacental bed, have provided evidence of the association between high-resistance waveform patterns and adverse outcomes, including pre-eclampsia, intrauterine growth restriction (IUGR) and placental abruption. Sixty to seventy per cent of women at 20–24 weeks' gestation with bilateral uterine notches will subsequently develop one or more of these complications. The pregnancies in such women will

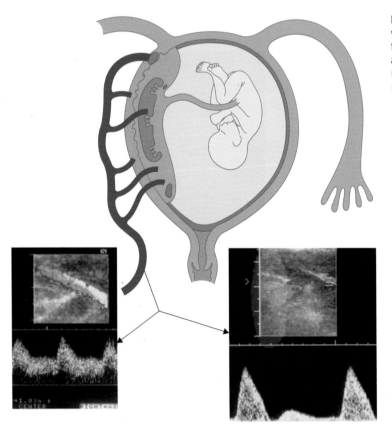

Figure 8.6 Left: a low-resistance waveform from the uterine artery; note the abundance of diastolic flow. Right: a high-resistance waveform from the uterine artery; note the notches and reduced diastolic flow.

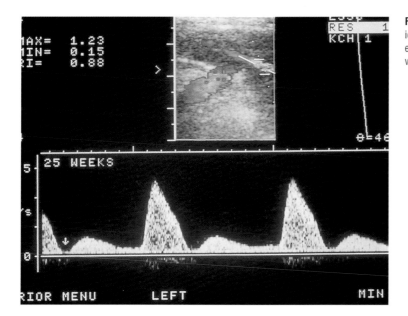

Figure 8.7 The uterine artery is easily identified crossing medial to the external iliac vein. A high resistance waveform is demonstrated.

therefore require close monitoring of the fetal growth rate and the possible development of maternal hypertension and proteinuria.

Measurement of cervical length

Cervical length measurement requires transvaginal scanning, but there is evidence that 50 per cent of women who deliver before 34 weeks will have a short cervix. The average length of the cervix at 23 weeks is 3.4 cm, and if the measurement is <1.5 cm, a recent study suggests that there is a 50 per cent chance of spontaneous preterm labour and delivery before 34 weeks' gestation.

The importance of the routine scan

The early and mid-pregnancy routine scans have assumed great importance in the effective management of pregnancy. They allow parental choice if a fetal abnormality is detected. For example, if an abnormality is lethal or will result in serious long-term handicap, parents can opt for termination of pregnancy. On some occasions, early diagnosis may allow the prenatal treatment of certain conditions, such as an obstructed fetal bladder, which can give rise to renal damage without insertion of a vesico-amniotic shunt. Even if the parents do not want a termination of pregnancy, it will allow arrangements to be made for delivery in a tertiary centre, to provide optimal care for the baby. A routine scan will also allow triaging of women for hospital care if high-risk factors are found, such as multiple gestation, abnormal uterine artery Doppler or a short cervix.

A routine scan is also the parents' first glimpse of their new baby. Much has been written about the importance of involving the parents in the examination as the scan is performed. This is indeed important, for it has been shown in randomized studies that parents bond with their baby much better if they can see the ultrasound image on the screen. As a consequence, the parents are more likely to comply with health recommendations, such as improving diet or reducing smoking and alcohol consumption.

The scan has now become a family event and it is important that the routine scan should be an informative and enjoyable experience. It should not be assumed that the parents wish to know the sex of their child, and the information should not be gratuitously given or officiously withheld. If a fetal abnormality is detected, this should be discussed with the parents at the end of the scan. Although parents can recognize anatomical features when they are pointed out, it is extremely rare for them to recognize an abnormality without it being demonstrated to them on the screen. The image of the anomaly should be videotaped and shown to the parents afterwards, for distressed parents can have exaggerated imaginings of fetal abnormalities and they cope much better when they see the apparent lesion on the screen. On many occasions, operators need a second opinion and may be uncertain as to whether there is an abnormality. It is always better to explain why a second opinion is required rather than give some reassuring but dishonest explanation, such as 'the baby is in a difficult position'. The doctor–patient and sonographer–patient relationships are based on trust, and it is important to tell parents that the recognition of fetal anomalies is not 100 per cent accurate and that false-positive and false-negative diagnoses are possible.

The impact of the mid-pregnancy routine scan is illustrated by the meta-analysis shown in Figure 8.8,

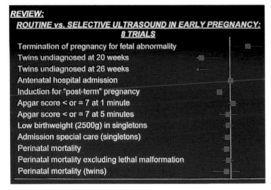

Figure 8.8 Meta-analysis of eight studies comparing routine and selective scanning. Routine ultrasound reduces the number of undiagnosed twins and unnecessary inductions of labour, and increases the number of terminations of pregnancy for fetal anomalies, but has not been shown to reduce prenatal mortality or morbidity.

where eight studies comparing random allocation of antenatal patients to routine scanning or scanning on indication are compared. In the routine scan group, there was a significant increase in the number of terminations of pregnancy for fetal abnormalities and a significant reduction in undiagnosed twins. Because ultrasound corrects mistakes in gestational age assigned from the LMP, there was also a significant reduction in the number of inductions for post-term pregnancy. These are all tangible benefits, but some criticism of the routine scan has been made because its introduction does not seem to have led to any change in the perinatal mortality rate, the incidence of low birth weight or the neonatal condition. This is, in fact, not surprising, as there is unlikely to be a change in these outcomes unless routine ultrasound causes a change in management. In future, we might anticipate improvements if triaging of care, based on the identification of high-risk pregnancies by uterine

artery Doppler or assessment of cervical length, can be made. Successful prophylactic treatment of pre-eclampsia or preterm labour can only be instituted if women at high risk are identified. This must be the future goal of the routine scan.

Ultrasound in the third trimester

The principal aims of ultrasound in the third trimester are:
- to assess fetal growth,
- to assess fetal well-being.

Assessing fetal growth and estimating fetal weight
The external dimensions of the fetus can be used to chart its growth rate in utero. The standard measurements used in the assessment of fetal growth/weight are the BPD, HC, abdominal circumference (AC) and FL (see Fig. 8.3). It is customary now to measure all these parameters when assessing fetal size, as they provide information about fetal symmetry. In addition, when combined in an equation, these measurements provide a more accurate estimate of fetal weight (EFW) than any of the parameters taken singly. All measurements can be immediately compared with a normal reference range taken from an unselected population.

In pregnancies at high risk of IUGR, serial measurements are plotted on the normal reference range (Fig. 8.9: see also Chapter 13). Growth patterns are helpful in distinguishing between different types of growth restriction (symmetrical and asymmetrical). Asymmetry between head measures (BPD, HC) and abdominal measure (AC) can be identified in IUGR, where a brain-sparing effect will result in a relatively large HC compared with the AC. The opposite would occur in a diabetic pregnancy, where the abdomen is disproportionately large due to the effects of insulin on the fetal liver and fat stores. Cessation of growth is an ominous sign of placental failure. However, the importance of serial measurements has lessened with more dynamic tests of fetal well-being such as umbilical and fetal Doppler and the antenatal cardiotocograph (CTG; see below).

Of all the parameters measured, the AC is the most accurate predictor of fetal weight because it is reduced in both symmetrical and asymmetrical IUGR. However, equations combining several parameters will reduce the random variation in the accuracy of the predictions. For example, by combining BPD, HC,

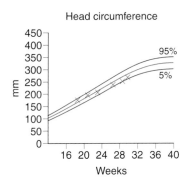

Head circumference

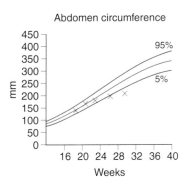

Abdomen circumference

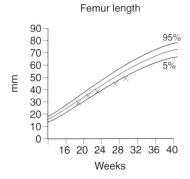

Femur length

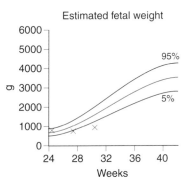

Estimated fetal weight

Figure 8.9 Growth pattern in a case of intrauterine growth restriction plotted on reference charts for head circumference, abdominal circumference, femur length and estimated fetal weight.

AC and FL, fetal weight will be predicted to within 150 g/kg of true weight. This is especially valuable in predicting the weight of small fetuses, such as growth-restricted preterm infants, to provide information as to their potential viability. For example, an estimated birth weight of <600 g would generally be considered non-viable. Birth-weight assessments, however, are less accurate with larger babies and, above 3 kg, ultrasound assessments are little better than estimates made by abdominal palpation. This is why routine screening in the third trimester to assess fetal size is not usually performed; the detection rate of the late small for gestational age (SGA) fetus on a single ultrasound scan is little better than that obtained by serial measurements of the symphysis–fundal height.

Placental morphology

The appearance of the placenta in the second and early third trimesters is one of a fairly uniform texture (echogenicity). Towards the end of the third trimester, the placenta develops a mature appearance, being distinctly lobular, with white echoes demarcating the cotyledons. While there is some evidence that premature maturation of the placenta is associated with impaired function, this is not strong enough to make it a useful test.

Ultrasound in the assessment of fetal well-being

Amniotic fluid volume

The amount of amniotic fluid in the uterus is a guide to fetal well-being in the third trimester. The influence of congenital abnormalities on amniotic fluid volume in early pregnancy has already been described. A precise evaluation cannot be made by ultrasound, as the fluid gathers in irregular pockets around the fetus; this is demonstrated on ultrasound as echo-free spaces. Two relatively crude methods are used as indicators of volume. The maximum vertical pool is measured after a general survey of the uterine contents. Measurements of <2 cm suggest oligohydramnios, and measurements >7 cm suggest polyhydramnios. The amniotic fluid index (AFI) is the sum of all the maximum vertical pool measurements from the four quadrants of the uterus, and provides a more useful measurement. The AFI alters throughout gestation, but in the third trimester it should be between 10 and 25 cm; values below 10 cm indicate a reduced volume and those below 5 cm indicate oligohydramnios, while values above 25 cm indicate polyhydramnios.

Amniotic fluid volume is decreased in fetal growth restriction, in association with redistribution of fetal blood away from the kidneys to vital structures such as the brain and heart; there is a consequent reduction in renal perfusion and urine output.

The cardiotocograph

Antenatal CTG uses external (and therefore indirect) methods of monitoring the fetal heart rate. The most widely used method for obtaining this information is ultrasound fetal CTG. This utilizes the physical principle of the Doppler effect to detect fetal heart motion. Signals can also be obtained from antenatal fetal electrocardiography, but this is more prone to failure. The interval between successive beats is measured, thereby allowing a continuous assessment of fetal heart rate. Most modern transducers have increased numbers of transmitting crystals and detectors, so that failure to detect signals from cardiac valve or wall movement is a relatively rare event.

The woman should be comfortable and in a left lateral or semi-recumbent position (avoiding compression of the maternal vena cava). An external ultrasound transducer for monitoring the fetal heart and a toco-dynometer (stretch gauge) for recording uterine activity are secured overlying the uterus. Recordings are then made for at least 30 minutes; the output from the CTG machine is conventionally an ink tracing of fetal heart rate and a second tracing of uterine activity (Fig. 8.10).

Fetal cardiac physiology

Fetal cardiac behaviour is regulated through sympathetic and parasympathetic signals and by vasomotor, chemoceptor and baroreceptor mechanisms. Pathological events such as fetal hypoxia modify these signals and also the fetal cardiac response.

Fetal heart rate variability

Under normal physiological conditions, the interval between successive heart beats (beat-to-beat) varies. This is called 'short-term variability' and increases with increasing gestational age. It is not visible on a standard CTG (although this information can be obtained from fetal electrocardiograms, see below). In addition to these beat-to-beat variations in heart rate, there are longer-term fluctuations in heart rate occurring between two and six times per minute. The preferred term for this variation in fetal heart rate is 'baseline variability'. Normal baseline variability reflects a normal fetal autonomic nervous system. As well as gestational age, baseline variability is modified by fetal sleep states and activity, and also by hypoxia, fetal infection, and drugs suppressing the fetal central nervous system, such as opioids, and hypnotics (all of these medications reduce baseline variability). Baseline variability is considered abnormal when

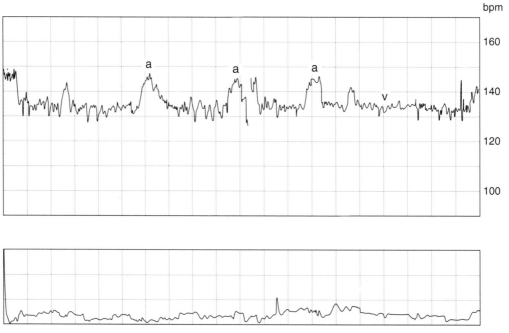

Figure 8.10 A normal fetal cardiotocograph showing a normal rate, normal variability (v), and the presence of several accelerations (a).

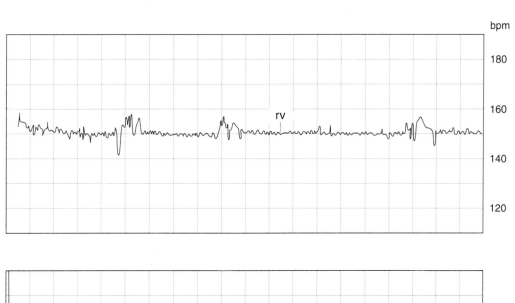

Figure 8.11 A fetal cardiotocograph showing a baseline of 150 beats per minute (bpm) but with reduced variability (rv).

it is <10 beats per minute (bpm; Fig. 8.11). As fetuses display deep sleep cycles of 20–30 minutes at a time, baseline variability may be normally reduced for this length of time, but should be preceded and followed by a period of trace with normal baseline variability if the CTG is continued for a sufficient duration.

Baseline fetal heart rate

The baseline fetal heart rate falls with advancing gestational age as a result of maturing fetal parasympathetic (vagal) tone. It is best determined over a period of 5–10 minutes. The normal fetal heart rate at term is 110–150 bpm, whilst prior to term 160 bpm is taken as the upper limit of normal. A rate lower than 110 bpm is termed a fetal bradycardia. If all other features of the CTG are normal, this is unlikely to represent fetal hypoxia unless the rate is <100 bpm. Fetal heart rates between 150 and 170 bpm are again unlikely to represent fetal compromise if the trace is otherwise normal (normal baseline variability in the presence of accelerations and in the absence of decelerations) and there are no antenatal risk factors. Fetal tachycardias can be due to congenital tachycardias and are also associated with maternal or fetal infection,

acute fetal hypoxia, fetal anaemia and drugs such as adrenoceptor agonists (ritodrine).

Fetal heart rate accelerations

These are increases in the baseline fetal heart rate of at least 15 bpm, lasting for at least 15 seconds. The presence of two or more accelerations on a 20–30-minute CTG defines a reactive trace. The importance of accelerations is that they are only observed very rarely in the presence of fetal hypoxia, i.e. normally they are a good sign of fetal health. Accelerations can be so frequent as to suggest a fetal tachycardia (Fig. 8.12), and this emphasizes the need to interpret CTG tracings carefully in the light of the overall clinical picture.

Fetal heart rate decelerations

These are transient reductions in fetal heart rate of 15 bpm or more, lasting for more than 15 seconds. Occasional decelerations are frequently seen on otherwise normal CTG tracings. Decelerations that occur in the presence of other abnormal features (Table 8.2) such as reduced variability or baseline tachycardia are more likely to reflect fetal hypoxia. When baseline variability is reduced, decelerations can be <15 bpm from baseline and still be highly significant (Fig. 8.13).

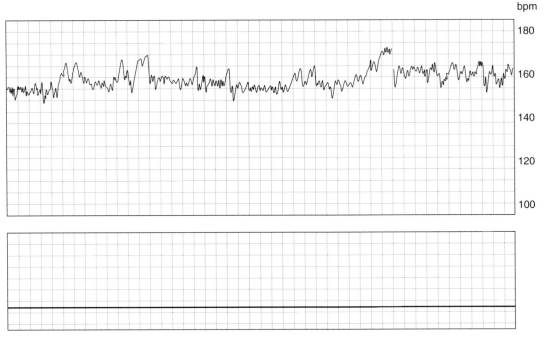

Figure 8.12 A fetal cardiotocograph from a term pregnancy. The true baseline is about 150 beats per minute (bpm), as seen at the start of the trace. This baby was very active and the apparent raised baseline rate for the majority of the tracing is due to almost continuous accelerations.

Table 8.2 – Cardiotocography: summary of fetal heart rate patterns and their implications

Normal
Baseline rate 110–150 bpm
Variability 10–25 bpm
Two accelerations in 20 min
No decelerations

Suspicious
Absence of accelerations (important), +
Abnormal baseline rate (<110 or >150 bpm)
Reduced variability (<10 bpm)
Variable decelerations

Abnormal
No accelerations and two or more of the following:
• abnormal baseline rate

• abnormal variability
• repetitive late decelerations
• variable decelerations with ominous features
features (duration >60 s, late recovery
baseline, late deceleration component,
poor variability between/during
decelerations)

Others
Sinusoidal pattern
Prolonged bradycardia
Shallow decelerations with reduced variability in
a non-reactive trace

From the above descriptions, a normal antepartum fetal CTG can therefore be defined as a baseline of 110–150 bpm, with baseline variability exceeding 10 bpm, and with more than one acceleration being seen in a 20–30-minute tracing. Reduced baseline variability, absence of accelerations and the presence of decelerations are all suspicious features. A suspicious CTG must be interpreted in clinical context. If many antenatal risk factors have already been identified, a suspicious CTG may warrant delivery of the baby, although where no risk factors exist, a repeated investigation later in the day may be more appropriate.

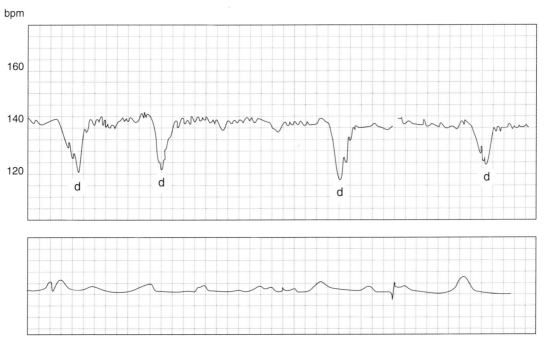

Figure 8.13 An admission cardiotocograph from a term pregnancy. Although the baseline fetal heart rate is normal, there is reduced variability, an absence of fetal heart rate accelerations, and multiple decelerations (d). The decelerations were occurring after uterine tightenings and are therefore termed 'late'.

Stress and non-stress cardiotocography

An antenatal CTG performed with the mother positioned comfortably is called a non-stress test. In this situation, the 'stress' of the title refers to what the fetus is experiencing (not the mother). Although not popular in the UK, in the USA fetuses that demonstrate sub-optimal non-stress CTG tracings may be subjected to contraction stress tests. These tests are carried out in the same way as non-stress tests except that an oxytocin infusion is administered intravenously to induce uterine contractions. Oxytocin has no direct effect on fetal cardiac activity. A positive test result is fetal cardiac decelerations in response to uterine contractions, and is abnormal. The test has not been adopted in the UK, as it is thought to be a poor predictor of fetal outcome, have unacceptably high false-positive and uterine hyperstimulation rates (5–10 per cent each) and be too time consuming and invasive. An alternative to oxytocin infusion that can be used for inducing uterine activity is repetitive nipple stimulation. Whilst less invasive, this technique does not overcome the problems of poor prediction of fetal outcome. Fetal provocation using acoustic, light or exercise stimuli has been documented, but again has not been shown to improve the detection of the at-risk fetus.

The computerized cardiotocograph

The basis of fetal CTG is pattern recognition, and this leads to differences in interpretation amongst different clinicians. Computerized CTG interpretation packages have been developed. These packages have been shown to be equal (or superior) to human interpretation in differentiating normal from abnormal outcome.

One commonly used package relies on the computer's ability to calculate heart rate variability by measuring the variation in frequency of individual heart beats and assessing increased variability with fetal movements. In this way fetal heart rate accelerations are identified by a reduced interval between beats, and decelerations are identified from an increased interval. A sinusoidal trace can be recognized by short-term variation of more than two standard deviations below the mean value expected for a given gestation.

Several potential advantages of a computerized interpretation seem to exist. The computer is often able to declare a CTG normal after 10 minutes (rather than the more standard 30-minute tracing normally performed manually). Also, if signal contact is lost during the tracing, the machine alarms, requiring the Doppler transducer to be repositioned. The interactive nature of this monitoring also reduces the total duration of CTG recording and aids interpretation.

Biophysical profile
In an effort to refine the ability of fetal CTG to identify antenatal hypoxia, investigators have looked at additional fetal parameters. In experimental animals, fetal hypoxia can be induced by making the mother breathe hypoxic gas mixtures. Under these conditions, fetal biophysical variables, such as fetal breathing movements and forelimb movements, are abolished. This reduction in movement may persist even after the normal fetal oxygenation has been re-established. Similar changes in those active biophysical variables controlled by the central nervous system have been noticed in human fetuses that are acutely hypoxic. These include breathing movements, gross body movements, flexor tone and accelerations in fetal heart rate related to movements. If chronic fetal hypoxia occurs, there is an associated reduction in amniotic fluid volume, and fetal growth restriction is seen. By assigning each of the active variables, and also amniotic fluid volume and the CTG scores of either 2 (= normal) or 0 (= sub-optimal), it is possible to assign an individual fetus score of between 0 and 10. This is the basis of fetal biophysical profiling (Table 8.3).

The first prospective, blind clinical study using biophysical profile scores to predict fetal outcome was reported in 1980. Scores were recorded in 216 women but the data were not available to the clinicians managing the pregnancies. The perinatal mortality varied between 600/1000 when all five variables were abnormal and 0/1000 when all variables were considered to be normal. Intermediate scores were associated with intermediate mortality rates. This study did not allow an assessment of whether performing biophysical profiles was able to reduce perinatal mortality, as clinicians responsible for the care of individual women were unable to act on the results of this new and, at that time, unproven test. Larger studies, in which women at high risk for fetal hypoxia were delivered if biophysical scores were abnormal, suggested that delivery at a score of <6 was associated with a lower perinatal mortality than either high-risk pregnancies in which biophysical profiles were not performed or even low-risk pregnancies in which biophysical profiles were not performed. The implication from the latter observation was that, even in low-risk antenatal populations, some fetuses will be hypoxic with no apparent risk factors. These same large series have suggested that the false-negative rate for the test (a normal score with subsequent death of the fetus within 1 week of the test) is very low.

These results would appear to argue strongly in favour of the widespread and routine use of biophysical profiling for all pregnancies. However, such widespread use has not occurred in many countries, including the UK. There appear to be several reasons for this lack of implementation. Biophysical profiles can be time consuming. Fetuses spend approximately 30 per cent of their time in non-rapid eye movement (non-REM) sleep, during which time they are not

Table 8.3 – Biophysical profile scoring

Biophysical variable	Normal (score 2)	Abnormal (score 0)
Fetal breathing movements	>1 episode for 30 s in 30 min	Absent/<30 s in 30 min
Gross body movements	>3 body/limb movements in 30 min	<3 body/limb movements in 30 min
Fetal tone	>1 episode body/limb extension followed by return to flexion, open–close cycle of fetal hand	Slow or absent extension–flexion of body or limbs
Reactive fetal heart rate	>2 accelerations with fetal movements in 30 min	<2 accelerations or 1 + deceleration in 30 min
Qualitative amniotic fluid	>1 pool of fluid, at least 1 cm × 1 cm	Either no measurable pool or a pool <1 cm × 1 cm

very active and do not exhibit breathing movements. It is therefore necessary to scan them for long enough to exclude this physiological cause of a poor score. The longer individual ultrasound scans take to perform, the more machines and operators are required to apply the test to the whole antenatal population. This problem is compounded when the test is performed earlier and more frequently. Another problem with fetal biophysical profiles is that by the time a fetus develops an abnormal score prompting delivery, it is already severely hypoxic. Whilst delivery may reduce the perinatal death rate (death in utero, or within the first week of life), it may not be increasing long-term survival and, in particular, survival without significant mental and physical impairment.

Doppler investigation

The principles of Doppler have already been discussed. The umbilical artery has been the most extensively studied vessel, probably because signals can be obtained with inexpensive CW Doppler equipment. It should be regarded as a placental vessel, however, and only by studying fetal vessels with the more expensive colour Doppler machines can important information on the fetal response to hypoxia be obtained.

Umbilical artery

Waveforms from these vessels provide information on feto-placental blood flow and should be performed on high-risk mothers, for example with hypertension, or where there is an SGA fetus or an elevated uterine artery resistance index or notch. Normally, diastolic flow in the umbilical artery increases (i.e. placental resistance falls) throughout gestation. If the resistance index (RI = maximum umbilical artery systolic velocity − minimum umbilical end-diastolic velocity/maximum umbilical artery systolic velocity) measured in the umbilical artery rises above the 95th centile of the normal graph, this implies faulty perfusion of the placenta, which may eventually result in fetal hypoxia. Absent or reversed end-diastolic flow in the umbilical artery is a particularly serious development with a strong correlation with fetal distress and intrauterine death (Fig. 8.14). Meta-analysis of several randomized studies shows that umbilical Doppler monitoring will reduce perinatal mortality in high-risk pregnancies.

Fetal vessels

Falling oxygen levels in the fetus result in a redistribution of blood flow to protect the brain, heart, adrenals and spleen, and vasoconstriction in all other vessels. Several fetal vessels have been studied, and reflect this 'centralization' of flow. The middle cerebral artery will show increasing diastolic flow (falling pulsatility index) as hypoxia increases, while a rising resistance in the fetal aorta reflects compensatory vasoconstriction in the fetal body. When diastolic flow is absent in the fetal aorta, this implies fetal acidaemia (Fig. 8.15). Perhaps the most sensitive index of fetal acidaemia and incipient heart failure is demonstrated by increasing pulsatility in the central veins supplying the heart, such as the ductus venosus and inferior vena cava. When late diastolic flow is absent in the ductus venosus, delivery should be considered, as fetal death is imminent (Fig. 8.16). The significance of these findings is discussed in Chapter 13.

Ultrasound and invasive procedures

Ultrasound is used to guide invasive diagnostic procedures such as amniocentesis, chorion villus sampling

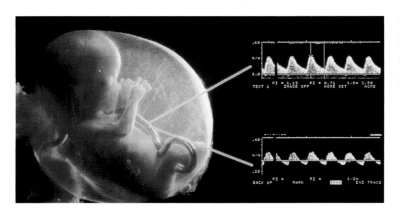

Figure 8.14 Normal (top) and abnormal (bottom) Doppler signals from the umbilical artery. Reversed flow in diastole indicates poor placental function and impending fetal demise.

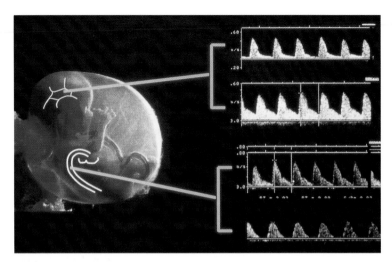

Figure 8.15 Normal and abnormal Doppler signals from the middle cerebral artery and thoracic aorta. Increasing flow in the middle cerebral artery and absence of diastolic flow in the aorta indicate fetal acidaemia.

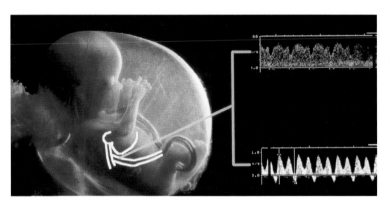

Figure 8.16 Normal and abnormal Doppler signals from the ductus venosus. There is progressive reduction of flow to the heart in late diastole (i.e. with atrial contraction), with increasing fetal acidaemia.

and cordocentesis, and therapeutic procedures such as the insertion of fetal bladder shunts or chest drains. If fetoscopy is performed, the endoscope is inserted under ultrasound guidance. This use of ultrasound has greatly reduced the possibility of fetal trauma, as the needle or scope is visualized throughout the procedure and guided with precision to the appropriate place.

New developments

Magnetic resonance imaging

This technique utilizes the effect of powerful magnetic forces on spinning hydrogen protons, which, when knocked off their axis by pulsed radio waves, produce radio frequency signals as they return to their basal state. The signals reflect the clinical composition of tissue (i.e. the

amount and distribution of hydrogen protons) and thus the images provide significant improvement over ultrasound in tissue characterization. The technique also has the advantage of providing sectional images in any plane. The main disadvantages are that magnetic resonance imaging (MRI) is many times more expensive than ultrasound and images are more likely to be affected by movement artefacts. Some centres sedate the mother prior to an examination to reduce fetal movement.

MRI does provide superb images of fetal anatomy and is extremely useful when ultrasound images are not diagnostic or when they are sub-optimal because of maternal obesity. An example of a fetal MRI scan is given in Figure 8.17.

Three-dimensional ultrasound

This technique may transform ultrasound imaging in the future. In conventional scanning, the ultrasound beam is swept electronically in a single plane across a flat

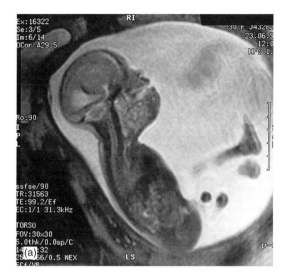
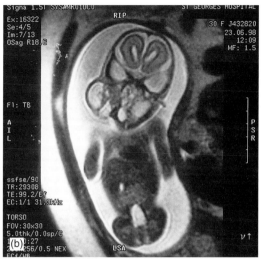

Figure 8.17 (a) and (b) Magnetic resonance imaging scan of fetus showing thyroid tumour.

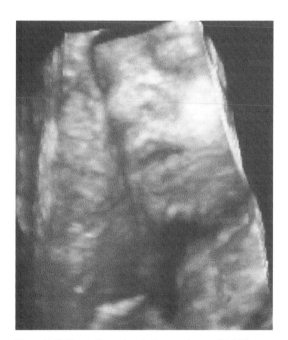

Figure 8.18 Three-dimensional ultrasound scan of fetal face.

transducer. In three-dimensional scanning, the beam is swept in two orthogonal planes to capture a block or volume of echoes that are digitally stored. The aim of the operator is to capture a volume from the region of interest, and this is normally completed in 5–15 seconds, depending on the required volume for diagnosis. After this, the volume of echoes can be re-sliced in any plane to provide the appropriate two-dimensional image. Furthermore, by surface or volume rendering, life-like three-dimensional reconstructions of surface features of the fetus, or particular organs, can be made, and surface or volume rendering can remove artefacts or structures that obscure the image. The advantages are that the scanning time can be drastically shortened and volumes can be stored for later analysis. In the future, volumes will be transferred electronically to tertiary centres for expert diagnosis. From the parents' perspective, the images, especially of the fetal face, have a life-like photographic quality (Fig. 8.18) and are likely to improve antenatal parental bonding. The images are at the moment static, but real-time three-dimensional imaging should be available within a few years. There is evidence that three-dimensional imaging improves the diagnosis of certain fetal abnormalities, such as cleft lip and palate.

� Key Points

- Abnormalities of fetal well-being are usually the result of impaired transfer of nutrients and oxygen across the placenta leading to the development of IUGR and chronic hypoxia.
- The fetal response to placental insufficiency is:
  - a reduction of growth rate in response to impaired transfer of nutrients and to conserve oxygen,
  - redistribution of the circulation to preferentially perfuse the brain, myocardium and adrenal gland, with a consequent reduction in blood flow to other organs: this

will lead to asymmetrical growth with relative brain sparing and oligohydramnios due to reduced renal perfusion,
- reduction of fetal activity to conserve oxygen and reduce anaerobic metabolism: this will result in a reduction of general body and breathing movements,
- modification of the autonomic control of the fetal heart with a reduction in baseline variability.
- Ultimately, as fetal acidaemia develops as a result of anaerobic glycolysis, there will be abnormal Doppler waveforms in the ductus venosus as a result of right heart failure, and decelerations in the fetal heart trace as a result of increased vagal tone.
- Most of these changes can now be documented by means of Doppler ultrasound and antenatal CTG. (A brief summary of the sequence of events in given in Figure 8.19.)
- The decision about when to deliver the baby will be taken by the obstetrician on the basis of an evaluation of several of these antenatal tests together with the maternal condition, e.g. the presence of pre-eclampsia or diabetes mellitus. For example, after 32 weeks, the decision to deliver might be

based on an SGA infant with oligohydramnios and evidence of circulatory redistribution. Before 32 weeks, delivery may be delayed in order to achieve greater fetal maturity; in this situation, tests of fetal cardiac function (ductus venosus and CTG) become critical.

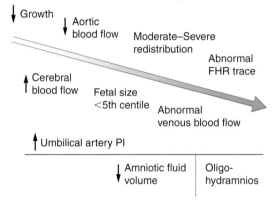

Figure 8.19 Sequential changes in tests of fetal well-being in uteroplacental failure. (FHR, fetal heart rate; PI, pulsatility index.)

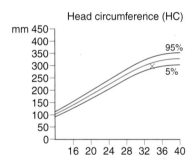

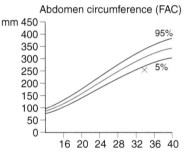

Figure 8.20 Plot of fetal head circumference and fetal abdominal circumference (FAC) for case history.

CASE HISTORY

An 18 year old in her first pregnancy attends for review at the antenatal clinic at 34 weeks' gestation. Her dates were confirmed by ultrasound at booking (12 weeks). She is a smoker. The midwife measures her fundal height at 30 cm. An ultrasound scan is performed because of the midwife's concern that the fetus is SGA, and the measurements are plotted in Figure 8.20.

Do the ultrasound findings support the clinical diagnosis of SGA?

Yes, because the fetal AC is below the 5th centile for gestation. This finding does not give an indication of the well-being of the fetus and is compatible with IUGR

secondary to placental insufficiency or a healthy, constitutionally small baby.

What additional features/measures on ultrasound assessment could give an indication of fetal well-being?

Liquor volume
Amniotic fluid volume is decreased in fetal growth restriction associated with fetal hypoxia with redistribution of fetal blood flow away from the kidneys to vital structures such as brain and heart, with a consequent reduction in renal perfusion and urine output.

Biophysical profile

In the presence of fetal hypoxia associated with IUGR, fetal biophysical variables such as gross body movements, flexor tone and fetal breathing movements are abolished. These can be observed using ultrasound.

Doppler ultrasound

Umbilical artery

Waveforms from the umbilical artery provide information on feto-placental blood flow and placental resistance. Diastolic flow in the umbilical artery increases (i.e. placental resistance falls) throughout gestation. If the RI in the umbilical artery rises above the 95th centile of the normal graph, this implies faulty perfusion of the placenta, which may eventually result in fetal hypoxia. Absent or reversed end-diastolic flow in the umbilical artery is a particularly serious development, with a strong correlation with fetal distress and intrauterine death.

Fetal vessels

Falling oxygen levels in the fetus result in a redistribution of blood flow to protect the brain, heart, adrenals and spleen, and vasoconstriction in all other vessels. The middle cerebral artery will show increasing diastolic flow as hypoxia increases, while a rising resistance in the fetal aorta reflects compensatory vasoconstriction in the fetal body. When diastolic flow is absent in the fetal aorta, this implies fetal acidaemia. Increasing pulsatility in the central veins supplying the heart, such as the ductus venosus and inferior vena cava, is an indicator of fetal acidaemia and impending heart failure; when late diastolic flow is absent in the ductus venosus, fetal death is imminent.

Cardiotocography

Fetal tachycardia, reduced variability in heart rate, absence of accelerations and presence of decelerations identified on a CTG are associated with fetal hypoxia.

Prenatal diagnosis

OVERVIEW

The aims of prenatal diagnosis relate to the identification of fetal abnormality in order to:
- reassure parents by reducing the likelihood of undiagnosed fetal abnormality,
- maximize the information available to parents if an abnormality is detected to assist in decision making,
- allow the parents of pregnancies in which an abnormality is identified to prepare for the birth of the child if they decide to continue with the pregnancy,
- enable parents at risk of inherited conditions to have healthy children by diagnosis of abnormality and termination of affected fetuses,
- allow appropriate perinatal management and intrauterine treatment.

Tests for fetal abnormality fall into two groups, namely screening and diagnostic. Screening tests are not diagnostic, but enable the selection of pregnancies to which diagnostic tests can be applied, allowing for the early detection of conditions whose identification at an earlier stage will allow more appropriate perinatal management or termination of pregnancy.

Although there are numerous congenital abnormalities, the overall prevalence of disorders is approximately 2 per 100 pregnancies. The classification and incidence of common congenital abnormalities are shown in Table 9.1.

Table 9.1 – Classification and incidence of common congenital abnormalities

Congenital abnormality	Example	Incidence per 1000 births
Structural	Congenital heart disease	4–6
	Neural tube defects	2–6
	Cleft lip/palate	1–2
	Talipes equinovarus	1
Chromosomal	Trisomy 21 (Down's syndrome)	1.5
	Monosomy X (Turner's syndrome)	0.3
	Other trisomies (13 and 18)	0.3

(continued)

Table 9.1 *(continued)*

Genetic	Cystic fibrosis	0.5
	Sickle-cell disease	Depends on ethnicity
Miscellaneous	Viral infection	0.2

Prenatal screening and diagnostic tests

The distinction between screening and diagnosis is often blurred in common usage (Table 9.2). Screening tests are performed on all women in order to identify a subset of patients who are at high risk of a disorder. They do not confer any risk to the pregnancy and are performed for disorders with a relatively high prevalence and for which there are accurate prenatal diagnostic tests. Diagnostic tests, on the other hand, are carried out on pregnancies that have been identified as high risk by a prior screening test. They are usually invasive and carry a small risk of miscarriage. Therefore the risks of being affected by the condition should be severe enough to warrant consideration for a diagnostic test.

Table 9.2 – Difference between prenatal screening and diagnostic tests

	Screening	Diagnostic tests
Population tested	All women	Women at 'high risk'
Purpose of test	Select a 'high-risk' group	To diagnose abnormality
Usual method of testing	Maternal history	Ultrasound
	Maternal biochemistry	Amniocentesis
	Maternal virology	Chorion villus sampling
	Ultrasound	Cordocentesis
Prerequisite to test	Diagnostic test available	Patient aware of potential risks
Risk of test	Anxiety of a 'screen-positive' result	Small risk of miscarriage from invasive test

Invasive diagnostic tests

A number of different tests exist to sample material of fetal origin (Table 9.3). The sample obtained can be used for cytogenetic, biochemical, enzymatic or DNA analysis to give a prenatal diagnosis. Generally these tests are invasive in nature and carry a small risk of miscarriage.

Amniocentesis
A thin needle is passed transabdominally under ultrasound guidance into the amniotic cavity (Fig. 9.1). A small amount of amniotic fluid is removed, which contains fetal fibroblasts. This test is usually performed at or after 15 weeks' gestation; its procedure-related miscarriage rate is 1 per cent. Although it is technically possible to perform amniocentesis at earlier gestations, this is generally avoided, as it is associated with a higher cell culture failure rate and a higher rate of miscarriage, neonatal talipes and respiratory difficulties.

Chorion villus sampling
A thin needle is passed transabdominally or transcervically under ultrasound guidance into the placenta

Table 9.3 – Details of prenatal diagnostic procedures

	Amniocentesis	Chorion villus sampling	Cordocentesis
Gestation (weeks)	15–40	10–40	20–40
Route	Transabdominal	Transabdominal/transcervical	Transabdominal
Cells sampled	Fetal fibroblasts	Trophoblast cells	Fetal white blood cells
Procedure-related risk of miscarriage (%)	1	1	1
Direct karyotype result	FISH for chromosomes 13, 18, 21 and XY 24–48 hours	24–48 hours	Not needed
Culture karyotype result	2–3 weeks	1–2 weeks	24–48 hours
Mosaicism rate on karyotype	None	1%	None

FISH, fluorescence in-situ hybridization.

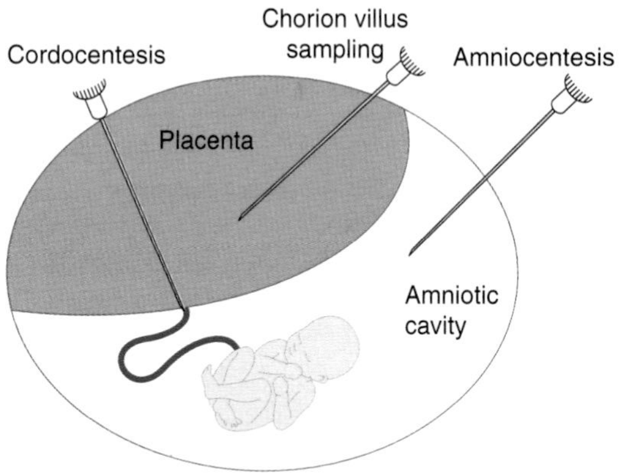

Figure 9.1 Diagram illustrating placement of the needle for amniocentesis, chorion villus sampling and cordocentesis.

(chorionic plate; Fig. 9.1). Chorionic villi, which are feto-placental in origin, are aspirated or biopsied through this needle. This test is usually performed at or after 10 weeks' gestation. Although the miscarriage rate after chorion villus sampling (CVS) is thought to be higher than that following amniocentesis (2–3 per cent), this is because the background spontaneous miscarriage rate of pregnancy is higher at 10 weeks. The procedure-related miscarriage rate of CVS is the same as for amniocentesis, 1 per cent. Although, it is technically possible to do CVS at earlier gestations, this is generally avoided, as it is associated with a higher rate of cleft lip/palate and digital amputation abnormalities.

Cordocentesis

A thin needle is passed transabdominally under ultrasound guidance into the umbilical cord to sample fetal blood (Fig. 9.1). This test is usually performed at or after 20 weeks' gestation; its procedure-related miscarriage rate is 1 per cent. Although it is technically possible to do this test at earlier gestations, this is generally avoided, as it is associated with a higher rate of miscarriage.

Laboratory analysis

Cytogenetic analysis

Cells obtained from invasive prenatal diagnostic tests are cultured until enough cells in mitosis are available to make a cytogenetic diagnosis. The more rapidly the tissue divides, the quicker the results are available. Hence the times for diagnosis for amniocentesis, CVS and cordocentesis are 2–3 weeks, 1–2 weeks and 24–48 hours, respectively.

With CVS, the sampled chorionic villi have so many cells already in mitosis that a 'direct' result may be available in 24–48 hours. In this instance, the quality of the diagnosis is adequate to exclude an aneuploidy (abnormal number of chromosomes). However, the direct preparation is usually not of sufficient quality to permit G-banding, hence chromosomal aberrations such as deletions or inversions cannot be effectively excluded.

The use of fluorescence in-situ hybridization (FISH) can facilitate rapid results with amniocentesis. The technique detects and localizes specific DNA sequences directly in interphase or metaphase, and hence cell culture is not required. It allows the rapid (24–48 hours) prenatal diagnosis of major aneuploidies for chromosomes 13, 18, 21 and XY.

DNA analysis

Fetal DNA obtained from invasive tests can be used for DNA probe (sickle-cell disease and cystic fibrosis), polymerase chain reaction (PCR) (fragile X syndrome, congenital toxoplasmosis and cytomegalovirus) or linkage analysis (fragile X syndrome).

Biochemical and enzymatic analysis

When DNA analysis is not possible, biochemical or enzymatic assays can be performed for specific diseases (congenital adrenal hypoplasia and mucopolysaccharidoses).

Diagnosis of structural abnormalities

Structural abnormalities constitute the majority of congenital abnormalities encountered in clinical practice. There are established screening programmes for fetal neural tube and cardiac defects; these are discussed in detail in this section. Other fetal structural malformations occur less commonly and are sporadic in nature.

The Royal College of Obstetricians and Gynaecologists in the UK has recommended a two-stage scan programme for screening for structural abnormalities: an initial scan at booking (11–14 weeks) and a further scan at or around 20 weeks. Details of these routine scans are provided in Chapter 8, along with details of the features that should be identified on the later scan.

Neural tube defects

Neural tube defects (NTDs) are among the most common major abnormalities. They occur due to defects in the formation of the neural tube during embryogenesis. The aetiology is multi-factorial, with well-defined environmental, genetic, pharmacological and geographical factors implicated.

Neural tube defects affecting the cranial vault present on ultrasound as anencephaly or encephalocele. The former is universally lethal, while the prognosis for encephalocele is related to the size of the defect. The remainder of NTDs, termed spina bifida, usually affect the spinal cord at the caudal end. The local effects of spina bifida (paralysis of the legs, urinary and faecal incontinence) depend on the spinal level and the number of spinal segments affected in the lesion. Spina bifida has previously been associated with impaired intellect due to progressive hydrocephalus and infection of ventriculo-peritoneal shunts. With modern imaging techniques and antibiotics, the intellectual prognosis for this condition is much improved.

Prenatal screening and diagnosis of neural tube defects

When a parent or previous sibling has had an NTD, the risk of recurrence is 5–10 per cent. Mid-trimester maternal serum alpha-fetoprotein (AFP) levels are increased in pregnancies affected by open NTDs. These were once used as the established screening tests for NTDs, with screen-positive women being referred for amniocentesis. The presence of acetylcholinesterase (a central nervous system neurotransmitter) in amniotic fluid was taken as being diagnostic of an open NTD. The need for a two-step screening/diagnosis process was quickly superseded by the development of high-resolution ultrasound. Anencephaly and encephaloceles are detectable on first trimester ultrasound if an adequate examination of the cranial vault is performed (Fig. 9.2). Spina bifida, on the other hand, requires the systematic detailed examination of the fetal spine (Fig. 9.3) at the routine 20-week anomaly scan. The diagnosis may be suspected from the visualization of the 'lemon' (shape of the skull) and 'banana' (absent cerebellum) signs in the fetal brain at this examination (Fig. 9.4). The sensitivity of ultrasound for both open and closed defects and NTDs is greater than 95 per cent. Other central nervous system abnormalities (not strictly NTDs), such as hydrocephalus, can also be detected at the 20-week scan (Fig. 9.5; Table 9.4).

Prevention of neural tube defects

Folate deficiency and drugs that interfere with folate metabolism (i.e. anti-epileptics) are implicated in about 10 per cent of NTD cases. Periconceptual folate

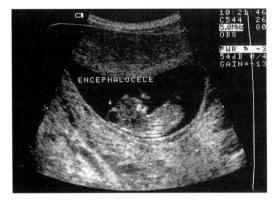

Figure 9.2 Fetal encephalocele detected at 12 weeks' gestation.

supplementation of the maternal diet reduces the risk of developing these defects by about half. Folic acid should be given for at least 3 months prior to conception and for the first trimester of pregnancy. The dosage of folic acid is 400 mcg for primary prevention and 4 mg for women wishing to prevent a recurrence of an NTD or with type 1 diabetes mellitus.

Congenital heart defects

Abnormalities of the heart and great arteries are another common group of congenital abnormalities. About half are either lethal or require major surgery and the remainder are asymptomatic. The aetiology of congenital heart defects (CHDs) is heterogeneous and includes genetic factors, environmental factors and viral infections. Gene mutations and chromosomal abnormalities account for less than 5 per cent of cases.

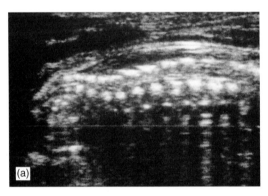
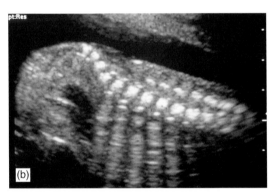

Figure 9.3 (a) Normal fetal spine showing posterior spinous process. (b) Abnormal fetal spine with spinous process absent in the sacral and 5th lumbar segments.

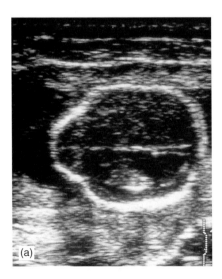
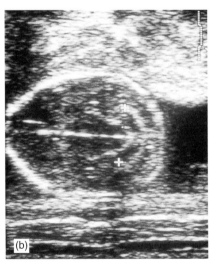

Figure 9.4 (a) Lemon-shaped skull and (b) curved (banana) cerebellum – typical cranial signs of spina bifida.

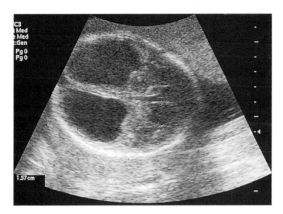

Figure 9.5 Enlarged cerebral ventricles at 22 weeks, diagnostic of hydrocephalus.

Table 9.4 – Some major structural abnormalities detectable by ultrasound at the mid-trimester scan

Body system	Example
Cranium	Anencephaly[a]
	Encephalocele[a]
	Hydrocephalus
Skeleton	Spina bifida
	Kyphoscoliosis
Thorax	Congenital heart disease
	Cystic adenomatoid malformation
	Diaphragmatic hernia
Abdomen	Gastroschisis
	Exomphalos[a]
	Renal agenesis
	Multi/polycystic disease
	Hydronephrosis
Limbs	Talipes equinovarus
	Polydactyly[a]

[a] Abnormalities that can often be detected at the first trimester scan.

Prenatal screening for congenital heart defects
When a previous sibling or father is affected by CHD, the risk is 2 per cent. When two siblings or the mother have CHD, the recurrence risk is 10 per cent. The second major group considered to be at high risk is the offspring of women with type 1 diabetes mellitus, for whom the incidence of CHD is doubled. However, more than 90 per cent of fetuses with CHD are from pregnancies without such risk factors.

Prenatal diagnosis of congenital heart defects
Although 90 per cent of major CHDs may be detected antenatally in specialist centres, in most units performing routine 20-week anomaly scans, this figure is closer to 30 per cent. As specialist fetal echocardiography cannot be performed on all pregnancies, the limiting factor in diagnosis is selection of cases for referral to these specialist units (Fig. 9.6).

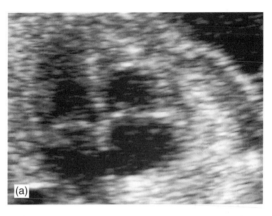

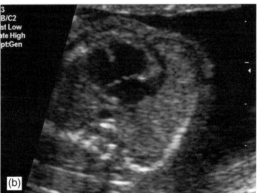

Figure 9.6 (a) Normal four-chamber fetal heart. (b) Abnormal heart with atrio-ventricular and septal defect.

Gastrointestinal abnormalities

Bowel obstruction
Bowel obstruction above the ileum, e.g. duodenal and oesophageal atresia, usually results in polyhydramnios and is easily visualized with ultrasound. Duodenal

atresia is characteristically associated with a 'double bubble' appearance on ultrasound. One-third of cases will be associated with Down's syndrome, and karyotyping should be considered.

Abdominal wall defects

Omphaloceles are due to a midline abdominal wall defect through which peritoneal sac herniates. This sac will contain varying amounts of abdominal contents, including small bowel and liver. Approximately 50 per cent of omphaloceles have associated cardiac or chromosomal abnormalities. In gastroschisis, the insertion of the umbilical cord is intact, but there are free loops of bowel in the amniotic cavity. In the majority of cases, the anomaly is isolated and there is no increased incidence of chromosomal anomalies.

Renal tract abnormalities

Major abnormalities of the renal tract such as renal agenesis will normally be detected by 20 weeks because of the associated oligohydramnios.

Renal pelvis dilatation

The commonest abnormality seen in the renal tract and identified on ultrasound is mild pelvicalyceal dilatation. This abnormality is found in approximately 2 per cent of fetuses on the second trimester scan, and the significance of the finding is controversial. Pelvicalyceal dilatation may be physiological or result from mild reflux or pelvi-ureteric junction obstruction. Postnatal renal ultrasonography is required to assess progression or regression. Failure of resolution increases the risk of urinary tract infections.

Other structural abnormalities

Cleft lip/palate

The typical cleft lip appears as a linear defect extending from the lip to the nostril, with the majority of cases (75 per cent) being unilateral. In about 50 per cent of cases, both the lip and palate are defective; in the remainder, either the lip or palate is involved. Cleft lip ($\pm$palate) is identifiable on ultrasound, whereas the diagnosis of isolated cleft palate is difficult. Associated abnormalities are found in about 15 per cent of fetuses with cleft lip/palate, usually because genetic or chromosomal abnormalities are implicated in the aetiology. Postnatally, because of cosmetic, feeding and respiratory problems, early surgical correction is usually advocated.

Talipes equinovarus

In talipes equinovarus, also known as clubfoot, the forefoot is supinated and the ankle is plantar flexed. The deformity is bilateral in 50 per cent of cases and affects twice as many males as females. The aetiology is sporadic and the condition is neurological in origin, with the skeletal malformation being secondary. The diagnosis is reliably established on ultrasound, except in positional talipes, a temporary malformation secondary to oligohydramnios. Talipes equinovarus is lethal in about 20 per cent of cases because of associated malformations, most commonly spina bifida.

Chromosomal abnormalities

The most common chromosomal abnormalities can be classified as either aneuploidies (usually trisomies) or sex chromosome abnormalities.

Aneuploidies

Trisomies occur in the majority of cases due to non-dysjunction in meiosis. This abnormality of gametogenesis is known to occur more frequently with advancing maternal age. Rarely, trisomies may occur due to unbalanced translocations (6 per cent) or mosaicism (4 per cent). Although any chromosome may be affected, the majority of trisomies result in first trimester miscarriage except for trisomies 13 (Patau's), 18 (Edward's) and 21 (Down's). Down's syndrome is associated with characteristic mental and physical features (Table 9.5). Trisomies 13 and 18 are associated with such major structural defects that their diagnosis is usually suspected on antenatal ultrasound. Since trisomies 13 and 18 have a very high intrauterine lethality (90–95 per cent), screening programmes are geared mainly towards the antenatal detection of Down's syndrome, which is the commonest chromosomal abnormality at birth.

Sex chromosome abnormalities

Unlike trisomies, the prevalence of sex chromosome abnormalities does not change with maternal age. The cumulative prevalence of Turner's (monosomy

Table 9.5 – Characteristic features of Down's syndrome

Intrauterine lethality	40% at 12–40 weeks
Mental effects	Mental retardation, deafness, short-sightedness
Physical effects	Flat facies, macroglossia, cardiac septal defects (40%), intestinal atresias
Postnatal outcome	Premature ageing, reduced immunity, leukaemia, reduced life-span

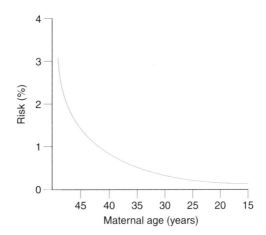

Figure 9.7 Down's syndrome risk and maternal age.

X or 45XO), Klinefelter's (47XXY) and other sex chromosome abnormalities is greater than that of Down's syndrome. Turner's syndrome individuals are infertile females of normal intellect and short stature. Klinefelter's syndrome individuals are infertile males with slightly reduced IQ, testicular dysgenesis and tall stature. As many of the characteristics of these conditions are mild, many affected individuals remain undiagnosed throughout their lifetime. Routine screening for these conditions is not available and the diagnosis is often made incidentally.

Fragile X

Fragile X syndrome is the most common inherited cause of mental retardation, explaining the excess of males affected by non-specific mental retardation in the population. The fragile X gene (*FMR1*) becomes hypermethylated with inactivated multiple repeats (>200). The estimated prevalence of the condition is 1:4000 males. Prenatal diagnosis is possible using PCR and Southern analysis, but only for male fetuses at present. As screening for fragile X in pregnancy is not feasible, prenatal testing is reserved for families in which one of the parents is known to be a carrier by virtue of a previous affected pregnancy.

Screening tests for Down's syndrome

Maternal age and history
The prevalence of Down's syndrome increases with advancing maternal age (Fig. 9.7). Because of this,

historically, women over the age of 35 were offered diagnostic testing for Down's syndrome. However, 90 per cent of pregnant women are younger than 35 years and, despite being at lower risk, they give birth to 75–80 per cent of Down's syndrome babies. Women who have already had a pregnancy affected by Down's syndrome are routinely offered prenatal diagnosis, based on their background risk for trisomy being slightly increased.

Maternal serum biochemistry
Measurement of maternal serum hormones during the second trimester (15–22 weeks' gestation) offers an alternative method of screening. The two main hormones of fetal origin that are commonly assayed are AFP and human chorionic gonadotrophin (hCG). In pregnancies complicated by a fetus with Down's syndrome, these levels are decreased and increased respectively. Based on maternal age, gestation and variation in hormone levels, an algorithm predicts the individual's risk for a Down's syndrome pregnancy. This is not diagnostic, but identifies a group at high risk (>1:250) who should be offered a diagnostic test such as amniocentesis. It is also important to remember that being assessed as low risk, based on biochemical screening, does not exclude an affected pregnancy.

First trimester screening uses two biochemical markers – pregnancy-associated plasma protein (PAPP-A), which is lowered in Down's syndrome, and β-hCG, which is elevated – in addition to maternal age to provide an individual risk, in a similar fashion to second trimester biochemical screening.

This approach identifies approximately 60 per cent of affected pregnancies, i.e. is similar to second trimester screening. The advantage of early screening is that termination of pregnancy, if required, may be performed as a day-case surgical procedure rather than by induction of labour, as is often required after second trimester serum screening.

Ultrasound

Nuchal translucency

A newer screening test for Down's syndrome involves the sonographic measurement of the subcutaneous collection of fluid in the nuchal (behind the neck) region of the fetus at 10–13 weeks' gestation. The nuchal translucency (NT) measurement is increased in the majority of aneuploid fetuses in the first trimester of pregnancy (Fig. 9.8; Table 9.6). Based on maternal age, gestation and NT measurement, an algorithm predicts the individual's risk for Down's syndrome in a similar way to the biochemical screening.

Combination of the NT measurement with first trimester maternal serum biochemical markers (see above) has been found to produce a sensitivity of up to 90 per cent for a screen-positive rate of 5 per cent.

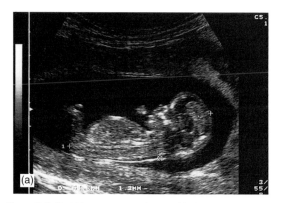 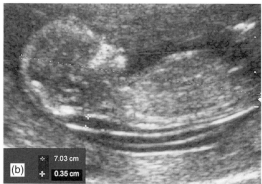

Figure 9.8 First trimester measurement of fetal nuchal translucency: (a) normal; (b) 3.5 mm (increased), suggestive of chromosome abnormality.

Table 9.6 – Screening tests for Down's syndrome

	Maternal age	Maternal serum biochemistry	Nuchal translucency
Method	History	Blood test	Ultrasound scan
Gestation	Any	10–14 weeks (PAPP-A, β-hCG) 15–22 weeks (AFP, β-hCG)	10–14 weeks
Sensitivity (%)	25	60–75	75–80
Advantages	Simple, cheap	Operator independent Screens for neural tube and abdominal wall defects	Early test Screens for all aneuploidy Applicable in multiple pregnancy
Disadvantages	Poor sensitivity	Late test Specific for Down's syndrome Requires dating scan	Operator dependent

PAPP-A, pregnancy-associated plasma protein; β-hCG, beta-human chorionic gonadotrophin; AFP, alpha-fetoprotein.

Other ultrasound anomalies

In addition to increased NT, other common abnormalities detected by ultrasound in Down's syndrome include brachycephaly and ventriculomegaly in the skull and brain, cardiac defects, echogenic chordae tendineae in the heart, echogenic bowel, mild hydronephrosis, short femur, abnormal hands and feet. At later gestations, fetuses may be small for gestational age.

Genetic disorders

There are numerous congenital abnormalities that exhibit a classical Mendelian pattern of inheritance. The commonest of these, cystic fibrosis and the haemoglobinopathies, are discussed below. Additionally, numerous genetic syndromes exist; the majority of these are sporadic, but some have recessive, dominant or sex-linked patterns of inheritance. The majority of conditions with recessive, dominant or sex-linked inheritance patterns have a relatively low frequency and are only screened for after the family has undergone genetic counselling regarding the disease, likelihood of recurrence, diagnostic tests and possible therapeutic interventions.

Cystic fibrosis

Cystic fibrosis is an autosomal recessive condition and the most common lethal genetic disease in Caucasians. The cystic fibrosis gene has been isolated to the long arm of chromosome 7 and there are more than 700 mutations identified to this region that are responsible for the disease. The commonest of these mutations is $\delta F508$, which is present in 68 per cent of cases. Multiple gene mutations and the cost of DNA testing for the population are the major reasons why parental screening has not been effective to date. At present, prenatal diagnosis is offered only to parents who are known carriers, usually because they have already had an affected child.

Haemoglobinopathies

Sickle-cell anaemia and thalassaemia are both autosomal recessive conditions with considerable disease heterogeneity. The carrier frequency may be as high as 20 per cent, especially in African (sickle-cell disease) and Mediterranean (thalassaemia) populations. Screening of at-risk populations is possible by haemoglobin electrophoresis. Sickle-cell mutations are limited in number and fairly well characterized, hence prenatal diagnosis is usually possible. As there are numerous thalassaemia mutations, parental studies are a prerequisite to establish whether a fetal diagnosis is possible. Prenatal diagnosis is made on fetal DNA, which can be obtained by any of the invasive techniques. As the risk of an affected pregnancy is high (25 per cent) for parents who are carriers, early testing through CVS is advocated.

Congenital viral and parasitic infections

Fetal infection with rubella, cytomegalovirus (CMV), *Toxoplasma* and parvovirus is known to have potentially serious deleterious effects (Table 9.7) and these are discussed in detail in Chapter 16. Maternal viral infections in pregnancy are relatively infrequent, with the likelihood of transplacental transfer and fetal infection increasing with gestational age. However, most infected fetuses (>95 per cent) remain unaffected. The risk of a congenitally infected fetus being affected is inversely proportional to the gestational age. Hence, although the chance of fetal infection is low in early pregnancy, if infected, the fetus is likely to be seriously affected and the pregnancy is doomed to miscarriage. Therefore, the most susceptible pregnancies are those infected at 12–18 weeks' gestation, when infected fetuses are likely to be seriously affected and yet survive.

Screening for congenital viral and parasitic infections

There is an established screening programme for rubella in pregnancy. Rubella-susceptible women are advised to avoid antenatal exposure to the virus and are vaccinated in the puerperium. Screening is not advocated for maternal CMV or toxoplasmosis infections in pregnancy because of the low incidence, the high false-positive rates, and the risk of miscarriage consequent on the invasive prenatal diagnostic tests necessary to confirm fetal infection. Additionally, confirming fetal infection does not necessarily indicate that the fetus has been affected.

Table 9.7 – Characteristics of congenital viral infection

	Rubella	Cytomegalovirus	Toxoplasmosis	Parvovirus
Source	Infected individuals	Infected individuals	Cat litter Under-cooked meat	Infected children
Features of congenital infection	Cataracts Heart defects Growth restriction Hepatomegaly Thrombocytopenia Mental retardation	Microcephaly Ventriculomegaly Cerebral calcification Heart defects Growth restriction Hepatomegaly Thrombocytopenia Mental retardation	Microcephaly Ventriculomegaly Cerebral calcification Heart defects Growth restriction Hepatomegaly Thrombocytopenia Mental retardation	Aplastic anaemia Hydrops

Prenatal diagnosis of congenital viral and parasitic infections

In cases of confirmed maternal viral infection, regular fetal ultrasound to detect the characteristic features of congenital infection is advocated. There is limited evidence that treatment of toxoplasmosis-infected mothers with spiramycin may prevent congenital fetal infection. Congenital parvovirus infection may result in a temporary fetal aplastic anaemia and hydrops. Supportive therapy with fetal intrauterine blood transfusions in these cases dramatically improves the prognosis.

New developments

Fetal cells in the maternal circulation
The presence of fetal cells in maternal blood is an established phenomenon. The methods for their isolation, identification and genetic analysis continue to be refined. Most investigators are focused on the isolation of fetal nucleated red blood or trophoblastic cells. The validation of a reliable technique for the safe, non-invasive acquisition of fetal cells will revolutionize prenatal diagnosis.

Pre-implantation genetic diagnosis
Couples at high risk of having pregnancies with inherited diseases may benefit from pre-implantation genetic diagnosis (PGD) in the early stages of human zygote/embryo development. The development of PGD allows parents to avoid the decision to terminate a pregnancy. PGD has evolved from the development of safe and effective techniques for embryo biopsy and the appropriate methods of genetic diagnosis by FISH or PCR.

Three-dimensional ultrasound
Advanced imaging technology has permitted the real-time three-dimensional reconstruction of data acquired by specially adopted ultrasound machines. This technology permits the increased resolution required for certain fetal malformations such as cleft lip/palate. Routine two-dimensional ultrasound requires the sonographer to 'reconstruct' the third dimension in a mental image. The real practical value of three-dimensional ultrasound technology is the potential to allow the remote acquisition of ultrasound data by technicians that can later be analysed by appropriate experts.

Fetal magnetic resonance imaging
The uses of prenatal magnetic resonance imaging (MRI) are being evaluated increasingly. The development of ultra-fast MRI sequences to overcome fetal movement artefact has resulted in significant improvement in the quality and usefulness of the image. MRI has the potential to become a powerful adjunct to the evaluation of the abnormal fetus discovered on ultrasound.

Key Points

- Although there are numerous congenital abnormalities, the overall prevalence of disorders is approximately 2 per 100 pregnancies.
- Tests for fetal abnormality fall into two groups, namely screening and diagnostic. Screening tests are not diagnostic, but enable the selection of pregnancies to which diagnostic tests can be applied and thus the early detection of conditions to allow appropriate management.
- A number of different tests exist to sample material of fetal origin (see Table 9.3). The sample obtained can be used for cytogenetic, biochemical, enzymatic or DNA analysis to give a prenatal diagnosis. Generally these tests are invasive in nature and carry a small risk of miscarriage.
- Ultrasound plays a major role in screening for a wide range of structural abnormalities of the fetus.
- Periconceptual folate supplementation of the maternal diet given for at least 3 months prior to conception and for the first trimester of pregnancy reduces by about half the risk of developing NTDs.
- In screening for Down's syndrome, an age-modified individual maternal risk can be calculated by the gestation-corrected assessment of second trimester maternal serum levels of AFP and hCG and by first trimester maternal serum levels of PAPP-A and hCG.
- The sonographic measurement of the subcutaneous collection of fluid in the nuchal region of the fetus (NT) at 10–13 weeks' gestation offers another approach to screening for Down's syndrome. Based on maternal age, gestation and NT measurement, an algorithm predicts the individual's risk of a Down's syndrome pregnancy, in a similar way to biochemical screening. NT can be combined with first trimester biochemical screening to improve the detection rate of Down's syndrome fetuses.

CASE HISTORY

A 24-year-old primigravida at 10 weeks' gestation attends the booking clinic. She has a friend who has a Down's syndrome child and is particularly anxious about knowing the chances of her baby having the condition. She has read about a 'blood test' for Down's syndrome in a magazine and wishes to discuss this along with other options for screening and diagnosis of Down's syndrome.

What issues would you wish to discuss with her?

Details of the 'blood test'
- When biochemical screening for Down's syndrome can be performed:
  - first trimester,
  - second trimester (15–20 weeks).
- A scan needs to be performed to confirm gestation (AFP, hCG and PAPP-A are gestation related).
- What is involved in the test (i.e. a maternal venous blood sample).
- How long the results take to be returned (usually within 24–48 hours).
- How she will receive the results.

What the test does
- It measures levels of pregnancy-associated hormones in the maternal circulation. In the first trimester PAPP-A and β-hCG and in the second trimester AFP and β-hCG (AFP typically low, hCG high and PAPP-A low compared to the population median in affected pregnancies).

- Combined with her age and gestation, an algorithm will give a personal risk of her having a Down's syndrome baby.
- This can be categorized as high (>1:250) or low (<1:250) risk.

What the test does not do
- It does not diagnose Down's syndrome and, if she is in the high-risk category, she will require further investigation to confirm the diagnosis, i.e. amniocentesis or CVS.
- Both of these diagnostic tests are invasive procedures associated with excess fetal loss.

Additional points
- If she is in the low-risk category, she can still have a baby with Down's syndrome.
- Measurement of nuchal thickness by ultrasound in the first trimester, either on its own or in combination with first trimester biochemical screening, is another option to screen for Down's syndrome.
- A detailed anomaly scan at 18–20 weeks may identify associated anomalies, e.g. cardiac abnormalities or other 'soft markers' in an affected fetus.
- She may wish to consider her actions if she had a Down's syndrome fetus, i.e. would she consider termination of pregnancy, as this may affect her decision as to whether or not to participate in the screening programme.

Second trimester miscarriage

OVERVIEW

Second trimester miscarriage complicates approximately 1 per cent of pregnancies. It is particularly distressing to the woman and her family because the pregnancy has become obvious abdominally and the mother may have started to notice fetal movements. There are many causes of second trimester miscarriage, some of which are amenable to treatment.

Definition

A 'late' or second trimester miscarriage occurs between 12 and 24 weeks' gestation. After 24 weeks' gestation, the baby is potentially viable and birth is referred to as a preterm delivery.

Prevalence

In the UK, as in most other countries, there is no formal record of miscarriages. The exact incidence of late miscarriages is unknown but is estimated to be approximately 1 per cent. 'Early' first trimester losses are far commoner, accounting for approximately 80 per cent of all miscarriages. Miscarriage can be associated with major haemorrhage and sepsis, and maternal death is a rare but recognized consequence. Infective sequelae may also lead to subsequent impairment of fertility.

Classification (Table 10.1)

As the interval between membrane rupture and delivery can occasionally be measured in weeks, some 'inevitable' second trimester miscarriages may result in preterm deliveries.

Aetiology

The likely aetiology behind second trimester losses varies with gestation. At 12–15 weeks, the predominant causes are those of first trimester miscarriage – fetal chromosomal and structural anomalies and possibly endocrine causes. At the latter part of the second trimester, between 19 and 23 weeks, the commonest factors underlying the miscarriage will be those linked to very preterm births; these include ascending genital tract infection, intrauterine bleeding and cervical weakness. The latter may be congenital or acquired

Table 10.1 – Classification of second trimester miscarriage

	Symptoms	Signs
Threatened	Bleeding Contractions Abnormal vaginal discharge	Minimal cervical dilatation Intact membranes
Inevitable	Any of the above *or* may be minimal	Cervical dilatation >3 cm Membranes ruptured
Missed	Usually none	Fetal death on ultrasound
Septic	Above + malaise	Fever, tachycardia, hypotension Uterine tenderness

through procedures such as cone biopsy or repeated cervical dilatation.

Epidemiological risk factors for second trimester miscarriage therefore draw from both first trimester loss and preterm delivery. They include poor socio-economic status, smoking, genital tract infections, previous miscarriage or premature birth and increasing maternal age. A specific risk factor for late miscarriage is mid-trimester amniocentesis. This procedure, commonly performed at 16–18 weeks' gestation, is associated with a 0.5 per cent chance of subsequent pregnancy loss.

P   Understanding the pathophysiology

Normal pregnancy
The uterus should be thought of as a distended sac filled with fluid, baby and placenta. There is one potential opening from it at the cervix. The cervix is usually at least 35 mm long and closed in mid-pregnancy (Fig. 10.1).

Uterine over-distension
The commonest cause of uterine over-distension is multiple gestation. Polyhydramnios has a similar effect. Over-stretching of the myometrium leads to increased contractile activity and premature shortening and opening of the cervix (Fig. 10.2).

Intrauterine bleeding
Disturbance at the uteroplacental interface may lead to intrauterine bleeding. The blood can track down behind the membranes to the cervix and be revealed. Alternatively, it may track away from the cervix and be concealed. Either way, the blood irritates the uterus, leading to contractions, and damages the membranes, leading to early rupture (Fig. 10.3).

Intrauterine infection
The uterine cavity is normally sterile but the vagina contains commensal bacteria. Depending on the bacterial load and cervical resistance, the bacteria may ascend through the cervix and reach the fetal membranes. This may activate the decidua, increase prostaglandin release and trigger contractions. Alternatively, it may weaken the membranes, leading to rupture (Fig. 10.4).

Abnormal cavity
A uterine cavity that is distorted by congenital malformation or fibroids in a low position may be less able to accommodate the developing pregnancy. However, fibroids are common and most pregnancies are successful despite their presence (Fig. 10.5).

Cervical weakness
Due to previous surgical damage or a congenital defect, the cervix may shorten and open prematurely. The membranes then prolapse and may be damaged by stretching or by direct contact with vaginal pathogens. Often referred to as cervical incompetence, weakness may be a better term. The evidence suggests that gradations of deficiency exist, rather than an 'all-or-nothing' phenomenon (Fig. 10.6).

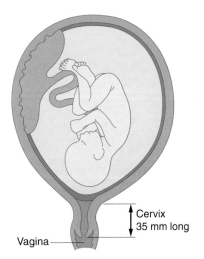

Cervix 35 mm long

Vagina

Figure 10.1 The uterus at 23 weeks' gestation.

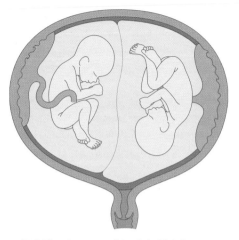

Figure 10.2 The uterus over-distended with twins or more.

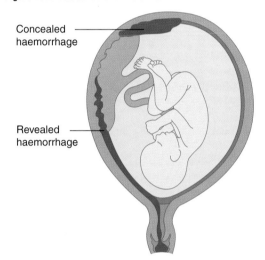

Concealed haemorrhage

Revealed haemorrhage

Figure 10.3 Retroplacental bleeding.

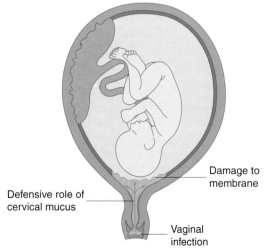

Damage to membrane

Defensive role of cervical mucus

Vaginal infection

Figure 10.4 Ascending genital tract bleeding.

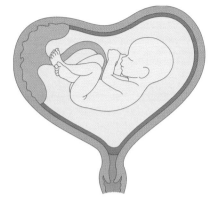

Figure 10.5 Abnormal uterine shape.

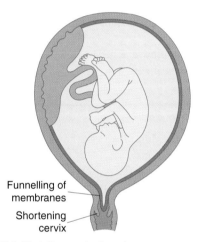

Funnelling of membranes

Shortening cervix

Figure 10.6 Weak (incompetent) cervix.

Clinical features

The clinical presentation of second trimester miscarriage is diverse. Commonly, there will be uterine cramping and bleeding. The membranes may be intact or ruptured. However, events may progress rapidly without significant pain, the mother complaining of relatively minor backache or abdominal discomfort. Some women report only a sudden increase in mucous vaginal discharge. In other cases, there may be clear evidence of membrane rupture with few other signs.

History

The presenting history may be of lower abdominal discomfort with backache, discomfort or pain from uterine contractions or vaginal loss. The vaginal loss may be mucus, blood or amniotic fluid. A history of being generally unwell with fever is also important. A history of previous miscarriage or preterm birth, cervical cerclage, an invasive prenatal diagnostic procedure, vaginal bleeding, fibroids or congenital uterine anomaly should be sought. Always enquire about any urinary or bowel symptoms. Fetal movements may be relevant in the late second trimester. Always check the dating of the pregnancy by reviewing the menstrual history and, if possible, any prior ultrasound examinations.

Examination

A brief general examination is important. Is the woman unwell? Check her pulse, blood pressure, temperature and state of hydration.

Perform a general abdominal examination, looking for evidence of renal tract infection or a gastrointestinal problem. Palpate the uterus for contractions, irritability or tenderness, either generalized or focal. Prior to 24 weeks, fetal parts cannot be reliably felt. A hand-held Doppler device (often referred to as a Sonicaid) should be used to auscultate the fetal heart.

Inspection of a sanitary towel or undergarments may give information about any vaginal loss. Initially, a speculum examination should be performed. A good light and proper positioning are important. A vaginal swab should be taken, especially if membrane rupture has occurred. The cervix should be visualized. It may have started to dilate and the membranes may be seen bulging through the external os. In this situation or after membrane rupture, digital examination should be avoided, as this may exacerbate any infection present. Any source of bleeding should be noted and loss of fluid from the uterus sought by asking the woman to cough during the examination.

Investigations

The following investigations should be considered in all women presenting with a possible second trimester miscarriage.
- Urine sample (midstream urine, MSU): infection.
- Cervico-vaginal swabs: infection.
- Full blood count: anaemia, leukocytosis.
- Blood group: anti-D may be required if rhesus negative and bleeding.

- Transabdominal ultrasound: to confirm gestation and viability, and assess amniotic fluid volume.
- Transvaginal ultrasound: for cervical length measurement.

Differential diagnosis

- Bowel disorders: constipation, colitis, gastroenteritis.
- Urinary disorders: infection, renal stone disease.
- Cervical disorders: ectropion, leucorrhoea, neoplasia.
- Uterine disorders: red degeneration of fibroids, round ligament stretching.

Treatment

Support

A holistic approach to the situation is essential. Sympathy, explanations, pain relief and reassurance are essential. The ideal place for women experiencing a second trimester loss is a purpose-designed area, away from a busy labour and delivery unit or gynaecological ward. Many hospitals now have a focus on pregnancy loss and there is often a specialist midwife co-ordinator for this. If the cervix has not already dilated, many women settle with supportive measures, and the pregnancy continues.

Pre-viable membrane rupture

If membrane rupture has occurred, the situation is more difficult. Precise diagnosis is crucial and membrane rupture should be confirmed by speculum examination and a follow-up ultrasound scan. At this gestation, if contractions and delivery do not ensue, membrane rupture with oligohydramnios carries a significant risk of fetal lung hypoplasia. This complication cannot be reliably predicted antenatally. If there are no contractions and no signs of infection, there is no urgency to interfere. The parents should be counselled as to the bleak prognosis. It is important that medical action only takes place when they are ready. Some may want to wait for nature to take its course; others may want more immediate action. In both cases, continuing support is important. No harm will come from conservatism as long as careful observation is made for signs of infection. Self-taken temperature and observation of changing vaginal discharge or lower uterine tenderness are recommended. This can be done at home until viability is reached. Established chorioamnionitis usually declares itself with contractions and delivery. Rarely do the membranes seal and fluid re-accumulate. This is usually only seen when membrane rupture follows amniocentesis.

Antibiotics

Antibiotics are given for identified or strongly suspected infection. Vaginal infection may be difficult to identify and there is some evidence that empirical antibiotics should be given, particularly with membrane rupture near viability. It seems that the best choice is erythromycin, possibly with clindamycin or metronidazole. This should be continued for 7 days. Great care must be exercised if there is already clinical evidence of chorioamnionitis. In these cases, delay in ending the pregnancy may lead to worsening infection and consequent morbidity. Augmenting the uterine contractions may be the most appropriate management.

Tocolytics

There is currently no place for tocolysis in the prevention of mid-trimester pregnancy loss. Even in later pregnancy, tocolytics are only used to secure short-term (i.e. 48-hour) prolongation of the pregnancy.

Emergency cervical cerclage

When a patient presents with an open cervical os and bulging membranes, the idea of passing a supporting 'stitch' around the cervix to close it seems logical. However, the results of emergency cervical cerclage are poor and are related to the cervical dilatation at insertion. A dilatation of more than 3 cm with an effaced cervix poses extreme difficulties, even for the most experienced operator. Every effort should be made to detect and treat other causes of the uterine instability. If persistent placental bleeding is leading to secondary opening of the cervix, closing the cervix with a stitch clearly does not address the primary

issue and is unlikely to be successful. Bleeding, contractions and infection are all contraindications to cerclage.

The procedure itself can be technically challenging. The membranes must first be reduced and there is a significant risk of membrane rupture while this is being achieved. Techniques used include a maternal head-down position and traction with ring forceps on the anterior and posterior cervical lips. A decompression amniocentesis is favoured by some. Often a transcervical Foley catheter is passed and the balloon inflated with 30–50 mL of water to hold the membranes above the internal os. As the suture is tied, the Foley catheter balloon is deflated and the catheter extracted. Depending on the initial dilatation of the cervix, the chance of the pregnancy proceeding beyond 26 weeks may be less than 50 per cent.

Augment contractions

When the option is taken to hasten the emptying of the uterus in an inevitable second trimester miscarriage, this is usually done by inducing contractions with prostaglandins, such as Cervagem or Cytotec. A high-dose oxytocin infusion may be necessary later in the process. Should the woman have undergone a previous Caesarean or other uterine surgery, special care should be taken when emptying the uterus. Consultation with experienced doctors is recommended.

Delivery

Adequate pain relief should be offered. These deliveries are usually quick, but there is no contraindication to epidural anaesthesia. Patient-controlled analgesia (PCA) also works well in this situation. Vaginal delivery will almost always occur, even if there is a transverse lie or fetal malformation. This is because of the relatively small size of the fetus. Unfortunately, retention of the placenta or part of it is more common under these circumstances, and manual removal under anaesthetic may be required.

Despite a gestational age of 23 weeks or less, some babies will show signs of life at delivery. The parents should be made aware of this beforehand to avoid unnecessary distress. Comfort care should be offered to all of these newborns. If there is any uncertainty as to the gestation or the pregnancy is close to 24 weeks, a paediatrician should be briefed and called to attend the delivery to assess viability at birth. The mother should view the fetus as a baby. She may want to touch or hold the baby, and this should be encouraged. Appropriate sensitivities should be exercised according to the choice of the woman and her partner. Follow-up by a senior member of staff and specialist midwife should be organized; this will lead to discussion about a future pregnancy. Contact details of local or national support groups, such as the Stillbirth and Neonatal Death Society (SANDS), should be given.

Later implications

During the follow-up discussion, any clues about the aetiology of the loss will need to be elucidated. The results of any investigations, such as placental pathology, should be reviewed. Many women are given the idea that mid-trimester loss is usually due to cervical weakness and the problem could be solved by cervical cerclage. Unfortunately, the issue is usually more complicated than this. Each potential cause must be considered in turn. If there was bleeding or the pregnancy was a multiple gestation, it is unlikely that a cervical suture will be helpful. Furthermore, the risk of recurrence is probably low. If infection seems to have played a prominent role, screening for genital tract pathogens and possibly antibiotics may be important in a future pregnancy.

If the pattern of the loss is compatible with cervical weakness, a prophylactic cervical suture may be appropriate in the next pregnancy.

Elective cerclage may be advised solely based on a woman's past obstetric history. Randomized trials suggest benefit when a woman has had three or more late miscarriages or very preterm deliveries. In this situation, the procedure is usually performed at 12–14 weeks' gestation. This is because the risk of first trimester miscarriage has passed and an initial assessment of fetal well-being can be performed with nuchal translucency. Cervical cerclage can be done under general or regional anaesthesia. The simplest and quickest procedure uses a purse-string suture (McDonald technique, Fig. 10.7).

The Mersilene tape suture (Mersilene RS22, Ethicon, Edinburgh; Fig. 10.8) is passed around the cervix, taking bites at all four quadrants. The problem with this type of suture is that it is rather low on the cervical canal (Fig. 10.9). However, removal later in pregnancy does not usually require an anaesthetic.

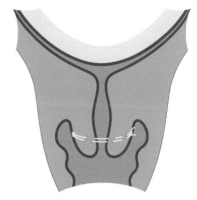

Figure 10.7 Cervical suture: McDonald technique.

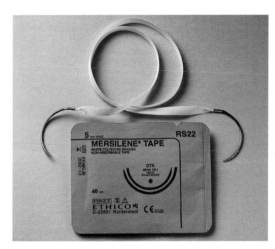

Figure 10.8 Mersilene tape with needles at each end.

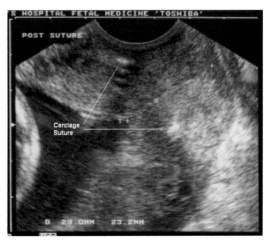

Figure 10.9 Ultrasound appearance of McDonald cerclage.

An experienced operator may use the Shirodkar technique (Fig. 10.10). Here, two small transverse incisions are made, one anteriorly at the cervico-vaginal fold and the second behind the cervix in the posterior fornix. Small tunnels are created upwards in front and behind the cervix and the Mersilene tape is then passed laterally between them, around the cervix. The vaginal skin incisions are then closed over the suture. This allows a much higher stitch placement (Fig. 10.11), resulting in an anatomical position close to the internal os. By virtue of its high position and being buried, it is also more distant from potentially infective vaginal secretions. However, a second anaesthetic is often required for removal. The suture is removed at 37 weeks' gestation or when the patient presents in labour or with membrane rupture, if this occurs preterm.

Selective cerclage is based upon serial transvaginal ultrasound measurements of cervical length, which is now commonly used to follow women known to be at high risk of cervical weakness. Various thresholds are used to define a weak cervix that may benefit from cerclage. Certainly the risk of very preterm delivery is substantial with cervical lengths less than 10–15 mm.

New developments

Bacterial infection
Study continues into the role of infection and, in particular, bacterial vaginosis. This condition should be diagnosed by microscopy, not culture.

Transvaginal ultrasound measurement of cervical length
Studies of the length of the cervix in the second trimester are being conducted on high-risk groups. A long cervical length offers considerable reassurance. Randomized studies concerning the management of women with short cervixes are yielding conflicting results at present.

Thrombophilias
Preliminary studies have suggested a role for various thrombophilias in late miscarriage, particularly when bleeding was involved.

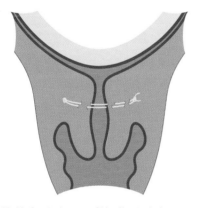

Figure 10.10 Cervical suture: Shirodkar technique.

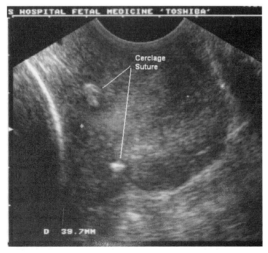

Figure 10.11 Ultrasound appearance of Shirodkar cerclage.

🔑 Key Points

- Second trimester miscarriage has many different presentations.
- Mid-trimester membrane rupture must be diagnosed with precision.
- Women with mid-trimester pregnancy loss require special consideration and treatment.
- All potential aetiologies must be considered to plan logical treatment.
- There is a role for antibiotics and cervical cerclage in selected cases.
- Sympathy and understanding are critical.

CASE HISTORY

Mrs M is 22 years old and pregnant for the second time. Her first pregnancy ended in miscarriage at 18 weeks after rupture of the membranes. According to her 12-week ultrasound scan, she is currently in her 20th week of gestation, and she has been admitted to the labour ward with low back pain, feeling warm and with slight vaginal blood loss followed by watery discharge.

What is the likely diagnosis?

The combination of a previous mid-trimester loss and a history of a temperature, backache and vaginal loss makes intrauterine infection (chorioamnionitis) and cervical dilatation a strong possibility.

What are the key points in the examination and investigation of Mrs M?

- Vital signs: may be tachycardic and pyrexial, hypotensive if shocked.
- Abdominal examination: uterus may be tender, suggesting chorioamnionitis.
- Speculum examination: pooling of amniotic fluid, cervical dilatation; cervico-vaginal swabs.
- MSU: exclude urinary tract infection.
- Ultrasound scan: document viability and confirm gestation; assess amniotic fluid volume.
- Full blood count: raised white cell count may represent infection.

Further management

On speculum examination, there were bulging membranes with some offensive amniotic fluid leaking. A high vaginal swab (HVS) was sent. Mrs M became unwell, with a temperature of 39.5 °C, a tachycardia of 130 bpm and a blood pressure of 85/50 mmHg. After counselling involving a neonatologist and obstetrician, a decision was made to terminate the pregnancy in the interests of maternal health, and a high-dose oxytocin infusion was commenced. Intravenous rehydration and broad-spectrum antibiotics were given and intensive maternal monitoring was commenced, including hourly urine output by indwelling catheter. The anaesthetist was closely involved in her management. Because of the risk of disseminated intravascular coagulation (DIC) and renal dysfunction, serial platelet counts, clotting profiles, fibrinogen and creatinine levels were sent. She received opiate analgesics by intravenous infusion.

Mrs M delivered a baby with no signs of life 8 hours after commencement of Syntocinon. She required an evacuation of retained products of conception (ERPC) under ultrasound guidance by the consultant, but bled heavily following this (approximately 2500 mL), requiring 8 units of blood and fresh frozen plasma. She developed severe DIC and, because of the combination of haemorrhage, DIC and sepsis, became anuric. Acute renal failure was diagnosed and she required dialysis for 3 months, eventually making a full recovery.

Termination of pregnancy

Unfortunately, termination of pregnancy (abortion) becomes necessary in some pregnancies. In the second trimester this may be due to fetal malformation, fetal death or some other compelling reason why the pregnancy cannot continue. In the UK it is done within the legislation of the Abortion Act (1967).

There are two options for this: medical termination or surgical termination. Surgical termination may not be available in some centres because it is a hazardous procedure requiring highly specialized skills. Although it is a short procedure requiring only a few hours in hospital, the family cannot see the fetal parts after the termination. Medical termination usually requires at least a day in hospital. However, the woman and her partner participate as in a labour and are able to see and hold the fetus if they wish. If it is a late medical termination beyond 22 weeks, the process should be commenced with a fetocide. Ideally, both procedures should be available and the woman given a choice.

Medical treatment

This now usually involves the initial use of the progesterone antagonist mifepristone. Over 48–72 hours, this drug enables the uterus to become more responsive to prostaglandins and significantly shortens the induction–delivery interval. The mother is usually admitted to hospital 2–3 days after mifepristone and then receives oral or vaginal prostaglandins. Many centres now use Cytotec for this. In most cases this leads to active contractions and provokes miscarriage within 12–18 hours. Pain relief is frequently by patient-controlled opiate pump. An ideal area for performing this procedure is often not available; it should be some form of transitional ward between obstetrics and gynaecology.

Surgical treatment

Surgical termination of pregnancy presents increasing hazards proportionate to the gestational age. This is because the fetal parts are bigger and therefore a greater degree of cervical dilatation is required. The risk of tearing the cervix or damaging the uterus during blind instrumentation is greater. The cervix should be prepared with a prostaglandin preparation or with Dilapan (Fig. 10.12), which absorbs moisture and swells up over 8–12 hours. The cervix is then already 12–14 mm dilated before the surgical procedure commences.

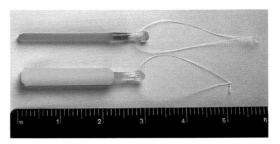

Figure 10.12 Dilapan before and after leaving in water for 12 hours.

The procedure should be performed with ultrasound available. This should be used to confirm the gestational age and guide insertion of the first instruments. It is also used at the end of the procedure to verify that the uterus is empty. Oxytocin is used to ensure the uterus is contracted after delivery.

Antenatal obstetric complications

OVERVIEW

There are a variety of maternal and fetal complications which can arise during pregnancy. Some of these conditions arise because the physiological changes of pregnancy exacerbate many irritating symptoms that in the normal non-pregnant state would not require specific treatment. These so-called 'minor' problems of pregnancy are not in any way dangerous to the mother but can be troublesome on a day-to-day basis; most are considerably improved by simple treatments. Some of the more major fetal and maternal complications are discussed in detail in other chapters. Here we discuss common complications, including malpresentation, rhesus disease and abnormalities of amniotic fluid production.

'Minor' problems of pregnancy

Backache

Backache is due to the laxity of spinal ligaments and weight of the pregnancy causing an exaggerated lumbar lordosis. Pregnancy can exacerbate the symptoms of a prolapsed intervertebral disc, occasionally leading to complete immobility. Advice should include maintenance of correct posture, avoiding lifting heavy objects (including children), avoiding high-heels, regular physiotherapy and simple analgesia (paracetamol or paracetamol–codeine combinations). Women often find swimming very soothing.

Symphysis pubis dysfunction

This is an excruciatingly painful condition usually occurring in the third trimester. The symphysis pubis joint becomes 'loose', causing the two halves of the pelvis to rub on one another when walking or moving. The condition will only improve after delivery, and the management revolves around simple analgesia and, under the physiotherapist's direction, a low stability belt may be worn.

Constipation

Constipation is usually blamed on the effect of progesterone in slowing gut motility, but the physical weight of the gravid uterus on the rectum may contribute, as may concomitantly administered iron tablets. A high-fibre diet should be encouraged, and a mild (non-stimulant) laxative such as lactulose may be suggested.

Hyperemesis gravidarum

Nausea and vomiting are often most pronounced in the first trimester, but by no means confined to it, and are also erroneously referred to as morning sickness. It is worse in a molar or multiple gestation and is probably related to high circulating human chorionic gonadotrophin (hCG) levels. Severe symptoms may lead to Mallory–Weiss tears, haematemesis, dehydration and even malnutrition. In this situation, admission to hospital is mandatory and anti-emetics such as metoclopramide or prochlorperazine are given on a regular basis. In addition, intravenous hydration support should be administered as long as the woman is vomiting. In the severest cases, total parenteral nutrition (TPN) is given, and parenteral B complex vitamins including thiamine are reported to reduce the mortality of the condition. A tapering course of steroids has been used with encouraging results in uncontrolled studies. In the very worst cases, termination of pregnancy may be considered if the mother is becoming malnourished and dehydrated.

Heartburn

This is very common. The symptoms are of burning in the chest or discomfort, often on lying down. Heartburn is caused by the weight effect of the pregnant uterus preventing stomach emptying and the general relaxation of the oesophageal sphincter due to progesterone. Management includes liquid antacid preparations, stopping smoking, reducing alcohol intake, frequent light meals and lying with the head propped up at night. Severe, refractory dyspeptic symptoms warrant gastroenterology referral just in case a stomach ulcer or hiatus hernia is being overlooked.

Varicose veins and piles

These both become worse in later pregnancy. Both are thought to be due to the relaxant effect of progesterone on vascular smooth muscle and the dependent venous stasis caused by the weight of the pregnant uterus on the inferior vena cava.

Neither condition should be treated surgically in pregnancy; piles may be improved with local anaesthetic/anti-irritant creams and a high-fibre diet. Never overlook the 'warning' symptoms of tenesmus, mucus, blood mixed with stool and back passage discomfort that may suggest rectal carcinoma; a rectal digital examination should be carried out if these symptoms are suggested.

Varicose veins of the legs may be symptomatically improved with support stockings, avoidance of standing for prolonged periods and simple analgesia. Thrombophlebitis may occur in a large varicose vein, more commonly after delivery. A large superficial varicose vein may bleed profusely if traumatized; the leg must be elevated and direct pressure applied. Vulval and vaginal varicosities are uncommon but symptomatically troublesome; trauma at the time of delivery (episiotomy, tear, instrumental delivery) may also cause considerable bleeding.

Carpal tunnel syndrome

Compression neuropathies occur in pregnancy due to increased soft-tissue swelling. The most common of these is carpal tunnel syndrome. The median nerve, where it passes through the fibrous canal at the wrist before entering the hand, is most susceptible to compression. The symptoms include numbness, tingling and weakness of the thumb and forefinger, and often quite severe pain at night. Diuretics are not advised; simple analgesia and splinting of the affected hand usually help, although there is no realistic prospect of cure until after delivery. Surgical decompression is very rarely performed in pregnancy.

Oedema

This is common, occurring to some degree in most pregnancies. There is generalized soft-tissue swelling and increased capillary permeability, which allows intravascular fluid to leak into the extravascular compartment. The fingers, toes and ankles are usually worst affected and the symptoms are aggravated by hot weather. Oedema is best dealt with by frequent periods of rest with leg elevation; occasionally, support stockings are indicated. Excessively swollen fingers may necessitate removal of rings and jewellery before they get stuck! It is important to remember that generalized (rather than lower limb) oedema may be a feature of pre-eclampsia, so remember to check the woman's blood pressure and urine for protein. More rarely, severe oedema may suggest underlying cardiac impairment or nephrotic syndrome.

Other common 'minor' disorders

- Itching
- Urinary incontinence
- Nose-bleeds
- Thrush (vaginal candidiasis)
- Headache
- Fainting
- Breast soreness
- Tiredness
- Altered taste sensation
- Insomnia
- Leg cramps
- Striae gravidarum and chloasma

Key Points

'Minor' disorders of pregnancy

The following are most common 'minor' disorders of pregnancy.

- Backache: usually low back, aggravated by movement.
- Heartburn: worst on lying down; better when sitting up.
- Varicose veins and piles: often co-exist, worse if pre-existing.
- Carpal tunnel syndrome: worse at night, may require splint.
- Oedema: worse in hot weather and when walking; better when resting with the feet up.

Problems due to abnormalities of the pelvic organs

Fibroids (leiomyomata)

Fibroids are compact masses of smooth muscle that lie in the cavity of the uterus (submucous), within the uterine muscle (intramural) or on the outside surface of the uterus (subserous). They may enlarge in pregnancy, and in so doing present problems later on in pregnancy or at delivery (Fig. 11.1). A large fibroid at the cervix or in the lower uterine segment may

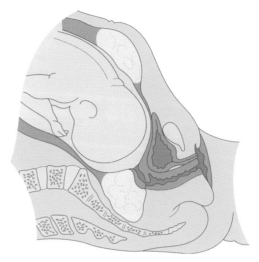

Figure 11.1 Fibroids complicating pregnancy. The tumour in the anterior wall of the uterus has been drawn up out of the pelvis as the lower segment was formed, but the fibroid arising from the cervix remains in the pelvis and will obstruct labour.

prevent descent of the presenting part and obstruct vaginal delivery.

Red degeneration is one of the commonest complications of fibroids in pregnancy. As it grows, the fibroid may become ischaemic, which manifests clinically as acute pain, tenderness over the fibroid and frequent vomiting. If these symptoms are severe, it may precipitate uterine contractions, causing miscarriage or preterm labour. Red fibroid degeneration requires treatment in hospital, with potent analgesics (usually opiates and intravenous fluids). The symptoms usually settle within a few days. The differential diagnosis of red degeneration includes acute appendicitis, pyelonephritis/urinary tract infection, ovarian cyst accident and placental abruption.

A subserous pedunculated fibroid may tort in the same way that a large ovarian cyst can. When this happens, acute abdominal pain and tenderness may make the two difficult to distinguish from one another. In this scenario, a pertinent history followed by ultrasound scan (transvaginal in the first trimester, transabdominal in the second and third) will clinch the diagnosis.

Retroversion of the uterus

Fifteen per cent of women have a retroverted uterus. In pregnancy, the uterus grows and a retroverted uterus will normally 'flip' out of the pelvis and begin to fill the abdominal cavity, as an anteverted uterus would. In a small proportion of cases, the uterus remains in retroversion and eventually fills up the entire pelvic cavity; as it does so, the base of the bladder and the urethra are stretched. Retention of urine may occur, classically at 12–14 weeks, and this is not only very painful but may also cause long-term bladder damage if the bladder becomes over-distended. In this situation, catheterization is essential until the position of the uterus has changed.

Congenital uterine anomalies

The shape of the uterus is embryologically determined by the fusion of the Mullerian ducts. Abnormalities of fusion may give rise to anything from a subseptate uterus through to a bicornuate uterus and even (very rarely) to a double uterus with two cervices. These findings are often discovered incidentally at the time of a pelvic operation such as a laparoscopy, or an ultrasound scan.

The problems associated with bicornuate uterus are:
• miscarriage,
• preterm labour,
• preterm prelabour rupture of membranes (PPROM),
• abnormalities of lie and presentation,
• higher Caesarean section rate.

Ovarian cysts in pregnancy

Ovarian cysts are common in pregnant women; fortunately, the incidence of malignancy is uncommon in women of childbearing age. The most common types of pathological ovarian cyst are serous cysts and benign teratomas. Physiological cysts of the corpus luteum may grow to several centimetres but rarely require treatment, therefore asymptomatic cysts may be followed up by clinical and ultrasound examination, but large cysts (for example dermoids) may require surgery in pregnancy.

Surgery is usually postponed until the late second or early third trimester, when there is the potential that if the baby were delivered, it would be able to survive. The major problems are of large (>8 cm) ovarian cysts in pregnancy, which may undergo torsion, haemorrhage or rupture, causing acute abdominal pain. The resulting pain and inflammation may lead to a miscarriage or preterm labour. Symptomatic cysts, most commonly due to torsion, will require an emergency laparotomy and ovarian cystectomy or even oophorectomy if the cyst is torted. A full assessment must include a family history of ovarian or breast malignancy, tumour markers (although these are of limited value in pregnancy) and detailed ultrasound investigation of both ovaries. Surgery is normally performed through a midline or paramedian incision; a low transverse suprapubic incision would not allow access to the ovary, as it is drawn upwards in later pregnancy.

Cervical cancer

Good pre-conception screening includes ensuring that a mother-to-be is up to date on cervical smears. Cervical abnormalities are much more difficult to deal with in pregnancy, partly because the cervix itself is more difficult to visualize at colposcopy, and also because any biopsy will cause considerable bleeding. Cervical carcinoma may most commonly arises in women with previous abnormal smears or in poor attenders for cervical screening. The disease may be asymptomatic, but a common presenting feature is vaginal bleeding (especially postcoital). Examination may reveal a friable or ulcerated lesion with bleeding and purulent discharge. The terrible prospect of cervical carcinoma in pregnancy leads to complex ethical and moral dilemmas concerning whether the pregnancy must be terminated (depending on the stage it has reached) and Wertheim hysterectomy performed. Cervical cancer is dealt with in greater detail in Chapter 12 of *Gynaecology by ten teachers*, 18th edition.

Urinary tract infection

Urinary tract infections (UTIs) are common in pregnancy. Eight per cent of women have asymptomatic bacteriuria; if this is untreated, it may progress to UTI or even pyelonephritis, with the attendant associations of low birth weight and preterm delivery.

The predisposing factors are:
• history of recurrent cystitis,
• renal tract abnormalities: duplex system, scarred kidneys, ureteric damage and stones,
• diabetes,
• bladder emptying problems, e.g. multiple sclerosis.

The symptoms of UTI may be different in pregnancy; it occasionally presents as low back pain and general malaise with flu-like symptoms. The classic presentation of frequency, dysuria and haematuria is not often seen. On examination, tachycardia, pyrexia, dehydration and loin tenderness may be present. Investigations should include a full blood count and midstream specimen of urine (MSU) sent for urgent microscopy, culture and sensitivities. If there is a strong clinical suspicion of UTI, treatment with antibiotics should start straightaway. The woman should drink plenty of clear fluids and take a simple analgesic such as paracetamol.

The commonest organism for UTI is *Escherichia coli*; less commonly implicated are streptococci, *Proteus*, *Pseudomonas* and *Klebsiella*. If more than 105 organisms are present at culture, this confirms a diagnosis of UTI. The commonly reported 'heavy mixed growth' is often associated with UTI symptoms and may be treated, or the MSU repeated after a week, depending on the clinical scenario. The first-line antibiotic for UTI is amoxycillin or oral cephalosporins.

Pyelonephritis is characterized by dehydration, a very high temperature ($>38.5\,°C$), systemic disturbance and occasionally shock. This requires urgent treatment including intravenous fluids, opiate analgesia and intravenous antibiotics (such as cephalosporins or gentamicin). In addition, renal function should be determined, with at least baseline urea and electrolytes, and the baby must be monitored with cardiotocography (CTG). An ultrasound scan may reveal a growth-restricted baby with oligohydramnios if the course of the infection has been subacute. It is a mistake, however, to deliver the baby without first resuscitating and treating the mother, because an anaesthetic might be dangerous in these circumstances, and fetal condition may improve as a result of treating the mother. The woman may require intensive therapy unit management, including inotropic support and oxygen should overwhelming sepsis occur. In this situation, fetal well-being is a secondary consideration.

Recurrent UTIs in pregnancy require MSU specimens to be sent to the microbiology laboratory at each antenatal visit, and low-dose prophylactic oral antibiotics may be prescribed. Investigation should take place after delivery, unless frank haematuria or other symptoms suggest that an urgent diagnosis is essential. Investigations might include a renal ultrasound scan, renal DMSA function scan, creatinine clearance, intravenous urogram and cystoscopy.

Abdominal pain in pregnancy

Abdominal pain is exceptionally common in pregnancy; the problem is in distinguishing pathological from 'physiological' pains. Most experienced obstetricians will remember women with ill-defined symptoms and signs for whom a diagnosis of acute appendicitis, pyelonephritis or lobar pneumonia was missed for crucial hours or days. This is not to excuse misdiagnosis, but with so many possibilities to exclude, a balance must be struck between over-investigation and complacency.

The causes listed in Table 11.1 are not exhaustive, but cover more than 95 per cent of possible diagnoses.

Table 11.1 – Abdominal pain in pregnancy: causes and clinical assessment

	Specific history	Key investigation
Extrauterine, non-pathological		
Ligament stretching (inguinal/round)		
Rib pain/costochondritis, 'wind'		
Constipation		
Heartburn	Relieved with food	
Extrauterine, pathological		
UTI	Frequency, dysuria, haematuria, hesitancy	MSU, microscopy culture and sensitivities
Pyelonephritis	As above, plus feverish	Blood culture, renal ultrasound

(continued)

Table 11.1 – *(continued)*

	Specific history	Key investigation
Renal stones	As above, but intermittent, spasmodic pains	Urine microscopy (haematuria, precipitated crystals), renal ultrasound, limited IVU
Cholecystitis	Nausea, temperature, vomiting	LFTs, ultrasound upper abdomen
Pancreatitis	Alcoholism, gallstones, autoimmune disease	Serum amylase, abdominal ultrasound, may require CT/MRI
Appendicitis	Often non-specific right-sided pain and tenderness	Temperature, white cell count, abdominal ultrasound
Intestinal obstruction	Bilious vomiting	Urea and electrolytes, abdominal X-ray
HELLP syndrome	Headache, blurred vision, bruising, bleeding gums	BP, urinalysis, LFTs, FBC, clotting, liver ultrasound
Fulminating pre-eclampsia	Headache, visual disturbance, oedema	As for HELLP syndrome
Uterine/fetoplacental		
Preterm labour	Intermittent pains, low backache, show	CTG for uterine activity
Placental abruption	Sudden severe abdominal pain, vaginal bleeding, reduced FM	CTG, FBC, clotting, senior obstetric input immediately
Fibroids (torsion, red degeneration)	Intermittent severe pain, nausea, vomiting	
Ovarian cysts (torsion, rupture)	As above	
Painful Braxton–Hicks contractions		
Medical conditions		
Diabetes	Weight loss, polydipsia, polyuria	Urinalysis (ketones, glucose), serum urea and electrolytes and glucose
Pneumonia (especially lower lobe)	Cough, temperature, chest pain	Examination, chest X-ray
Pulmonary embolus	Short of breath, haemoptysis, inspirational dyspnoea (possibly calf pain)	ECG, chest X-ray, blood gases, then ventilation/perfusion scan, spiral CT or pulmonary angiograph
Sickle-cell crisis	Ill-defined abdominal pain, temperature	Sickle status, % sickle Hb
Malaria	Recent travel in endemic area (within 1 year)	Urinalysis (protein, blood), thick film for parasites

UTI, urinary tract infection; MSU, midstream urine; IVU, intravenous urogram; LFTs, liver function tests; CT, computed tomography; MRI, magnetic resonance imaging; HELLP, haemolysis, elevated liver enzymes and low platelets; BP, blood pressure; FBC, full blood count; CTG, cardiotocography; FM, fetal movement; ECG, electrocardiography; Hb, haemoglobin.

The crucial point to make is that certain conditions are potentially so dangerous or debilitating (pneumonia, pulmonary embolus, renal stones, intestinal obstruction, pancreatitis) that obstetricians may have to perform X-rays and arrange invasive assessments to make a diagnosis. To avoid this, and risk not making an early diagnosis, means that women may not be treated appropriately for possibly very serious conditions.

Venous thromboembolism

Pulmonary embolus (PE) is the major cause of direct maternal death in the UK, and is responsible for approximately 11 fatalities per year. Pregnancy is a hypercoagulable state because of an alteration in the thrombotic and fibrinolytic systems. There is an increase in clotting factors VIII, IX, X and fibrinogen levels, and a reduction in protein S and anti-thrombin (AT) III concentrations. The net result of these changes is possibly nature's way of reducing the likelihood of haemorrhage following delivery.

These physiological changes predispose a woman to thromboembolism (the obstruction of a blood vessel by a blood clot), and any underlying preponderance to thrombosis may be unmasked in pregnancy. High levels of circulating oestrogen are associated with changes in clotting factors; the situation is in some ways analogous to that of women developing a deep vein thrombosis (DVT) while using the oral contraceptive pill. The additional factor that makes pregnancy a particular risk is venous stasis in the lower limbs due to the weight of the gravid uterus placing pressure on the inferior vena cava; this is compounded by immobility.

Pregnancy itself increases the risk of DVT by five times and Caesarean section by ten times. The risk of DVT after Caesarean section is probably around 1 per cent.

Risk factors for thromboembolic disease

Pre-existing
- Maternal age (>35 years)
- Thrombophilia
- Obesity (>80 kg)
- Previous thromboembolism
- Severe varicose veins
- Smoking
- Malignancy

Specific to pregnancy
- Multiple gestation
- Pre-eclampsia
- Grand multiparity
- Caesarean section, especially if emergency
- Damage to the pelvic veins
- Sepsis
- Prolonged bed rest

Thrombophilia

Some women are predisposed to thrombosis through changes in the coagulation/fibrinolytic system that may be inherited or acquired. Inherited thrombophilias include protein C, protein S and AT III deficiency. New thrombophilias are now being discovered at an alarming rate. One of the most common of these is resistance to activated protein C (APCR) caused by the Leiden mutation in the factor V gene. The incidence of this and other thrombophilias varies widely depending on ethnicity. For instance, APCR is commonest in Scandinavian countries but is present in less than 5 per cent of other European populations.

Acquired thrombophilia is most commonly associated with antiphospholipid syndrome (APS). APS is the combination of lupus anticoagulant with or without anti-cardiolipin antibodies, with a history of recurrent miscarriage and/or thrombosis. It may (or, more commonly, may not) be associated with other autoantibody disorders such as systemic lupus erythematosus (SLE).

It is crucial that women with a history of thrombotic events are screened for thrombophilia, even if this is first done in pregnancy (when protein S and AT III levels fall physiologically anyway and may complicate result interpretation). The presence of thrombophilia, with a history of thrombotic episode(s), means that prophylaxis should be considered for pregnancy.

Deep vein thrombosis

The commonest symptoms are pain in the calf with varying degrees of redness or swelling. Women's legs are often swollen during pregnancy; therefore unilateral symptoms should ring alarm bells. The signs are few, except that often the calf is tender to gentle touch. It is mandatory to ask about symptoms of PE (see later), as a woman with PE might present initially with a DVT. In any woman with suspicion of DVT, heparin or a low-molecular-weight heparin should be given in treatment doses until the diagnosis is confirmed or refuted. A firm diagnosis by one of the methods below is mandatory.

The two methods of diagnosing a DVT are venography and Doppler ultrasound. Venography is invasive, requiring the injection of contrast medium and the use of X-rays. It does, however, allow excellent visualization of veins both below and above the knee.

Colour Doppler ultrasound is now the preferred first-line method of investigating suspected DVT. It is widely available and allows non-invasive assessment of the deep veins between the knee and the iliac veins. Calf veins are often poorly visualized; however, it is known that a thrombus confined purely to the calf veins with no extension is very unlikely to give rise to a PE. The main advantage of colour Doppler is in allowing a dynamic assessment of the femoral and iliac veins.

Pulmonary embolus

It is crucial to recognize PE, as missing the diagnosis could have fatal implications. The classic presentation of inspiratory chest pain and breathlessness, with a pleural 'rub', hypoxia and S1QT3 changes on electrocardiograph (ECG) is rarely seen. The most common presentation is of mild breathlessness, or inspiratory chest pain, in a woman who is not cyanosed but may be slightly tachycardic (>90 bpm) with a mild pyrexia (37.5 °C). Rarely, massive PE may present with sudden cardiorespiratory collapse (see Chapter 19, p. 282).

Clinical suspicion, together with risk factors for PE, makes immediate full anticoagulation and confirmation of the diagnosis (preferably within 24 hours) not merely advisable, but essential. Ventilation/perfusion imaging can be safely performed in pregnancy, as the radiation to the fetus is minimal.

D-dimer is now commonly used as a screening test for thromboembolic disease in non-pregnant women, in whom it has a high negative predictive value. Outwith pregnancy, a low level of D-dimer suggests the absence of a DVT or PE, and no further objective tests are necessary, while an increased level of D-dimer suggests that thrombosis may be present and an objective diagnostic test for DVT and/or PE should be performed. In pregnancy, however, D-dimer can be elevated due to the physiological changes in the coagulation system, limiting its clinical usefulness as a screening test in this situation.

Anticoagulants

Heparin prolongs the activated partial thromboplastin time (APTT) – otherwise known as the kaolin cephalin time (KCT). The activity of low-molecular-weight

> ### Initial management of a non-moribund woman with suspected pulmonary embolism
>
> *History* (ask about risk factors)
> - Examine: pulse, blood pressure, temperature; examine calves, percuss and auscultate lung fields.
> - Investigate: arterial blood gases, chest X-ray, ECG, oxygen saturation monitor, baseline coagulation screen and blood count.
> - Don't forget to ask about the pregnancy and monitor the fetus (pre-eclampsia or chorioamnionitis might predispose to a PE).
>
> *If a pulmonary embolism is suspected*
> - Give oxygen.
> - Heparinize immediately (full anticoagulant dosage i.v.: 36 000 iu/24 h with a bolus dose).
> - Call for senior help (anaesthetic/medical/ cardiothoracic).
> - Definitive diagnosis: ventilation/perfusion scan or pulmonary angiography.
> - Further management: life-threatening PE may warrant thrombolytic drugs or surgery; this is rarely the case, however.

heparin derivatives is assessed by factor X assay. Both are given intramuscularly or intravenously. They do not cross the placenta, are not teratogenic and the effect can be stopped within hours by withholding further doses. They are regarded as relatively safe; maternal thrombocytopenia is a rare idiosyncratic reaction and osteoporosis is a risk if treatment is prolonged (>6 months).

Warfarin is given orally and prolongs the prothrombin time (PT). It crosses the placenta and can cause limb and facial defects in the first trimester, and fetal intracerebral haemorrhage in the second and third trimesters. Its use is largely confined to women at highest risk of thromboembolism requiring full anticoagulation; if it is used, exposure should be limited to the second and third trimesters.

Prophylaxis and treatment issues

These are controversial and the examples below are given as a guide.
- Women with risk factors for DVT (e.g. a woman aged 43, weighing 105 kg) should receive subcutaneous heparin prophylaxis and wear

Table 11.2 – Risk assessment at Caesarean section and recommendations for prophylaxis

Low risk	Medium risk	High risk
Elective Caesarean section	Age >35 years	Three or more moderate risk factors
Uncomplicated pregnancy	Weight >80 kg	Extended surgery, e.g. Caesarean
No other risk factors	Para 4 or more	section, hysterectomy
	Gross varicose veins	A personal history of deep venous
	Current infection	thrombosis, pulmonary embolism,
	Pre-eclampsia	thrombophilia
	Immobility prior to	Family history of deep venous
	surgery >4 days	thrombosis, pulmonary embolism,
	Major current illness	thrombophilia
	Emergency Caesarean section	Antiphospholipid antibody
	in labour	
Thromboprophylaxis		
Early mobilization and	Subcutaneous heparin or	Heparin and leg stockings
hydration	stockings	

Continue prophylaxis to the fifth postoperative day. May also use pneumatic or anti-thromboembolism boots.

elasticated stockings if admitted to hospital or undergoing a surgical procedure such as Caesarean section.

- Those with a previous history of thromboembolism in pregnancy or whilst taking the combined oral contraceptive pill may require prophylactic subcutaneous heparin throughout the pregnancy.
- Some women require full anticoagulation throughout pregnancy, e.g. those with artificial heart valves, women having had a PE in their current pregnancy and women with APS having had recurrent DVTs.

The Royal College of Obstetricians and Gynaecologists (RCOG) has issued a recommendation with respect to thromboembolism and Caesarean section (Table 11.2).

Antepartum haemorrhage

This is defined as vaginal bleeding from 24 weeks to delivery of the baby. The causes are placental or local. Placental causes are obviously the most worrying, as potentially the mother's and/or fetus' life is in danger. These include placental abruption, placenta praevia and vasa praevia. Local causes include cervicitis,

cervical 'erosion', cervical carcinoma, vaginal trauma or vaginal infection.

Antepartum haemorrhage must always be taken seriously, and any woman presenting with a history of fresh vaginal bleeding must be investigated promptly and properly. The key question is whether the bleeding is placental, and is compromising the mother and/or fetus, or whether it has a less significant cause. Normally, it will be obvious from looking at the woman whether the situation is in extremis or not. A pale, tachycardic woman looking anxious with a painful, firm abdomen, underwear soaked in fresh blood and reduced fetal movements needs emergency assessment and management for a possible placental abruption (see Chapter 19). A woman having had a small postcoital bleed with no systemic signs or symptoms represents a different end of the spectrum.

History

- How much bleeding?
- Triggering factors (e.g. postcoital bleed).
- Associated with pain or contractions?
- Is the baby moving?
- Last cervical smear (date/normal or abnormal)?

Examination

- Pulse, blood pressure.
- Is the uterus soft or tender and firm?
- Fetal heart auscultation/CTG.
- Speculum vaginal examination, with particular importance placed on visualizing the cervix (having established that placenta is not a praevia, preferably using a portable ultrasound machine).

Investigations

- Depending on the degree of bleeding, full blood count, clotting and, if suspected praevia/abruption, cross-match 6 units of blood.
- Ultrasound (fetal size, presentation, amniotic fluid, placental position and morphology).

Placental abruption

The premature separation of the placenta is termed abruption. The bleeding is maternal and/or fetal and abruption is acutely dangerous for both the mother and fetus (Figs 11.2 and 11.3; see Chapters 13 and 19).

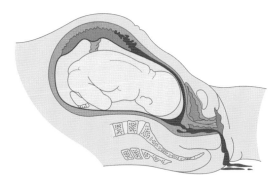

Figure 11.2 Placental abruption with revealed haemorrhage.

Placenta praevia

A placenta covering or encroaching on the cervical os may be associated with bleeding, either provoked or spontaneous. The bleeding is from the maternal not fetal circulation and is more likely to compromise the mother than the fetus (Fig. 11.4).

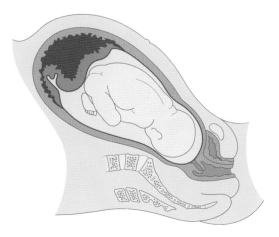

Figure 11.3 Placental abruption with concealed haemorrhage.

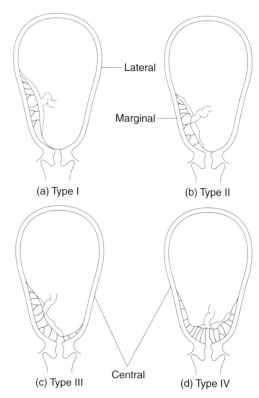

(a) Type I   (b) Type II

(c) Type III   Central   (d) Type IV

Lateral

Marginal

Figure 11.4 Classification of degrees of placenta praevia. a = lateral; b = marginal; c and d = central.

Risk factors for placenta praevia

- Multiple gestation
- Previous Caesarean section
- Uterine structural anomaly
- Assisted conception

Key Points

- Placenta praevia is most dangerous for the mother.
- Placental abruption is more dangerous for the fetus than the mother.

Further management

If there is minimal bleeding and the cause is clearly local vaginal bleeding, symptomatic management may be given (for example antifungal preparations for candidiasis), as long as there is reasonable certainty that cervical carcinoma is excluded by smear history and direct visualization of the cervix. Placental causes of bleeding are a major concern. A large-gauge intravenous cannula is sited, blood sent for full blood count, clotting and cross-match, and appropriate fetal and maternal monitoring instituted. If there is major fetal or maternal compromise, decisions may have to be made about immediate delivery irrespective of gestation; an attempt at maternal steroid injection should still be made. If this is the situation, and bleeding is continuing, emergency management is required (see Chapter 19). If bleeding settles, the woman must be admitted for 48 hours, as the risk of re-bleeding is high within this time frame. Rhesus status is important: if the mother is rhesus negative, send a Kleihauer test (to determine whether any, or how much, fetal blood has leaked into the maternal circulation) and administer anti-D.

Substance abuse in pregnancy

Drug dependence

Addiction to hard drugs is unfortunately becoming more common throughout the Western world. It is crucial to have a high index of suspicion about drug abuse if there are subtle or not so subtle signs. The picture of an 'addict' depends upon her degree of compensation and ability to adapt and may range from the very top to the lowest socio-economic groups. The classic dishevelled, thin, malnourished woman with venous access scars visible up her arm represents the very severest end of the spectrum.

Problems frequently encountered amongst drug addicts

- Social problems: housing, crime, other children in care or abused.
- Co-existent addictions: alcohol and smoking.
- Malnutrition: especially iron, vitamins B and C.
- Risk of viral infections, e.g. human immunodeficiency virus (HIV) or hepatitis B.
- Fetal and neonatal risks (Table 11.3).

Management becomes more complex once drug addiction is identified. The aims of management are to stabilize the mother's drug-taking habits and ensure contact with social/care workers and psychiatric/drug

Table 11.3 – Effects of some drugs of abuse on the fetus and neonate

	Fetal effects	Neonatal effects
Opiates	Preterm labour	Neonatal withdrawal syndrome
	Small for gestational age	Higher risk of sudden infant
	Anaemia	death syndrome
	Multiple gestation	Higher perinatal mortality
Cocaine and derivatives	Placental abruption	Increased cerebral infarction risk
	Preterm delivery	
	Small for gestational age	
Cannabis	Preterm delivery	
	Theoretical risk of chromosome damage	

liaison services as appropriate. It is important not to try to reduce the opiate dose too rapidly in pregnancy, as this can easily precipitate acute withdrawal in both the mother and fetus; the principle is to administer the lowest effective dose of methadone liquid in three divided doses every day.

Screening for infections such as hepatitis B and human immunodeficiency virus (HIV) is routinely offered in the UK. In many cases, multi-disciplinary case conferences should be held to make arrangements and decisions for when the baby is delivered.

Alcohol

There is much debate about what a 'safe' dose of alcohol is during pregnancy. What is likely is that an intake of <100 g per week (approximately two drinks per day, e.g. two medium glasses of wine or one pint of beer) is not associated with any adverse effects. Doses greater than this have been related to intrauterine growth restriction (IUGR). Massive doses, in excess of 2 g/kg of body weight (17 drinks per day), have been associated with fetal alcohol syndrome. However, the syndrome is not seen consistently in infants born to women who are heavy consumers of alcohol, and occurs only in approximately 30–33 per cent of children born to women who drink about 2 g/kg of body weight per day (equivalent to approximately 18 units of alcoholic drink per day). The differing susceptibility of fetuses to the syndrome is thought to be multifactorial and reflects the interplay of genetic factors, social deprivation, nutritional deficiencies, tobacco and other drug abuse, along with alcohol consumption.

If alcohol abuse is suspected, it may be necessary to involve social workers and arrange for formal psychiatric/addiction assessment. It is extremely difficult to 'test' for alcohol abuse, as even markers such as mean corpuscular volume and gamma GT are not reliable in pregnancy. Malnutrition is very likely in heavy alcohol abuse and requires (in addition to a change in basic diet) B vitamin supplements and iron; the problem is that the majority of such patients not only do not take their medicines but also default antenatal appointments.

Smoking and pregnancy

Smoking is not advisable in pregnancy. Although smokers have a lower incidence of pre-eclampsia than non-smokers, overall perinatal mortality is increased, babies are smaller at delivery, there is a higher risk of antepartum haemorrhage and there is some evidence of a link between antenatal maternal smoking and later development of leukaemia in childhood. It is estimated that a baby will weigh less than its target weight by a multiple of 15 g times the average number of cigarettes a woman smokes per day; smoking fewer than five cigarettes per day has a barely discernible obstetric effect. Smoking acutely reduces placental perfusion; this probably contributes to the IUGR. Consequently, all women should be counselled regarding smoking cessation at their booking visit.

Oligohydramnios and polyhydramnios

Amniotic fluid is produced almost exclusively from fetal urine from the second trimester onwards. It serves a vital function in protecting the developing baby from pressure or trauma, allowing limb movement, hence normal postural development, and permitting the fetal lungs to expand and develop through breathing.

Oligohydramnios

Too little amniotic fluid (oligohydramnios) is commonly defined as amniotic fluid index <5th centile for gestation. The amniotic fluid index (AFI) is an ultrasound estimation of amniotic fluid derived by adding together the deepest vertical pool in four quadrants of the abdomen. The AFI (in cm) is therefore associated with some degree of error. In general, however, it is possible to differentiate subjectively on ultrasound between 'too much', 'too little' and 'normal looking'.

Oligohydramnios may be suspected antenatally following a history of clear fluid leaking from the vagina; this may represent preterm prelabour rupture of the membranes (PPROM, see Chapter 14, p. 174). Clinically, on abdominal palpation, the fetal poles may be very obviously felt and 'hard', with a small for dates uterus. The possible causes of oligohydramnios and anhydramnios (no amniotic fluid) are described in the box.

The fetal prognosis depends on the cause of oligohydramnios, but both pulmonary hypoplasia and limb deformities (contractures, talipes) are common to severe early-onset (<24 weeks) oligohydramnnios.

Renal agenesis and bilateral multicystic kidneys carry a lethal prognosis, as life after birth is impossible without functioning kidneys. In this situation, the fetal lungs would probably be hypoplastic; this may also be true of severe urinary tract obstruction. Oligohydramnios due to IUGR/uteroplacental insufficiency is usually of a less severe degree and less commonly causes limb and lung problems.

Possible causes of oligohydramnios and anhydramnios	
Too little production	**Diagnosed by**
Renal agenesis	Ultrasound: no renal tissue, no bladder
Multicystic kidneys	Ultrasound: enlarged kidneys with multiple cysts, no visible bladder
Urinary tract abnormality/obstruction	Ultrasound: kidneys may be present, but urinary tract dilatation
IUGR and placental insufficiency	Clinical: reduced SFH, reduced fetal movements, possibly abnormal CTG Ultrasound: IUGR, abnormal fetal Dopplers
Maternal drugs (NSAIDs)	Withholding NSAIDs may allow amniotic fluid to re-accumulate
Post-dates pregnancy	
Leakage	**Diagnosed by**
PPROM	Speculum examination: pool of amniotic fluid on posterior blade
(SFH, symphysis–fundal height; NSAIDs, non-steroidal anti-inflammatory drugs.)	

Polyhydramnios

Polyhydramnios is the term given to an excess of amniotic fluid, i.e. AFI >95th centile for gestation on ultrasound estimation. It may present as severe abdominal swelling and discomfort. On examination, the abdomen will appear distended out of proportion to the woman's gestation (increased SFH). Furthermore, the abdomen may be tense and tender and the fetal poles will be hard to palpate. The condition may be caused by maternal, placental or fetal conditions.

Maternal
- Diabetes.

Placental
- Chorioangioma
- Arterio-venous fistula.

Fetal
- Multiple gestation (in monochorionic twins it may be twin-to-twin transfusion syndrome)
- Idiopathic
- Oesophageal atresia/tracheo-oesophageal fistula
- Duodenal atresia
- Neuromuscular fetal condition (preventing swallowing)
- Anencephaly.

The management of polyhydramnios is directed towards establishing the cause (hence determining fetal prognosis), relieving the discomfort of the mother (if necessary by amniodrainage), and assessing the risk of preterm labour due to uterine over-distension. The last-mentioned may require assessment of cervical length by ultrasound. If prior to 24 weeks following amniotic fluid drainage the cervical length is less than 25 mm, consideration might be given to cervical suture insertion.

Polyhydramnios due to maternal diabetes needs urgent investigation, as it often suggests high maternal blood glucose levels. In this context, polyhydramnios should correct itself when the mother's glycaemic control is optimized.

Twin-to-twin transfusion syndrome is a rare cause of acute polyhydramnios in the recipient sac of monochorionic twins. It is associated with oligohydramnios and a small baby in the other sac. The condition may be rapidly fatal for both twins; amniodrainage and removal by laser of the placental vascular connections are two therapeutic modalities employed in dealing with this condition. This is further discussed in Chapter 12.

Breech presentation, oblique and transverse lie at term

Breech presentation occurs in 40 per cent of babies at 26 weeks, 20 per cent at 30 weeks and 3 per cent at term. Similarly, oblique and transverse positions are not uncommon antenatally. They only become a problem if the baby (or first presenting baby in a multiple gestation) is not cephalic by 37 weeks. There are three types of breech: the commonest is extended (frank) breech (Fig. 11.5); less common is a flexed (complete) breech (Fig. 11.6); and least common is footling breech, in which a foot presents at the cervix. Cord and foot prolapse are risks in this situation.

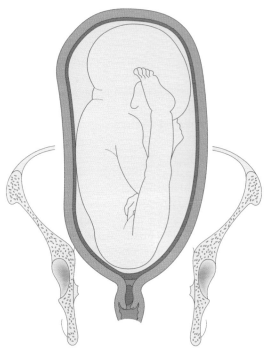

Figure 11.5 Frank breech (also known as extended breech) presentation with extension of the legs.

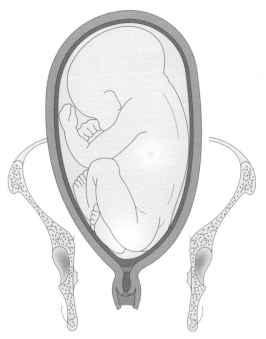

Figure 11.6 Breech presentation with flexion of the legs.

Predisposing factors for abnormal lie or breech presentation

Uterine
- Fibroids
- Congenital abnormalities, e.g. susceptible uterus
- Uterine surgery
- Oligohydramnios
- Polyhydramnios

Fetal
- Multiple gestation
- Abnormality, e.g. anencephaly or hydrocephalus
- Neuromuscular condition

Abnormal presentation or unstable lie at term

Any woman presenting at term with a transverse or oblique lie is at potential risk of cord prolapse following spontaneous rupture of the membranes, and prolapse of the hand, shoulder or foot once in labour. In most cases, the woman is multiparous with a lax uterus and abdominal wall musculature, and gentle version of the baby's head in the clinic or on the ward will restore the presentation to cephalic. If this does not occur, or the lie is unstable (alternating between transverse, oblique and longitudinal), it is important to think of possible uterine or fetal causes of this (see box, as for breech presentation).

The diagnosis of transverse or oblique lie might be suspected by abdominal inspection: the abdomen often appears asymmetrical. The SFH may be less than expected, and on palpation the fetal head or buttocks may be in the iliac fossa. Palpation over the pelvic brim will reveal an 'empty' pelvis.

It goes without saying that a woman in labour with the baby's lie anything other than longitudinal will not be able to deliver vaginally; this is one situation in which if Caesarean section is not performed both the mother and baby are at considerable risk of morbidity and mortality. The only exception to this is for exceptionally preterm or small babies, where vaginal delivery may occur irrespective of lie or presentation.

A woman with an unstable lie at term should be admitted to the antenatal ward. The normal plan would be to deliver by Caesarean section if the presentation is not cephalic in early labour or if spontaneous rupture of the membranes occurs. In a multiparous woman, an unstable lie will often correct itself in early labour (as long as the membranes are intact).

Assessment of a woman with a breech baby

Until recently, there were no reliable data concerning the perinatal mortality associated with breech versus cephalic delivery at term. Most obstetricians suspected that vaginal delivery was probably safer for the mother and less safe for the baby, and vice versa for Caesarean section. A recent large multi-centre trial confirmed that planned vaginal delivery of a breech presentation is associated with a 3 per cent increased risk of death or serious morbidity to the baby. Although this trial did not evaluate long-term outcomes for child or mother, it has led to the recommendation that *the best method of delivering a term breech singleton is by planned Caesarean section.* Despite this, either by choice (the factors which increase/decrease the likelihood of a successful vaginal delivery are detailed below) or as a result of precipitous labour, a small proportion of women with breech presentations will deliver vaginally. It therefore remains important that clinicians and hospitals are prepared for vaginal breech delivery. This is described in detail in Chapter 18.

Factors that strengthen recommendations for a Caesarean section

- Large or small baby (ultrasound estimated weight >3.5 or <2.5 kg)
- Small pelvis on pelvimetry or very flat sacrum
- Primigravid
- Previous Caesarean section
- Extended neck

Factors that increase the likelihood of a successful vaginal breech delivery

- Normal-size baby (2.5–3.5 kg)
- Good pelvimetry
- Flexed neck
- Multiparous
- Breech deeply engaged
- Positive mental attitude of woman and partner
- Obstetric unit with staff familiar with breech delivery

External cephalic version

The most common situation arises when a woman with an otherwise uncomplicated pregnancy presents in the antenatal clinic at 36 weeks' gestation with a breech baby. If there are no contraindications (see box below), an external cephalic version (ECV) may be performed at 36–37 weeks. ECV is a relatively straightforward and safe technique and has been shown to reduce the number of Caesarean sections due to breech presentations.

Contraindications to ECV

- Placenta praevia
- Oligohydramnios or polyhydramnios
- History of antepartum haemorrhage
- Previous Caesarean or myomectomy scar on the uterus
- Multiple gestation
- Pre-eclampsia or hypertension
- Plan to deliver by Caesarean section anyway

The procedure is mildly uncomfortable, and is usually carried out by a senior obstetrician at or near delivery facilities. The woman lies comfortably and, under ultrasound guidance, the baby is gently manipulated into the cephalic position. The technique is easier to perform in multiparous women where the uterus is already relatively lax. Alternatively, it can be performed following the administration of tocolytics such as nifedipine. ECV is much more difficult in women who are overweight or have fibroids, and deep engagement of the breech makes any manipulation more difficult. A fetal heart rate trace must be performed before and after the procedure. If the procedure fails, or becomes difficult, it is abandoned. Approximately two-thirds of babies can be turned to cephalic using this method (Fig. 11.7).

Risks of ECV

- Placental abruption
- Premature rupture of the membranes
- Cord accident
- Transplacental haemorrhage (remember anti-D administration to rhesus-negative women)
- Fetal bradycardia

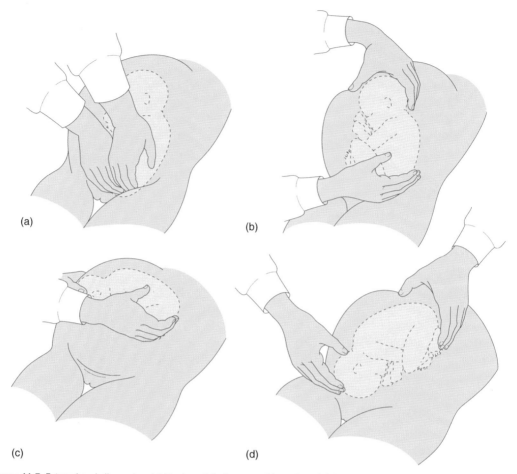

(a)

(b)

(c)

(d)

Figures 11.7 External cephalic version. (a) The breech is disengaged from the pelvic inlet. (b) Version is usually performed in the direction that increases flexion of the fetus and makes it do a forward somersault. (c) On completion of version, the head is often not engaged for a time. (d) The fetal heart rate should be checked after the external version has been completed.

⚷ Key Points

Breech presentation

- ECV should be offered at 36–37 weeks in selected women.
- Elective Caesarean section is safer than vaginal delivery for a baby presenting by the breech at or close to term.
- Planned or unexpected vaginal breech deliveries should be attended by experienced clinicians.

Post-term pregnancy

Term, by definition, is 37–42 weeks' gestation. A very small proportion (<5 per cent) of pregnancies would proceed beyond 42 weeks if left alone. It should be said at the outset that the definition of post-term pregnancy for a woman depends on her accurate dates, and preferably a first-trimester ultrasound estimation of crown–rump length.

Post-term pregnancy is a problem because at this gestation the baby is at its maximum size, and the placenta is becoming more calcified, less efficient and more prone to failure. There are no known tests that can predict fetal outcome post-term; an ultrasound scan may give temporary reassurance if the amniotic fluid and fetal growth are normal. Similarly, a CTG should be performed at and after 42 weeks. Some women wish to wait for their labour to start naturally, and in these cases it is usually reasonable to wait a day or two over 42 weeks as long as appropriate surveillance is carried out and the woman is aware of the increased risk of stillbirth or neonatal death.

Immediate induction of labour or delivery post-dates should take place if:

- there is reduced amniotic fluid on scan,
- fetal growth is reduced,
- there are reduced fetal movements,
- the CTG is not perfect,
- the mother is hypertensive or suffers a significant medical condition.

Induction of labour is discussed further in Chapter 17.

When counselling the parents regarding waiting for labour to start naturally after 42 weeks, it is important that the woman is aware that no test can guarantee the safety of her baby, and that perinatal mortality is increased (at least two-fold) beyond 42 weeks. A labour induced post-term is more likely to require Caesarean section; this may partly be due to the reluctance of the uterus to contract properly, and the possible compromise of the baby leading to abnormal CTG.

Rhesus iso-immunization

Blood group is defined in two ways. First, there is the ABO group, allowing four different permutations of blood group (O, A, B, AB). Second, there is the rhesus system, which consists of C, D and E antigens. The importance of these blood group systems is that a mismatch between the fetus and mother can mean that when fetal red cells pass across to the maternal circulation, as they do to a greater or lesser extent during pregnancy, sensitization of the maternal immune system to these fetal 'foreign' red blood cells may occur.

ABO blood group iso-immunization may occur when the mother is blood group O and the baby is blood group A or B. Anti-A and anti-B antibodies are present in the maternal circulation naturally, and hence do not require prior sensitization in order to be produced. This means that ABO incompatibility may occur in a first pregnancy. In this situation, anti-A or anti-B antibodies may pass to the fetal circulation, causing fetal haemolysis and anaemia. ABO incompatibility causes mild haemolytic disease of the baby, but may sometimes explain unexpected jaundice in an otherwise healthy term infant.

The rhesus system is more commonly associated with severe haemolytic disease. Of all the antibodies (C, D and E), the D antigen is associated most commonly with severe haemolytic fetal disease; however, this can only occur if the mother is D rhesus negative and the baby is D rhesus positive. Both anti-C and anti-E antibodies may also be associated with haemolytic disease requiring intrauterine fetal blood transfusion, but are much less commonly implicated.

Rare antibodies such as those listed below may unusually be associated with haemolytic disease.

The aetiology of rhesus disease

Rhesus disease does not affect a first pregnancy. The mother must have had exposure to D rhesus-positive fetal cells in a previous pregnancy and then developed an immune response that has lain dormant until a following pregnancy of a D rhesus-positive baby. In the subsequent pregnancy, when maternal re-sensitization occurs (rhesus-positive red cells pass from the baby to the maternal circulation; Fig. 11.8), IgG antibodies cross from the mother to the fetal circulation. If these antibodies are present in sufficient quantities, fetal haemolysis may occur, leading to such severe anaemia that the fetus may die unless a transfusion is performed. It is for this reason that rhesus-negative women have frequent antibody checks in pregnancy; an increasing titre of atypical antibodies may suggest an impending problem. It is important to note, however, that although the amount of D antibodies must be over a certain threshold limit (see below), absolute measure of the antibodies does not correlate well with the degree of fetal anaemia. It is for this reason that invasive and non-invasive assessments of the fetus are indicated in risk situations to determine whether the fetus is becoming anaemic.

Potential sensitizing events for rhesus disease

- Miscarriage
- Termination of pregnancy
- Antepartum haemorrhage
- Invasive prenatal testing (chorion villus sampling, amniocentesis and cordocentesis)
- Delivery

However, the other two rhesus antigens (C and E) may also be associated with haemolytic disease of the fetus or neonate; these are inherited in exactly the same way as D.

The problem of iso-immunization occurs when fetal cells have caused a maternal antibody response,

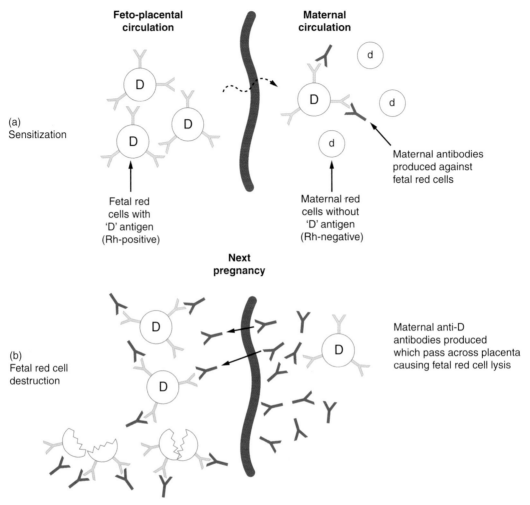

Figure 11.8 The mechanism of rhesus sensitization (a) and fetal red cell destruction (b).

and IgG antibodies are produced which cross the placenta and destroy fetal red cells, leading to fetal anaemia. Once a mother is sensitized to a fetal red cell antigen, the sensitization cannot be lost and the response will magnify with successive exposure, for instance in subsequent pregnancies.

The genetics of rhesus disease (Fig. 11.9)

- Rhesus-negative mother, rhesus-negative father (homozygote).
- Rhesus-negative mother, rhesus-positive father (heterozygote).
- Rhesus-negative mother, rhesus-positive father (homozygote).

Antibodies associated with haemolytic disease

- ABO
- Rhesus (C, D, E)
- Kell
- Duffy
- c (known as 'little c')
- S

Prevalence of rhesus disease

The prevalence of D rhesus negativity is 15 per cent in the Caucasian population, but lower in all other ethnic

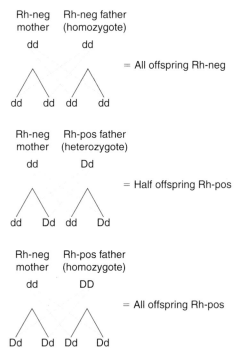

Rh-neg mother dd   Rh-neg father (homozygote) dd

= All offspring Rh-neg

dd   dd   dd   dd

Rh-neg mother dd   Rh-pos father (heterozygote) Dd

= Half offspring Rh-pos

dd   Dd   dd   Dd

Rh-neg mother dd   Rh-pos father (homozygote) DD

= All offspring Rh-pos

Dd   Dd   Dd   Dd

Figure 11.9 Parental genotype determinants of rhesus group.

groups. It is very uncommon in Orientals. Rhesus disease is commonest in countries where anti-D prophylaxis is not widespread, such as the Middle East and Russia.

Preventing rhesus iso-immunization

The process of iso-immunization can be 'nipped in the bud' by the intramuscular administration of anti-D immunoglobulins to a mother, preferably within 72 hours of exposure to fetal red cells. Anti-D immunoglobulins 'mop up' any circulating rhesus-positive cells before an immune response is excited in the mother. The practical implications of this are that anti-D immunoglobulin must be given intramuscularly as soon as possible after any potentially sensitizing event (see p. 141). It is normal practice to administer anti-D after any of these events; the exact dose is determined by the gestation at which sensitization has occurred and the size of the feto-maternal haemorrhage.

In the first trimester of pregnancy, because the volume of fetal blood is so small, it is unlikely that sensitization would occur, and a 'standard' dose of anti-D (the exact dose varies from country to country) is given;

this will more than cover even the largest feto-maternal transfusion. In the second and third trimesters, fetal blood volume is greater and because there is a possibility of a feto-maternal transfusion of several millilitres, a larger dose is given and a Kleihauer test performed. A Kleihauer is a test of maternal blood to determine the proportion of fetal cells present (relying on their ability to resist denaturation by alcohol or acid); it will allow calculation of the amount of extra anti-D immunoglobulin required should a large transfusion have occurred.

In many countries, rhesus-negative women are given anti-D at 28 and/or 34 weeks routinely. This is based on the finding that a small number of rhesus-negative women become sensitized during pregnancy despite the administration of anti-D at delivery and without a clinically obvious sensitizing event. The likelihood is that a small feto-maternal haemorrhage occurs without any obvious clinical signs; therefore, prophylactic anti-D would reduce the risk of iso-immunization from this event.

Signs of fetal anaemia

Note: clinical and ultrasound features of fetal anaemia do not usually become evident unless fetal haemoglobin is >5 g/dL less than the mean for gestation. Usually, features are not obvious unless the fetal haemoglobin is <6 g/dL.

- Polyhydramnios.
- Enlarged fetal heart.
- Ascites and pericardial effusions.
- Hyperdynamic fetal circulation (can be detected by Doppler ultrasound by measuring increased velocities in the middle cerebral artery or aorta).
- Reduced fetal movements.
- Abnormal CTG with reduced variability, eventually a 'sinusoidal' trace.

The spectrum of rhesus disease

(Mildest) …
- Normal delivery at term; mild jaundice requiring phototherapy.
- Preterm delivery of an anaemic fetus requiring exchange transfusion.
- Delivery of a fetus at 34 weeks following fortnightly blood transfusions from 26 weeks' gestation.

- Stillbirth or neonatal death due to rhesus (earlier gestation = worse prognosis).
… (Severest).

The management of rhesus disease

This depends on the clinical scenario.
- The woman is D rhesus negative, as is her partner. In this situation, there is no risk that the baby will be D rhesus positive (assuming that the woman's partner is the father of the baby). There is therefore no chance of rhesus disease.
- The woman is D rhesus negative and her partner is rhesus positive. She has no (or a very low titre of) D rhesus antibodies and it is either her first pregnancy or she has not had a pregnancy previously affected by D rhesus disease. Monitor atypical antibody levels at booking, 24 and 36 weeks. An increase in antibody titre to >10 iu/mL requires review in a fetal medicine centre so that early signs of fetal anaemia can be detected by ultrasound and, if appropriate, invasive assessment performed.
- The woman is D rhesus negative and she has been sensitized to the D rhesus antigen, manifesting itself in an adverse pregnancy outcome. Once a woman is sensitized to the D rhesus antigen, no amount of anti-D will ever turn back the clock. In this situation, there is therefore no role whatsoever for anti-D. Depending on her history (see 'The spectrum of rhesus disease', above), close surveillance is necessary. Begin by monitoring atypical antibodies every 2–4 weeks from booking. If the antibodies are at a low level (<10–15 iu/mL), the baby is unlikely to become infected. If the antibodies rise by <15 iu/mL, and/or there are features of fetal anaemia, a fetal medicine opinion must be sought urgently, as the baby may be very anaemic.

If a previous pregnancy resulted in a stillbirth or neonatal death, fetal blood sampling by cordocentesis may be performed at 10 weeks, before the onset of previous clinical disease. For example, if in a previous pregnancy a stillbirth occurred at 34 weeks due to previously unrecognized rhesus disease, in the next pregnancy fetal blood sampling should be performed from 24 weeks for estimation of fetal haemoglobin and possible intrauterine transfusion of blood into the umbilical vein. In some units, the bilirubin concentration of amniotic fluid is determined optically to give an indirect measure of fetal haemolysis; this avoids the risks to the baby from cordocentesis should the baby not require transfusion. The most severely affected fetuses may require repeat transfusions every 7–10 days; after 34 weeks, the risks of cordocentesis (fetal bradycardia, cord tamponade or haemorrhage, fetal death; see Chapter 9) outweigh the risks of prematurity, and delivery of the baby is normally undertaken. Prior to 24 weeks, intraperitoneal transfusion may be performed.

Blood transfusion

Blood may be given to the baby by a needle introduced through the mother's abdomen. Blood is given either intravascularly (into the umbilical vein or heart) or intraperitoneally. The first method is preferable, as blood enters the fetal circulation directly and severely anaemic fetuses may be saved. Intraperitoneal transfusion is reserved for cases of technical difficulty, or if the gestation is less than 22 weeks. If blood is taken from the fetus, the haemoglobin, fetal blood group and karyotype are usually checked. Clearly, if the baby is D rhesus negative, it will not develop D rhesus disease.

Blood transfused to the fetus must be:
- concentrated (Hb normally 22–24 g/dL)
- cytomegalovirus negative
- rhesus negative
- irradiated (to reduce the risk of graft-versus-host disease).

At delivery

If the baby is known to be anaemic or has had multiple transfusions, a neonatologist must be present at delivery should exchange transfusion be required. Blood must therefore always be ready for the delivery. All babies born to rhesus-negative women should have cord blood taken at delivery for a blood count, blood group and indirect Coomb's test.

D rhesus disease
- Rhesus disease gets worse with successive pregnancies.
- If the father of the fetus is rhesus negative, the fetus cannot be rhesus positive.
- If the father of the fetus is rhesus positive, he may be a heterozygote (50 per cent likelihood that the baby is D rhesus positive) or a homozygote (100 per cent likelihood).
- Anti-D is given only as prophylaxis and is useless once sensitization has occurred.
- Prenatal diagnosis for karyotype, or attempts at determining fetal blood group by invasive testing (e.g. chorion villus sampling), may make the antibody levels higher in women who are already sensitized.

CASE HISTORY

Ms W is 38 years old and at 22 weeks' gestation in her second pregnancy. She experienced severe nausea and vomiting earlier in her pregnancy, for which she required hospital admission. She has presented to the casualty department with severe retrosternal pain on lying down, and finds it difficult to eat and drink, saying that her 'stomach is burning'. She also occasionally brings up bloodstained vomitus and is losing weight.

What is the most likely diagnosis?

The symptoms sound like heartburn; however, this is simply the description of a symptom and it is quite possible that her hyperemesis earlier in the pregnancy was associated with gastro-oesophageal reflux, gastro-oesophagitis or even ulceration.

How would you manage Ms W?

You must concentrate on making a diagnosis, and alleviating her symptoms, allowing her to eat and drink. Severe upper gastrointestinal symptoms causing weight loss may warrant upper gastrointestinal endoscopy; at the very least, a gastroenterologist should be consulted. At the same time, remember that the following conditions can all present with vomiting and even weight loss in pregnancy, so the appropriate investigations should be carried out:
- urinary tract infections (send midstream urine sample to the laboratory),
- multiple gestation or triploidy/partial molar pregnancy (perform ultrasound if not done already),
- liver disease (send liver function tests).

The most likely diagnosis is mild reflux with heartburn, so provide a liquid antacid preparation to be taken three times daily and possibly an H2 blocker. Advise her to eat frequent small meals and to avoid spicy foods, smoking, caffeine and alcohol. Depending on her hydration and nutritional status, you may need to admit her to the antenatal ward, commence intravenous rehydration and give protein 'build-up' drinks.

Additional reading

James DK, Steer PJ, Weiner CP, Gonik B. *High risk pregnancy*, 2nd edn. London: WB Saunders 1999.
Lewis G (ed.) *Why mothers die 1997–1999. The Confidential Enquiries into Maternal Deaths in the United Kingdom*. London: RCOG Press, 2001. http://www.cemach.org.uk/publications/ CEMDreports/cemdrpt.pdf

Chapter 12

Twins and higher multiple gestations

OVERVIEW

In 1–2 per cent of pregnancies there is more than one fetus. The chances of miscarriage, fetal abnormalities, poor fetal growth, preterm delivery and intrauterine or neonatal death are considerably higher in twin than in singleton pregnancies. In about two-thirds of twins the fetuses are non-identical, or dizygotic, and in one-third they are identical, or monozygotic. In all dizygotic pregnancies there are two separate placentas (dichorionic). In two-thirds of monozygotic pregnancies there are vascular communications within the two placental circulations (monochorionic) and in the other one-third of cases there is dichorionic placentation. Monochorionic, compared to dichorionic, twins have a much higher risk of abnormalities and death. The maternal risks are also increased in multiple gestations, including adverse symptoms such as nausea and vomiting, tiredness and discomfort, and risks of serious complications, including hypertensive and thromboembolic disease and antepartum and postpartum haemorrhage.

Definitions

In general terms, multiple pregnancies consist of two or more fetuses. There are rare exceptions to this, such as twin gestations made up of a singleton viable fetus and a complete mole. Twins make up the vast majority (97–98 per cent) of multiple gestations. Pregnancies with three or more fetuses are referred to as 'higher multiples'.

Prevalence

In the UK, twins currently account for approximately 1.5 per cent of all pregnancies. Higher multiples occur in 1 in 2500 pregnancies.

Risk factors for multiple gestation include assisted reproduction techniques (both ovulation induction and in-vitro fertilization or IVF), increasing maternal age, high parity, black race and maternal family history.

Since the mid-1980s, the incidence of multiple pregnancy has been increasing. Traditionally, the expected incidence was calculated using Hellin's rule. Using this rule, twins were expected in 1 in 80 pregnancies, triplets in 1 in 80^2 and so on. Based upon the number of births in the UK in 2001, 7361 twins could have been predicted. In fact, 8484 were delivered, a 15 per cent increase. The figures for triplets are even more dramatic: 92 sets may have been expected but in actuality 211 were delivered. This represents a 130 per cent increase. Similar but more exaggerated figures are reported from the USA. In comparison to the expected numbers, the incidence of twin deliveries has increased by 50 per cent and triplets by 400 per cent.

The reasons for the increase in multiple gestations correspond to two related and overlapping trends. First, delay in childbearing results in increased maternal age at conception. Second, the increased use of infertility treatments, often by older women, also contributes.

Classification

The classification of multiple pregnancy is based on:
- number of fetuses: twins, triplets, quadruplets, etc.,
- number of fertilized eggs: zygosity,
- number of placentas: chorionicity,
- number of amniotic cavities: amnionicity.

Non-identical or fraternal twins are dizygotic, having resulted from the fertilization of two separate eggs.

Although they always have two functionally separate placentas (dichorionic), the placentas can become anatomically fused together and appear to the naked eye as a single placental mass. They always have separate amniotic cavities (diamniotic) and the two cavities are separated by a thick three-layer membrane (fused amnion in the middle with chorion on either side). The fetuses can be either same-sex or different-sex pairings.

Identical twins are monozygotic – they arise from fertilization of a single egg and are always same-sex pairings. They may share a single placenta (monochorionic) or have one each (dichorionic). If dichorionic, the placentas can become anatomically fused together and appear to the naked eye as a single placental mass, as mentioned above. The vast majority of monochorionic twins have two amniotic cavities (diamniotic) but the dividing membrane is thin, as it consists of a single layer of amnion alone. Monochorionic twins may occasionally share a single sac (monoamniotic). Figure 12.1 shows the relative contributions of the different types of twins to a hypothetical random selection of 1000 twin pairs.

Key Points

- Not all dichorionic pregnancies are dizygotic.
- All monochorionic pregnancies are monozygotic.

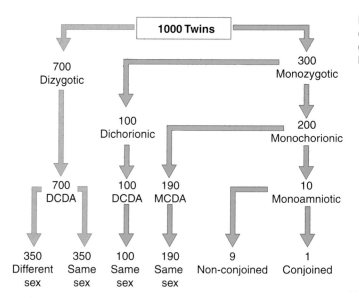

Figure 12.1 Incidence of monozygotic and dizygotic twin pregnancies. (DCDA, dichorionic diamniotic; MCDA, monochorionic diamniotic; MCMA, monochorionic monoamniotic.)

Aetiology

Dizygotic twins may arise spontaneously from the release of two eggs at ovulation. This tendency to release more than one egg can be familial or racial in origin and increases with maternal age. Ovulation induction treatments may also cause the release of more than one egg. With assisted conception techniques such as IVF, two or more embryos fertilized in the laboratory are replaced in the uterus.

Monozygotic twins arise from a single fertilized ovum that splits into two identical structures. The type of monozygotic twin depends on how long after conception the split occurs. When the split occurs within 3 days of conception, two placentas and two amniotic cavities result, giving rise to a dichorionic diamniotic (DCDA) pregnancy. When splitting occurs between days 4 and 8, only the chorion has differentiated and a monochorionic diamniotic (MCDA) pregnancy results. Later splitting after the amnion has differentiated leads to both twins developing in a single amniotic cavity, a monochorionic monoamniotic (MCMA) pregnancy. If splitting is delayed beyond day 12, the embryonic disc has also formed, and conjoined or 'Siamese' twins will result.

The incidence of monozygotic or identical twins is generally accepted to be constant at 1 in 250. It is not influenced by race, family history or parity. Recent evidence suggests a small increase in monozygotic twinning may be seen after IVF, for reasons that are unclear.

Other physiology

Maternal

All the physiological changes of pregnancy (increased cardiac output, volume expansion, relative haemodilution, diaphragmatic splinting, weight gain, lordosis, etc.) are exaggerated in multiple gestations. This results in much greater stresses being placed on maternal reserves. The 'minor' symptoms of pregnancy may be exaggerated. However, for women with pre-existing health problems, such as cardiac disease, a multiple pregnancy may substantially increase their risk of morbidity.

Fetal

Monochorionic placentas have the unique ability to develop vascular connections between the two fetal circulations. These anastomoses carry the potential for complications, discussed in the next section.

Complications relevant to twin pregnancy

Miscarriage and severe preterm delivery

General
Spontaneous preterm delivery is an ever-present risk in any twin pregnancy (Fig. 12.2) where the average gestation at delivery is 37 weeks. Therefore about half of all twins deliver preterm. As most babies born from 32 weeks onwards do very well, births at 34 or 35 weeks carry little clinical significance. In contrast, almost all babies born at 23 weeks or less die, with rates of mortality and handicap steadily falling between 24 and 31 weeks. Therefore, the clinical outcomes that should attract the most interest are late miscarriages (delivery between 12 and 23 weeks) or very preterm births (delivery between 24 and 32 weeks). In singleton pregnancies, the frequency of late miscarriage or very preterm birth is about 1 per cent each.

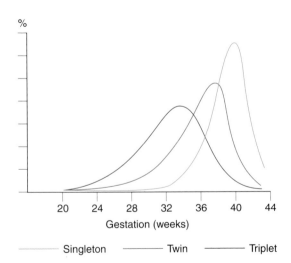

Figure 12.2 Gestational age distribution at delivery of singleton, twin and triplet pregnancies.

Table 12.1 – Common pregnancy complications in twin pregnancies according to chorionicity, compared with singleton pregnancies

Complication	Singleton (%)	Twins dichorionic (%)	Monochorionic (%)
Miscarriage at 12–23 weeks	1	2	12
Delivery at 24–32 weeks	1	5	10
Growth restriction	5	10	20
Fetal defects	1	2	8

Dichorionic/monochorionic differences

In a dichorionic pregnancy, the chance of late miscarriage is 2 per cent. In 5 per cent of cases, delivery will be very preterm. With two babies resulting from each preterm twin delivery, multiple gestations account for at least 10 per cent of special care baby unit admissions.

For monochorionic twins, the chance of early birth is increased even further, with 12 per cent born before viability and 10 per cent delivering between 24 and 32 weeks (Table 12.1).

Perinatal mortality in twins

General

The overall perinatal mortality rate for twins is around six times higher than for singletons. The biggest contributor to this high rate is complications related to preterm birth.

Dichorionic/monochorionic differences

As preterm delivery is most common in monochorionic twins, their perinatal mortality secondary to this is twice as high as in dichorionic twins. Monozygotic twins also have both additional risks and unique complications that further increase their chance of death and handicap, as discussed below.

Death of one fetus in a twin pregnancy

General

After the first trimester, the intrauterine death of one fetus in a twin pregnancy may be associated with a poor outcome for the remaining co-twin. Maternal complications such as disseminated intravascular coagulation have been reported, but the incidence of this appears to be very low.

Dichorionic/monochorionic differences

In dichorionic twins, the second or third trimester intrauterine death of one fetus may be associated with the onset of labour. However, in some cases the pregnancy may continue uneventfully and even result in delivery at term. Careful fetal and maternal monitoring is required. By contrast, fetal death of one twin in monochorionic twins may result in immediate complications in the survivor. These include death or brain damage with subsequent neurodevelopmental handicap. Acute hypotensive episodes, secondary to placental vascular anastomoses between the two fetuses, result in haemodynamic volume shifts from the live to the dead fetus. Death or handicap of the co-twin occurs in up to 25 per cent of cases.

Intrauterine growth restriction

General

Compared to singletons, the risk of poor growth is higher in each individual twin alone and substantially raised in the pregnancy as a whole.

When a fetus is growth restricted, the main aims of antenatal care become prediction of the severity of impaired fetal oxygenation and selecting the appropriate time for delivery. In singletons, this is a balance between the relative risks of intrauterine death versus the risk of neonatal death or handicap from elective preterm delivery. The situation is much more complicated in twin pregnancies. The potential benefit of expectant management or elective delivery for the small fetus must also be weighed against the risk of the same policy for the normally grown co-twin.

Dichorionic/monochorionic differences

In a dichorionic pregnancy, each fetus runs twice the risk of a low birth weight and there is a 20 per cent chance that at least one of the fetuses will suffer poor growth. The chance of poor fetal growth for monochorionic twins is almost double that for dichorionic twins (see Table 12.1).

In dichorionic twin pregnancies where one fetus has intrauterine growth restriction (IUGR), elective preterm delivery may lead to iatrogenic complications of prematurity in the previously healthy co-twin. In general, delivery should be avoided before 32 weeks, even if there is evidence of imminent intrauterine death of the smaller twin. However, this may not be applicable in the management of monochorionic twins. The death of one of a monochorionic twin pair may result in either death or handicap of the co-twin because of acute hypotension secondary to placental vascular anastomoses between the two circulations (see earlier discussion under 'Death of one fetus in a twin pregnancy'). As the damage potentially happens at the moment of death of the first twin, the timing of delivery may be a very difficult decision. Below 32 weeks' gestation, the aim is to prolong the pregnancy as far as possible without risking the death of the growth-restricted twin.

Fetal abnormalities

General

Compared to singletons, twin pregnancies carry at least twice the risk of the birth of a baby with an anomaly. However, there are important differences in both risk and management, based upon chorionicity.

Dichorionic/monochorionic differences

Each fetus of a dichorionic twin pregnancy has a risk of structural anomalies, such as spina bifida, that is similar to that of a singleton. Therefore, the chance of finding an anomaly within a dichorionic twin pregnancy is twice that of a singleton. In contrast, each fetus in a monochorionic twin pregnancy carries a risk for abnormalities that is four times that of a singleton. This is presumably due to a higher risk of vascular events during embryonic development (see Table 12.1).

Multiple gestations with an abnormality in one fetus can be managed expectantly or by selective fetocide of the affected twin. In cases where the abnormality is non-lethal but may well result in handicap, the parents may need to decide whether the potential burden of a handicapped child outweighs the risk of loss of the normal twin from fetocide-related complications, which occur after 5–10 per cent of procedures. In cases where the abnormality is lethal, it may be best to avoid such risk to the normal fetus, unless the condition itself threatens the survival of the normal twin. Anencephaly is a good example of a lethal abnormality that can threaten the survival of the normal twin. At least 50 per cent of pregnancies affected by anencephaly are complicated by polyhydramnios, which can lead to the spontaneous preterm delivery of both babies.

Fetocide in monochorionic pregnancies carries increased risk and requires a different technique. As there are potential vascular anastomoses between the two fetal circulations, intracardiac injections cannot be employed. Methods have evolved that employ cord occlusion techniques. These require significant instrumentation of the uterus and are therefore associated with a higher complication rate.

Chromosomal defects and twinning

General

In twins, as in singletons, the risk for chromosomal abnormalities increases with maternal age. The rate of spontaneous dizygotic twinning also increases with maternal age. Many women undergoing assisted conception techniques (which increase the chance of dizygotic twinning) are also older than the mean maternal age. Chromosomal defects may be more likely in a multiple pregnancy for various reasons, and couples should be counselled accordingly.

Dichorionic/monochorionic differences

Monozygotic twins arise from a single fertilized egg and therefore have the same genetic make-up. It is clear that in monozygotic twin pregnancies, chromosomal abnormalities such as Down's syndrome affect neither fetus or both. The risk is based upon maternal age.

In dizygotic twins, the maternal age-related risk for chromosomal abnormalities for each individual twin remains the same as for a singleton pregnancy. Therefore, at a given maternal age, the chance that at least one of the twin pair is affected by a chromosomal defect is twice as high as for a singleton pregnancy. For example, a 40-year-old woman with a singleton pregnancy has a fetal risk of trisomy 21 of 1 in 100. If she has a dizygotic twin pregnancy, the risk that one fetus would be affected is 1 in 50 (1 in 100 plus 1 in 100).

Complications unique to monochorionic twinning

In all monochorionic twin pregnancies there are placental vascular anastomoses present which allow communication between the two feto-placental circulations. In some monochorionic twin pregnancies, imbalance in the flow of blood across these arteriovenous communications results in twin-to-twin transfusion syndrome (TTTS). The development of mild, moderate or severe TTTS depends on the degree of imbalance. The donor fetus suffers from both hypovolaemia due to blood loss and hypoxia due to placental insufficiency, and may become growth-restricted and oliguric. As fetal urine is the major component of amniotic fluid, this fetus develops oligohydramnios. The recipient fetus becomes hypervolaemic, leading to polyuria and polyhydramnios. There is a risk of myocardial damage and high output cardiac failure. Severe disease may become apparent at 18–24 weeks of pregnancy. The mother often complains of a sudden increase in abdominal girth associated with extreme discomfort. Clinical examination shows tense polyhydramnios and ultrasound confirms the diagnosis.

More than 90 per cent of pregnancies complicated by TTTS end in miscarriage or severe preterm delivery, due either to the polyhydramnios or to intrauterine death of one or both fetuses. With treatment, one or both babies survive in about 70 per cent of pregnancies.

A common method of treatment is amniocentesis every 1–2 weeks with the drainage of large volumes of amniotic fluid. Exactly how this treatment improves the underlying pathophysiology is uncertain, but it appears to prolong the pregnancy and improve survival. More recently, some centres have used fetoscopically guided laser coagulation to disrupt the placental blood vessels that connect the circulations of the two fetuses.

Complications unique to monoamniotic twinning

Monoamniotic twins share a single amniotic cavity, with no dividing membrane between the two fetuses. They are at increased risk of cord accidents, predominantly through their almost universal cord entanglement. Many clinicians advocate elective delivery by Caesarean section at 32–34 weeks' gestation, as this complication is usually acute, fatal and unpredictable.

Differential diagnosis

The differential diagnosis of a multiple gestation includes all the other causes of a 'large for dates' uterus: polyhydramnios, uterine fibroids, urinary retention and ovarian masses.

Antenatal management

Routine antenatal care for all women involves screening for hypertension and gestational diabetes. These conditions occur more frequently in twin pregnancies and there is also a higher risk of other problems (such as antepartum haemorrhage and thromboembolic disease). However, the management is the same as for a singleton. Due to the increased feto-placental demand for iron and folic acid, many would recommend routine (as opposed to selective) supplementation in multiple pregnancies. Minor symptoms of pregnancy are more common, but management is again unchanged compared to singletons.

Elements of antenatal care that have specific importance in multiple pregnancies include the following.

Determination of chorionicity

As described, there are important differences in risk and outcome between dichorionic and monochorionic pregnancies. Therefore, determination of chorionicity is critical to 'good' management, and this is done most reliably by ultrasound in the late first trimester. In dichorionic twins, there is a V-shaped extension of placental tissue into the base of the inter-twin membrane, referred to as the 'lambda' or 'twin-peak' sign. In monochorionic twins, this sign is

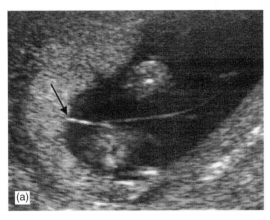

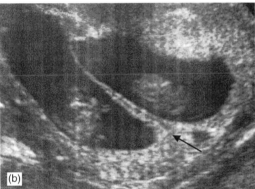

Figure 12.3 Ultrasound appearance of monochorionic (a) and dichorionic (b) twin pregnancies at 12 weeks' gestation. Note that in both types there appears to be a single placental mass, but in the dichorionic type there is an extension of placental tissue into the base of the inter-twin membrane forming the lambda sign.

absent and the inter-twin membrane joins the uterine wall in a T-shape (Fig. 12.3).

Assessment of chorionicity later in pregnancy is less reliable and relies upon the assessment of fetal gender, number of placentas and characteristics of the membrane between the two amniotic sacs. The 'lambda' sign becomes less accurate, and membrane thickness must be utilized. Different-sex twins must be dizygotic and therefore dichorionic. In same-sex twins, two separate placentas mean dichorionic, although the babies may still be monozygotic. However, monozygotic dichorionic twins do not carry the additional risks of vascular anastomoses.

Screening for fetal abnormalities

Screening for trisomy 21 using maternal serum biochemistry (see Chapter 9) is not effective in multiple gestations. This is because the relative contributions from each twin to each serum marker cannot be isolated. The optimal method of screening twins is by ultrasound. The measurement of nuchal translucency at 12 weeks' gestation allows each fetus to have an individualized assessment of risk. If prenatal diagnosis is required (see Chapter 9), knowledge of chorionicity is essential. Monochorionic twins are monozygotic and therefore only one sample is needed for karyotyping.

Both amniocentesis and chorion villus sampling (CVS) can be performed in twin pregnancies, but in dichorionic pregnancies, it is essential that both fetuses are sampled. As the placentas are often fused together, CVS has special challenges. With amniocentesis, dye-injection techniques have previously been used to prevent sampling the same sac twice. However, many practitioners now rely on direct puncture of the inter-twin membrane to avoid this.

Screening for fetal structural anomalies is done using second trimester ultrasound, with optimal detection rates seen at 20 weeks' gestation. More time must be allowed for each appointment. As monochorionic twins have a significantly increased risk of fetal anomalies, many argue that they should be screened within specialized fetal medicine units.

Monitoring fetal growth and well-being

Measurement of symphysis–fundal height and maternal reporting of fetal movements are unreliable, as once again the individual contribution of each twin cannot be assessed. Monitoring for fetal growth and well-being in twins is principally by ultrasound scan. Each assessment should include fetal measurements, fetal activity, fetal lies and amniotic fluid volumes. In monochorionic twins, features of TTTS should be sought, including discordances between fetal size, fetal activity, bladder volumes, amniotic fluid volumes and cardiac size. In any twin pregnancy, when one or both fetuses are small, additional information about fetal well-being can be obtained from Doppler assessment of the fetal circulations and cardiotocography (CTG). Specialized twin monitors should be used to ensure both twins' heart rates are sampled.

It is reasonable to plan 4–6-weekly ultrasound scans in dichorionic twins, but, due to the increased risks in monochorionic pregnancies, fortnightly ultrasound is appropriate. These are approximate guidelines that should be modified around individual pregnancy circumstances.

Threatened preterm labour

As in singleton pregnancies, neither bed rest nor prophylactic administration of tocolytics is useful in preventing preterm delivery. Despite this, screening for preterm birth may be worthwhile. Antenatal strategies in those identified as at high risk may include screening for bacterial vaginosis (treatment may eliminate a co-factor for spontaneous preterm labour), screening for group B *Streptococcus* (GBS; intrapartum antibiotics reduce neonatal infection), maternal steroid therapy to enhance fetal lung maturation, supplementary education as to the signs and symptoms of preterm labour, advance planning regarding intrapartum care and additional medical and midwifery support.

At present, transvaginal cervical ultrasound shows the most promise as a predictor of very preterm delivery (see Chapter 14). As regular ultrasound examination is already part of the care of multiple pregnancy, there is little impact on healthcare resources. Once preterm labour is diagnosed, neonatal unit staff must be promptly involved. The use of tocolytic drugs in this situation, particularly the beta-agonists, carries risks of serious maternal morbidity.

Multiple pregnancy support groups

Twin pregnancies are associated with a number of financial, personal and social costs for families that continue long beyond the neonatal period. A significant contribution to these costs comes from the increased incidence of handicap, largely secondary to preterm delivery. Several specialized support groups for multiple pregnancy exist. In the UK, these include the Twins and Multiple Birth Association (TAMBA) and the Multiple Birth Foundation. All parents expecting twins should be given contact details for such resources locally.

Intrapartum management

Preparation

This should begin long before labour, with antenatal education and an intrapartum care plan. A twin CTG machine should be used for fetal monitoring and a portable ultrasound machine should be available during the delivery. A standard oxytocin solution for augmentation should be prepared, run through an intravenous giving-set and clearly labelled 'for augmentation', for use for delivery of the second twin, if required. A second high-dose oxytocin infusion should also be available for the management of postpartum haemorrhage. However, it is advisable to keep this separate, not run through a giving-set until needed and clearly labelled 'for postpartum use only'. It is essential that two neonatal resuscitation trolleys, two obstetricians and two paediatricians are available and that the special care baby unit and anaesthetist are informed well in advance of the delivery.

The management of twin deliveries is discussed in Chapter 18.

Postpartum haemorrhage

The risk of postpartum haemorrhage is increased in twin pregnancies due to the larger placental site and uterine over-distension. For that reason, all multiple gestations should have an intravenous line and blood grouped and saved during labour.

Management is generally no different from that of postpartum haemorrhage complicating singleton delivery (see Chapter 19). However, ideally, the third stage should be actively managed and a high-dose oxytocin infusion commenced following delivery as prophylaxis.

Higher multiples

A consequence of the widespread introduction of assisted reproductive techniques has been an exponential increase in the incidence of higher multiple gestations, mostly triplets. At least 75 per cent of triplet pregnancies are secondary to assisted conception. They are associated with increased risks of miscarriage, perinatal death and handicap. The median gestational age at birth is 33 weeks and long-term complications are primarily a consequence of extremely preterm delivery. Although the demands on maternal physiology are greater still, antenatal care is essentially no different from that for a twin gestation. Caesarean section is usually advocated for delivery due to the difficulties of intrapartum fetal monitoring. However, the evidence to support this strategy is weak, and several

CASE HISTORY

Miss O is a 32-year-old woman who is unmarried but in a stable relationship. She works as a research scientist. She has a high body mass index (35) but is otherwise fit and well. She required ovulation induction with clomiphene and was discovered to have a triplet pregnancy on a transvaginal scan at 8 weeks' gestation. She is now 12 weeks' gestation and the pregnancy has been classified as trichorionic triamniotic. All fetuses appear structurally normal and all have nuchal measurements that represent a considerable reduction in her age-related risk of Down's syndrome.

Was Miss O's gynaecological treatment successful?

The incidence of multiple pregnancy is increased after ovulation induction. Although most commonly twins, triplets and higher multiples are all more frequent. The pregnancy achieved is immediately 'high risk'. Pregnancy in the obese carries increased maternal risks, such as hypertension; these risks are multiplied with multiple pregnancy. The chances of operative delivery are substantially elevated, secondary to both maternal size and the multiple pregnancy. The risks of surgical and postoperative complications are significant in overweight patients. Although her treatment was successful, her long-term health interests may have been better served by weight reduction.

What obstetric risks does Miss O face?

The risks of miscarriage and extremely preterm delivery are far higher with a triplet pregnancy. The mean gestation at delivery is approximately 33 weeks, and perinatal morbidity and mortality are much increased over a singleton pregnancy. Maternal complications such as pre-eclampsia and venous thromboembolism are slightly more frequent in multiple gestation. She will suffer much more from the 'minor' conditions of pregnancy: backache, varicose veins, heartburn and anaemia particularly.

Might embryo reduction be considered?

This is an option that should be considered. The ethical views of the parents will be an important influence. The scientific evidence suggests the overall chance of miscarriage and preterm delivery before 28 weeks is halved.

Is there any way of predicting her risk of severe preterm delivery?

Transvaginal ultrasound cervical length assessment at 20–24 weeks may be useful. However, there is no clear treatment that reduces the chances of an early birth in those identified as high risk. Nevertheless, a negative test may offer reassurance and minimize the risk of inappropriate medical intervention.

How often should Miss O be seen at the hospital?

She should be booked for full hospital care, ideally in a specialized multidisciplinary clinic for multiple pregnancies. She will require a detailed structural ultrasound survey of all three fetuses at 20 weeks, and growth scans every 3 weeks thereafter.

What other antenatal measures should be taken?

Many would argue that iron supplements should be given routinely to women with multiple gestation due to their increased requirements. The mother should be given contact numbers for the local multiple birth support groups. If identified as at high risk of very preterm delivery, screening for GBS colonization, prophylactic steroids for fetal lung maturity, an intrapartum care plan and a neonatal consultation may all be helpful.

case series of vaginal birth have reported comparable neonatal outcomes.

In an attempt to reduce the morbidity and mortality associated with extremely preterm delivery, the procedure of multi-fetal reduction was introduced. Iatrogenic fetal death is achieved by the ultrasound-guided puncture of the fetal heart and injection of potassium chloride. Although it is technically feasible to perform reduction from as early as 7 weeks' gestation, it is usually delayed until around 11–12 weeks. This allows for spontaneous reduction to occur and for the screening and diagnosis of major fetal abnormalities and chromosomal defects. Following reduction, there is gradual resorption of the dead fetuses and their placentas.

A triplet pregnancy managed expectantly has a 20 per cent chance of loss prior to 24 weeks and an 8 per cent risk of extremely preterm delivery between 24 and 28 weeks. After multi-fetal reduction, usually to twins, the risks of both mid-trimester loss and extremely preterm birth are halved. However, the risks of subsequent miscarriage and extremely preterm delivery have been found to increase with the number of fetuses reduced.

New developments

- Transvaginal ultrasound measurement of cervical length at 20–24 weeks may be used to assess the risk of very preterm delivery.
- The interrelated phenomena of delayed childbearing and increased use of assisted conception techniques have dramatically increased the incidence of multiple pregnancy.
- The optimal way to screen for Down's syndrome in multiple pregnancy is by nuchal translucency at 12 weeks' gestation. Chorionicity can also be reliably determined at this time.
- Multi-fetal reduction is increasingly accepted as improving overall outcomes in higher multiples.

Key Points

- Twins account for about 1.5 per cent of pregnancies but for more than 10 per cent of special care baby unit admissions.
- Perinatal mortality rate in twins is about six times higher than in singletons, primarily due to spontaneous preterm births.
- Both serious maternal complications and minor discomforts are increased in multiple gestation.
- The determination of chorionicity is very important – the highest risks are seen in monochorionic twins.

Disorders of placentation

OVERVIEW

The development of the human placenta and the maintenance of a successful pregnancy are dependent on the proliferation, migration and invasion of trophoblast into the maternal decidua and myometrium in early pregnancy. The process of trophoblast invasion leads to the transformation of the spiral arteries supplying the intervillous space. These small, narrow calibre arteries are gradually converted into large sinusoidal vessels, as the endothelium and the internal elastic lamina are replaced by trophoblast. These changes transform the vascular supply to a low-pressure, high-flow system, allowing an adequate blood flow to the placenta and fetus.

The Confidential Enquiry into Maternal Deaths has repeatedly identified pre-eclampsia and eclampsia as leading causes of maternal death in pregnancy. Furthermore, pre-eclampsia is frequently accompanied by intrauterine growth restriction, which is responsible for considerable perinatal mortality and morbidity. Although fetal growth is determined by a number of factors, including genetic predisposition, maternal nutritional status and ability of the placenta to allow nutrient exchange, it is now apparent that the origins of both pre-eclampsia and much of the fetal growth restriction seen in clinical practice lie in defective placentation. A further condition frequently related to impaired trophoblast invasion is abruptio placentae, or premature separation of a normally sited placenta, which is usually of sudden onset and associated with a high fetal mortality and substantial maternal mortality and morbidity. Knowledge of the early events in the invasion of the maternal uterine wall by placental trophoblast cells is therefore helpful in understanding the aetiology of these important clinical conditions.

The placenta

The placenta is usually regarded as a fetal organ, although it contains maternal and fetal vascular beds that are juxtaposed. It receives the highest blood flow of any fetal organ (40 per cent of fetal cardiac output) and, towards the end of pregnancy, competes with the fetus for maternal substrate, consuming the major fraction of glucose and oxygen taken up by the gravid uterus.

The functional unit of the placenta is the fetal cotyledon, and the mature human placenta has about 120 cotyledons, which are grouped into visible lobes. Each cotyledon contains a primary villus stem arising from the chorionic plate and supplied by primary branches of fetal vessels. The primary stems divide to form secondary and tertiary stems from which arise the terminal villi, where maternal–fetal exchange takes place. The fetal cotyledons appear to develop around the entries of the maternal spiral arteries from the decidual plate, and the centre of each cotyledon is hollow, where the pulsatile jet of blood from the spiral artery enters the intracotyledonary space (Fig. 13.1). Blood from the spiral arteries rises high to the chorionic plate, then disperses laterally between and over the surface of the terminal villi, becoming increasingly desaturated of oxygen and nutrients and picking up carbon dioxide and waste products. The blood then

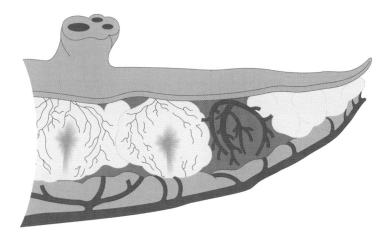

Figure 13.1 Diagram of placenta showing the arrangement of fetal cotyledons and the maternal and fetal vascular systems.

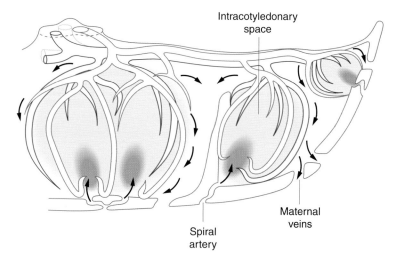

Intracotyledonary space

Spiral artery

Maternal veins

Figure 13.2 Diagram showing the direction of maternal blood flow through the fetal cotyledons.

filters into narrow venous channels between the cotyledons, before falling back to the maternal decidual plate, where the maternal veins return the desaturated blood to the maternal circulation (Fig. 13.2). Maternal and fetal blood is separated by three microscopic tissue layers: trophoblastic tissue, connective tissue and the endothelium of the fetal capillaries. However, microscopic examination of the terminal villi surrounding the intracotyledonary space shows numerous vasculosyncytial membranes where the fetal capillaries and trophoblast fuse to form a very thin membrane, where most of the transfer of nutrients and blood gases takes place (Fig. 13.3).

Normal placentation

The maternal blood flow to the placenta increases throughout pregnancy from 50 mL/min in the first trimester to 600 mL/min at term. This twelve-fold

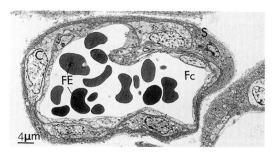

Figure 13.3 A terminal villus in cross-section, showing the vasculo-syncytial membrane (arrow). (FE, fetal erythrocyte; Fc, fetal capillary.)

increase in perfusion can only be accomplished by an anatomical conversion of the maternal spiral arteries by trophoblast, from narrow, tortuous, muscular vessels to wide-bore, flaccid vessels. In the first 12 weeks, the decidual segments of the spiral arteries are invaded and replaced by trophoblast and fibrinoid. At the end of this period, the trophoblast plugs, which occupy the lumen of the spiral arteries, are released and this is associated with a sudden increase in blood flow to the intervillous space. Following this, the trophoblast invasion of the intramyometrial segment of the spiral arteries occurs, which further reduces resistance to blood flow to the placenta and is associated with a mid-trimester fall in the maternal blood pressure. This process should be complete by 20 weeks. These flaccid transformed spiral arteries not only permit increased perfusion but, because they lack smooth muscle, are also less likely to respond to vasoactive compounds (Fig. 13.4).

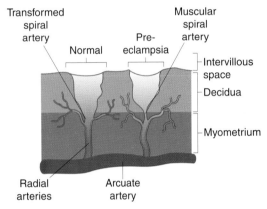

Figure 13.4 The transformation of spiral arteries.

Abnormal placentation

Pre-eclampsia, intrauterine growth restriction (IUGR) and abruptio placentae are clinical manifestations of total or patchy failure of trophoblast invasion of the myometrial segments of the spiral arteries. In terms of the aetiology of the condition, there are still more questions than answers. It is still not clear why trophoblast invasion fails and why this pathological maladaption can produce a pregnancy with pre-eclampsia or IUGR or abruptio placentae, or all three. It is likely that the more complete the failure of trophoblast invasion, the more likely that pre-eclampsia will supervene. There are other general conditions associated with impaired perfusion of the placenta, such as collagen vascular disease, antiphospholipid syndrome, severe diabetes mellitus and chronic hypertension. All of these result in a small placenta with gross morphological changes. The most serious of these changes are:

- infarcts (Fig. 13.5)
- basal haematomas (Fig. 13.6).

An infarct represents an area of ischaemic necrosis of a cotyledon resulting from spiral artery occlusion, usually by thrombosis. A placenta with multiple infarcts is significantly associated with intrauterine fetal death and growth restriction. Closely associated with infarcts are placental haematomas, which consist of a mass of blood in the centre of the fetal cotyledon due to rupture of a damaged spiral artery. This lesion is also associated with maternal hypertension and increased perinatal mortality. These serious pathological lesions should not be confused with calcification or fibrin deposition in the placenta, which can often give it an 'unhealthy' appearance, but are benign.

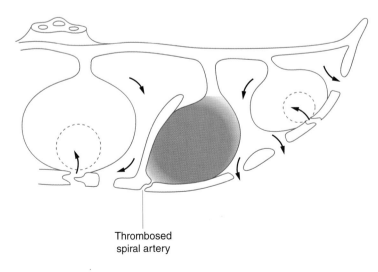

Figure 13.5 Diagram showing how an infarct occurs due to thrombosis of a spiral artery.

Thrombosed
spiral artery

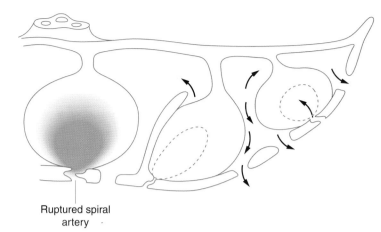

Figure 13.6 Diagram showing the formation of a massive haematoma.

Ruptured spiral
artery

Pre-eclampsia

Definition

In the past, the diagnostic criterion for pre-eclampsia has varied. This has led to difficulty in comparing studies on treatments, or outcomes, in different populations. There is now a widely accepted classification system of hypertensive disorders in pregnancy, which defines *pre-eclampsia* as hypertension of at least 140/90 mmHg recorded on two separate occasions at least 4 hours apart and in the presence of at least 300 mg protein in a 24-hour collection of urine, arising de novo after the 20th week of gestation in a previously normotensive women and resolving completely by the sixth postpartum week.

S Symptoms of pre-eclampsia

- May be asymptomatic
- Headache
- Visual disturbances
- Epigastric and right upper abdominal pain

Signs of pre-eclampsia

- Elevation of blood pressure
- Fluid retention (non-dependent oedema)
- Brisk reflexes
- Ankle clonus (more than three beats)
- Uterus and fetus may feel small for gestational age

Chronic hypertension with or without renal disease, and existing prior to pregnancy, is of a different aetiology from pre-eclampsia (see Chapter 15), although it can predispose to the later development of superimposed pre-eclampsia.

Gestational hypertension alone, i.e. hypertension arising for the first time in the second half of pregnancy and in the absence of proteinuria, is not associated with adverse pregnancy outcome and as such should be clearly distinguished from pre-eclampsia.

Eclampsia is a serious and life-threatening complication of pre-eclampsia. It is defined as convulsions occurring in a woman with established pre-eclampsia, in the absence of any other neurological or metabolic cause. It is an obstetric emergency and the management of this condition is discussed further in Chapter 19.

Incidence

Pre-eclampsia complicates approximately 3 per cent of pregnancies, but the incidence varies depending on the exact definition used and the population studied. Eclampsia is relatively rare in the UK, occurring in approximately 1:2000 pregnancies. In the most recent Confidential Enquiry (1997–1999) there were 15 maternal deaths due to pre-eclampsia, making this the second commonest cause of death in late pregnancy and the puerperium. Worldwide, it is a far greater problem, with an estimated 72 000 deaths annually.

Epidemiology

Pre-eclampsia is more common in primigravid women. It is thought that the normal fetal–maternal transfusion that occurs during pregnancy, and particularly during delivery, exposes the mother to products of fetal (and hence paternal) genome, protecting her in subsequent pregnancies. In keeping with this concept, prolonged exposure to paternal antigens (e.g. through unprotected sex) prior to conceiving appears to reduce the risk of pre-eclampsia and, conversely, the protective effect of first pregnancy is partially lost if a woman has a child with a new father. There also appears to be a maternal genetic predisposition to pre-eclampsia, as there is three–four-fold increase in the incidence of pre-eclampsia in the first-degree relatives of affected women. Finally, there are a number of general medical conditions and pregnancy-specific factors that predispose to the development of pre-eclampsia.

Risk factors for pre-eclampsia

Predisposing factors for the development of pre-eclampsia include:

- conditions in which the placenta in enlarged (multiple gestation, diabetes, hydrops)
- pre-existing hypertension or renal disease
- pre-existing vascular disease (such as in diabetes or autoimmune vasculitis)

Aetiology

Pre-eclampsia only occurs in pregnancy, but has been described in pregnancies lacking a fetus (molar pregnancies) and in the absence of a uterus (abdominal pregnancies, see Chapter 8 in *Gynaecology by ten teachers*, 18th edition), suggesting that it is the trophoblast tissue that provides the stimulus for the disorder. Placental bed biopsies have demonstrated that in pre-eclampsia, trophoblast invasion is patchy, and the spiral arteries retain their muscular walls. This is thought to prevent the development of a high-flow, low-impedance uteroplacental circulation. The reason why trophoblast invades less effectively in these pregnancies is not known. However, extravillous trophoblast cells from placental bed biopsies taken from pre-eclamptic pregnancies do not show the normal adhesion molecule switch characteristic of invasive trophoblast, although the reason for this also remains poorly understood.

It is widely believed that defective trophoblast invasion results in relative under-perfusion of the placenta and that this releases a factor(s) into the maternal circulation that targets the vascular endothelium (Fig. 13.7). The nature of this factor has not yet been identified, although numerous candidates have been proposed, including a variety of growth factors, cytokines and products of abnormal lipid metabolism.

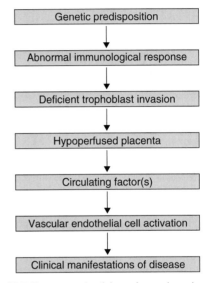

Figure 13.7 The proposed aetiology of pre-eclampsia.

Pathophysiology

There is abundant evidence that the clinical picture of pre-eclampsia is due to an activation or dysfunction of vascular endothelial cells. The concentration of cell surface makers for endothelial cell damage (including fibronectin, adhesion molecules and von Willebrand factor) is increased in the plasma of women with pre-eclampsia.

Normal pregnancy is characterized by marked peripheral vasodilatation (see Chapter 5, p. 50), resulting in a fall in total peripheral resistance despite an increase in cardiac output and circulating volume. This peripheral vasodilatation is accomplished through a reduced vascular sensitivity to vasoconstrictors such as angiotensin, and possibly by enhanced vasodilator production by vascular endothelial cells. In pre-eclampsia, the insensitivity to vasoconstrictors is lost and vessels in vivo and in vitro show reduced sensitivity to vasodilators and enhanced sensitivity to vasoconstrictors.

Vasospasm and endothelial cell dysfunction, with subsequent platelet activation and micro-aggregate formation, account for many of the pathological features of pre-eclampsia seen in almost every major organ system.

Organ-specific changes associated with pre-eclampsia

Cardiovascular
- Generalized vasospasm
- Increased peripheral resistance
- Reduced central venous/pulmonary wedge pressures

Haematological
- Platelet activation and depletion
- Coagulopathy
- Decreased plasma volume
- Increased blood viscosity

Renal
- Proteinuria
- Decreased glomerular filtration rate
- Decreased urate excretion

Hepatic
- Periportal necrosis
- Subcapsular haematoma

Central nervous system
- Cerebral oedema
- Cerebral haemorrhages

Loss of endothelial cell integrity results in an increase in vascular permeability and contributes to the formation of generalized oedema, which is often found in women with pre-eclampsia. Dependent oedema of the feet is very common in healthy pregnant women. However, rapidly progressing oedema of the face and hands is suggestive of pre-eclampsia.

In the kidney, a highly characteristic lesion (called glomeruloendotheliosis) is seen. This consists of endothelial and mesangial cell swelling, basement membrane inclusions, but little disruption of renal epithelial podocytes. This is relatively specific for pre-eclampsia and is associated with the development of proteinuria, reduced renal clearance of uric acid and oliguria. It is not seen with hypertension due to other causes.

In the liver, subendothelial fibrin deposition is associated with elevation of liver enzymes. This can be associated with haemolysis and a low platelet count due to platelet consumption (and subsequent widespread activation of the coagulation system). The presence of these findings is called the HELLP syndrome (**h**aemolysis, **e**levation of **l**iver enzymes and **l**ow **p**latelets). The HELLP syndrome is a particularly severe form of pre-eclampsia. It occurs in approximately 2–4 per cent of women with pre-eclampsia and is associated with a fetal loss rate of up to 60 per cent if occurring antenatally and a maternal mortality of up to 24 per cent. The management of HELLP syndrome is discussed further in Chapter 19.

Vasospasm and cerebral oedema have both been implicated in the cerebral manifestations of pre-eclampsia and the progression to eclampsia. Retinal haemorrhage, exudates and papilloedema are characteristic of hypertensive encephalopathy and are rare in pre-eclampsia, suggesting that hypertension alone is not responsible for the cerebral pathology.

Within the vasculature of the placental bed, the characteristic lesion seen in pre-eclampsia is acute atherosis of the spiral arteries, with platelet microaggregates and larger thromboses.

Screening tests

More than 160 substances have been shown to be increased in the circulation of women with pre-eclampsia. Unfortunately, this has not yet led to the development of a sensitive and specific screening blood test.

The ability of Doppler ultrasound uterine artery waveform analysis to identify women at risk of pre-eclampsia and other adverse pregnancy outcome has been investigated with varying success. In pregnancies with inadequate or incomplete trophoblast invasion of the spiral arteries, a characteristic 'notch' can been seen in the waveform pattern (Fig. 13.8; see also Chapter 8). Such screening may have a place in women already identified as being at risk of pre-eclampsia because of their medical or past obstetric history. However, it has limited diagnostic potential for adverse pregnancy-related complications in a low-risk population.

Screening has been criticized on the basis that it will cause unnecessary alarm in pregnant women when there are no proven methods of preventing pre-eclampsia. The most commonly used preventive therapy is low-dose aspirin (at 75 mg daily), on the basis that this dose will inhibit platelet activation and the

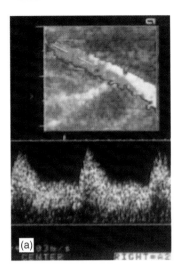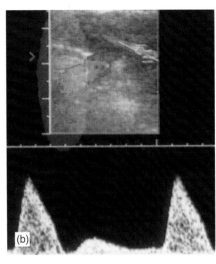

Figure 13.8 Uterine artery Doppler showing (a) normal waveform and (b) 'notched' waveform associated with pregnancies destined to be complicated by pre-eclampsia or intrauterine growth restriction.

release of vasoactive compounds such as thromboxanes without impairing the synthesis of vasodilating prostaglandins produced by the vascular endothelium. Two large placebo-controlled studies have failed to show any significant benefit of aspirin therapy in preventing pre-eclampsia. However, there is some evidence that aspirin may be more effective if given to a more targeted group at high risk of developing the disease, if given at night, and if given in doses that affect bleeding times (e.g. 150 mg daily). This is why the development of early and effective screening tests for this condition is so important. There are other reasons for developing such tests. The accurate prediction of women at risk of developing pre-eclampsia will facilitate targeting of increased antenatal surveillance whilst allowing women at low risk of the condition to participate in community-based antenatal care.

Management and treatment

The mainstay of treatment for pre-eclampsia remains ending the pregnancy by delivering the fetus (and the placenta). This can be a significant problem for the baby if pre-eclampsia occurs at 24–28 weeks' gestation; thus many strategies have been proposed to delay the need for delivery.

The principles of management of pre-eclampsia are:
- early recognition of the symptomless syndrome,
- awareness of the serious nature of the condition in its severest form,

- adherence to agreed guidelines for admission to hospital, investigation and the use of antihypertensive and anticonvulsant therapy,
- well-timed delivery to pre-empt serious maternal or fetal complications,
- postnatal follow-up and counselling for future pregnancies.

A diagnosis of pre-eclampsia usually requires admission of the patient for more intensive investigations and monitoring of her condition. When the blood pressure is only mildly elevated (i.e. a diastolic blood pressure of 90–95 mmHg) and there is minimal proteinuria with normal haematological and biochemical parameters, it may be possible to monitor the patient's condition as an outpatient, attending for regular fetal and maternal assessment.

In the presence of higher blood pressure values, greater proteinuria or abnormal haematological and biochemical parameters, admission is mandatory. Investigations indicated in the further management of this condition are listed in the box below.

Investigations for pre-eclampsia

These investigations will be repeated at intervals depending on the overall clinical picture.
- Urinalysis by dipstick (quantitatively inaccurate).
- 24-hour urine collection (total protein and creatinine clearance).
- Full blood count (platelets and haematocrit).

(continued)

- Blood chemistry (renal function, protein concentration).
- Plasma urate concentration.
- Liver function.
- Coagulation profile.
- Ultrasound assessment:
  - fetal size
  - amniotic fluid volume
  - maternal and fetal
  - Dopplers.

The aim of antihypertensive therapy is to lower the blood pressure and reduce the risk of maternal cerebrovascular accident without reducing uterine blood flow and compromising the fetus. There is a variety of antihypertensives used in the management of pre-eclampsia in the UK. Labetolol is an alpha-blocking and beta-blocking agent. It can be given orally or intravenously and has a good safety record in pregnancy. Methyldopa is a centrally acting antihypertensive agent. It, too, has a long-established safety record in pregnancy, but can only be given orally and takes upwards of 24 hours to take effect. Nifedipine is a calcium-channel blocker with a rapid onset of action. It can, however, cause severe headache that may mimic worsening disease.

In severe cases of fulminating disease, an intravenous infusion of hydralazine/labetolol can be titrated rapidly against changes in the blood pressure. The drug of choice for the treatment of eclampsia is magnesium sulphate. This is given intravenously and has been shown to reduce the incidence of further convulsions in women with eclampsia. The role of magnesium sulphate in the prevention of eclampsia is less certain and is the subject of several ongoing trials.

Most of the maternal deaths related to pre-eclampsia are due to a failure to recognize a deteriorating condition after delivery and result from multiple organ failure, including disseminated intravascular coagulation (DIC), adult respiratory distress syndrome and renal failure. The importance of involving clinicians from other specialties (intensive care, haematology) cannot be overstated.

Additional points in management

Iatrogenic premature delivery of the fetus is often required in severe pre-eclampsia. This necessitates optimizing the fetal condition prior to delivery. Dexamethasone (12 mg intramuscularly, twice, 12 hours apart) should be given to the mother to reduce the chance of neonatal pulmonary insufficiency. If the patient's condition permits, she should be transferred to a tertiary centre prior to delivery, to improve both her own management and the facilities for her baby. Delivery before term is usually by Caesarean section. Such patients are at particularly high risk for thromboembolism and should be given prophylactic subcutaneous heparin and issued with anti-thromboembolic stockings. In the case of spontaneous or induced labour and if clotting studies are normal, epidural anaesthesia is indicated as it helps control blood pressure. Ergometrine is avoided in the management of the third stage as it can significantly increase blood pressure.

New developments

Several groups are investigating the genetics of pre-eclampsia, although the variable phenotype of the condition within a couple suggests the cause is unlikely to relate to a single gene. Several studies on the therapeutic role of vitamins C and E (major anti-oxidants) in the prevention and treatment of pre-eclampsia are now in progress.

CASE HISTORY

Mrs A is a 41-year-old married doctor, a non-smoker who weighs 90 kg. She is gravida 1, with no notable past history. At her antenatal booking visit at 11 weeks, she was well, with a blood pressure measurement of 120/75 mmHg. She had ultrasound nuchal screening for Down's syndrome, her dates were confirmed and she was found to be at low risk of aneuploidy. Her pregnancy continued normally until 30 weeks'

gestation, when her blood pressure was found to be 150/95 mmHg and urinalysis revealed ++ proteinuria.

How should this patient be managed?

Mrs A had a positive screen for pre-eclampsia in the clinic. She should have her blood pressure taken again several times to ensure it is not simply related to attending the clinic. She should also be screened for urinary tract infection, a common cause of proteinuria. Assuming her blood pressure is elevated, she should be admitted for bed rest, 24-hour urine collection (quantify protein and creatinine clearance), baseline platelet count and renal and hepatic function, and she should have a scan to assess fetal growth, liquor volume and possibly fetal Doppler studies.

Should she be commenced on medications?

At this blood pressure, there is no proven advantage to commencing antihypertensives. This situation is not analogous to chronic elevated blood pressure, and the only aim of treatment is the prevention of an acute episode such as cerebrovascular accident (CVA). As she is overweight and has been admitted for bed rest, she should be commenced on heparin prophylaxis against thromboembolism. As she may require delivery in the near future, she should be given a course of dexamethasone to promote fetal lung maturation.

If delivery is the main treatment for pre-eclampsia, when should this be carried out?

The decision to deliver must balance the beneficial effect on the mother's health against detrimental effects on the baby's prognosis. Many women with pre-eclampsia run a chronic course, and prolonging gestation will improve fetal maturity. There is no correct answer to this question. The decision to deliver must be based on frequent repetition of investigations into maternal and fetal health, and will occur at a time when it is felt that either maternal health is becoming compromised by further delay to delivery or the fetus can be better looked after ex utero than in utero.

Intrauterine growth restriction

There is a variety of reasons why a fetus may be small, including congenital anomaly, fetal infections and chromosomal abnormality. However, the majority of fetuses which appear to be small are either constitutionally small (i.e. born to small parents and fulfilling their genetic potential) or are small secondary to abnormal placental function.

Significance

Intrauterine growth restriction is a major cause of neonatal morbidity and mortality. It has a significant cost in terms of the facilities required to look after these infants. In addition, there is a growing appreciation that certain adult diseases (including hypertension and diabetes) are related to IUGR.

Definitions and incidence

Intrauterine growth restriction is defined as failure of the fetus to achieve its genetic growth potential. This usually results in a fetus that is small for gestational age (SGA), and babies born below a particular centile weight for gestation (e.g. below the 3rd or 5th centile) are frequently classified as IUGR. While this is convenient and makes it simple to calculate the incidence of IUGR (3 per cent if the 3rd or 5 per cent if the 5th centile is chosen), the terms SGA and IUGR are not synonymous. The term SGA implies that the fetus or neonate is below a certain defined centile of weight or size for a particular gestational age, and some SGA fetuses are constitutionally small due to normal genetic influences. IUGR indicates that a particular pathological process is operating to modify the intrinsic growth potential of the fetus by reducing its growth rate. Indeed, some IUGR fetuses may not fall into any definition of SGA, but will have failed to achieve their full growth potential.

Aetiology

There are many causes of IUGR (Table 13.1). They are best grouped into two main categories: factors that directly affect the intrinsic growth potential of the fetus and external influences that reduce the support for fetal growth. Postnatal 'catch-up' growth is more likely to occur in fetuses in the latter category than in the former (Fig. 13.9).

Chromosome abnormalities, genetic syndromes, infections and drugs can alter intrinsic fetal growth potential. Many chromosome abnormalities, such as trisomy 18 and triploidy, and single-gene defects, such as Seckel's syndrome, will alter the genetic potential of the fetus, as will some multi-factorial structural abnormalities such as anencephaly and renal agenesis. Viral infections, such as cytomegalovirus and

Table 13.1 – Causes of intrauterine growth restriction

Investigations	Cause
Reduced fetal growth potential	Chromosome defects, e.g. trisomy 18, triploidy
	Single-gene defects, e.g. Seckel's syndrome
	Structural abnormalities, e.g. renal agenesis
	Infections, e.g. cytomegalovirus, toxoplasmosis
Reduced fetal growth support	*Maternal factors*
	Under-nutrition, e.g. poverty, eating disorders
	Maternal hypoxia, e.g. altitude, cyanotic heart disease
	Drugs, e.g. cigarette smoke, alcohol, cocaine
	Placental factors
	Reduced uteroplacental perfusion, e.g. inadequate trophoblast invasion, antiphospholipid syndrome, diabetes mellitus, sickle-cell disease, multiple gestation
	Reduced feto-placental perfusion, e.g. single umbilical artery, twin–twin transfusion syndrome

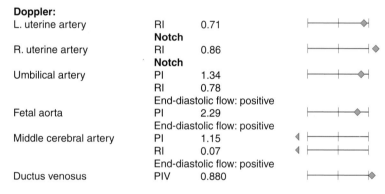

Doppler:

L. uterine artery	RI	0.71	
	Notch		
R. uterine artery	RI	0.86	
	Notch		
Umbilical artery	PI	1.34	
	RI	0.78	
	End-diastolic flow: positive		
Fetal aorta	PI	2.29	
	End-diastolic flow: positive		
Middle cerebral artery	PI	1.15	
	RI	0.07	
	End-diastolic flow: positive		
Ductus venosus	PIV	0.880	

Diagnosis: Stable moderate redistribution. Increased DV PI.

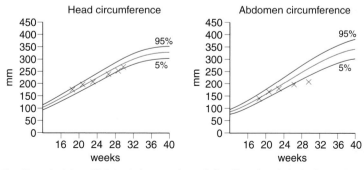

Figure 13.9 The growth pattern of a fetus with intrauterine growth restriction. Note the relative brain-sparing effect, with head circumference less affected than abdominal circumference. The Doppler chart demonstrates high resistance and notches in the uterine artery. There is fetal hypoxia, as demonstrated by low resistance waveforms in the fetal brain (low pulsatility index) and probable acidaemia due to the high pulsatility in the ductus venosus. (RI, resistance index; PI, pulsatility index; PIV, pulsatility index for veins; DV, ductus venosus.)

rubella, and protozoal infections, such as toxoplasmosis, can also affect fetal growth potential.

External influences that affect fetal growth can be subdivided into maternal systemic factors and placental insufficiency. Maternal under-nutrition is globally the major cause of IUGR and, even in developed countries, it is now recognized that maternal eating disorders, such as anorexia or bulimia, can significantly affect fetal growth. Low maternal oxygen saturation, which can occur with cyanotic heart disease, chronic respiratory disease or at high altitude, will reduce fetal P_{O_2} levels and fetal metabolism. Smoking, by increasing the amount of carboxyhaemoglobin in the maternal circulation, effectively reduces the amount of oxygen available to the fetus, thus causing growth restriction. A wide variety of drugs other than tobacco can affect fetal growth: alcohol, marijuana, heroin and cocaine are all associated with fetal growth restriction, probably through multiple mechanisms affecting fetal enzyme systems, placental blood flow and maternal substrate levels.

In developed countries, the most common cause of IUGR is poor placental function, secondary to inadequate trophoblast invasion of the uterine decidua and myometrial spiral arteries. This results in reduced perfusion of the intracotyledonary space, which leads to abnormal development of the terminal villi and impaired transfer of oxygen and nutrients to the fetus. Less frequently, reduced perfusion can occur from other conditions, such as a severe diabetes mellitus, the antiphospholipid syndrome and sickle-cell disease. Multiple gestation usually results in a sharing of the uterine vascularity, which causes a relative reduction in the blood flow to each placenta. On the fetal side of the placental circulation, abnormalities of the umbilical cord, such as a single umbilical artery, is associated with IUGR, as are the intraplacental vascular connections found in monochorionic twinning.

Pathophysiology

Intrauterine growth restriction fetuses are frequently described as symmetrical or asymmetrical in terms of their body proportions. Symmetrically small fetuses are usually associated with factors that directly impair the intrauterine growth potential of the fetus (i.e. chromosome abnormalities, viral infections, etc.), while asymmetrical growth restriction is classically associated with uteroplacental insufficiency. The cause of fetal

asymmetry follows upon the reduced oxygen transfer to the fetus and impaired excretion of carbon dioxide by the placenta. The resulting fall in P_{O_2} and rise in P_{CO_2} in the fetal blood will induce a chemoreceptor response in the fetal carotid bodies, with resulting vasodilatation in the fetal brain, myocardium and adrenal glands and vasoconstriction in the kidneys, splanchnic vessels, limbs and subcutaneous tissues. The liver circulation is also severely reduced. Normally, 50 per cent of the well-oxygenated blood in the umbilical vein passes to the right atrium through the ductus venosus, eventually to reach the fetal brain, with the remainder going to the portal circulation in the liver. When there is fetal hypoxia, more of the well-oxygenated blood from the umbilical vein is diverted through the ductus venosus, which means that the liver receives less. The result of all these circulatory changes is an asymmetrical fetus with relative brain sparing, reduced abdominal girth and skin thickness. The vasoconstriction in the fetal kidneys results in impaired urine production and oligohydramnios. The fetal hypoxaemia also leads to severe metabolic changes in the fetus reflecting intrauterine starvation. Antenatal fetal blood sampling has shown reduced levels of nutrients such as glucose and amino acids (especially essential amino acids) and of hormones such as thyroxine and insulin. There are increased levels of corticosteroids and catecholamines, which reflect the increased perfusion of the adrenal gland. Haematological changes also reflect the chronic hypoxia, with increased levels of erythropoietin and nucleated red blood cells.

The fetal hypoxia eventually leads to fetal acidaemia, both respiratory and metabolic, which if prolonged can lead to intrauterine death if the fetus is not removed from its hostile environment. IUGR fetuses are especially at risk from profound asphyxia in labour due to the further compromise of the uteroplacental circulation caused by the uterine contractions.

Investigation

The prediction and detection of the IUGR fetus are the principal aims of antenatal care, and the earlier the diagnosis is made, the better the chance of improving the outlook for the fetus. On the premise that most IUGR fetuses are SGA, most antenatal screening programmes for IUGR judge their efficacy on the ability to predict the birth weight of an infant below the

5th centile birth weight for gestation. The detection of an SGA infant contains two elements: first, the accurate assessment of gestational age, and second, the recognition of fetal smallness.

As described in Chapter 6, early measurement of the fetal crown–rump length before 12 weeks or the biparietal diameter between 12 and 20 weeks is routinely carried out in most hospitals and provides the most accurate assessment of gestational age. If there is any discrepancy between the assessments made at 12 weeks and 20 weeks, the prediction from the earlier measurement should be accepted. The most precise method of detecting fetal smallness is by ultrasound biometry, in particular, measurement of the biparietal diameter, head circumference, abdominal circumference and femur length. It is logistically impossible to repeat these measurements in all pregnancies, so serial ultrasound biometry is usually performed on the following groups.

- Pregnant mothers who have had a previous SGA fetus, who are of low pre-pregnancy weight (<40 kg), who are heavy smokers and/or drug abusers, have a medical condition such as hypertension, antiphospholipid syndrome or diabetes, or who give a history of eating disorders or persistent hyperemesis.
- Pregnancies where twins have been diagnosed at the first or second trimester scan.
- Pregnancies where there are abnormal uterine artery waveforms at the mid-pregnancy scan (this is only performed in a few hospitals).
- Pregnancies where the symphysis–fundal height measurement, which is made at each visit to the antenatal clinic, is more than 3 cm below the expected size for the gestational age.

When a diagnosis of SGA has been made, the next step is to establish whether this represents IUGR or whether the fetus is 'small normal'. A careful ultrasound scan of the fetal anatomy should be made to detect whether there are any fetal abnormalities to explain fetal smallness that may have been missed on the second trimester scan. Even if the anatomy is normal, if the fetal head and femur are disproportionately small or if there is an increased amount of amniotic fluid, this would raise the suspicion of a fetal genetic defect and, under these circumstances, an amniocentesis and rapid fetal karyotype should be offered. Features suspicious of uteroplacental insufficiency would be an asymmetrical fetus with a relatively small abdominal circumference, oligohydramnios and a high umbilical artery resistance.

Management

At present, there are no widely accepted treatments available for growth restriction related to placental dysfunction. Obvious adverse factors such as smoking, alcohol and drug abuse should be stopped and the health of the woman should be maximized (optimize control of diabetes, thyroid dysfunction, etc.). When growth restriction is severe, and the fetus is considered too immature to be delivered, bed rest in hospital is usually advised in an effort to maximize placental blood flow. The aim of these interventions is to gain as much maturity as possible before delivering the fetus, thereby reducing the morbidity associated with prematurity. A growth-restricted baby weighing 1 kg and delivered at 32 weeks' gestation usually has a less stormy neonatal course than does a normally grown baby delivered at 28 weeks' gestation with the same birth weight.

Timing delivery to maximize gestation without the baby dying in utero involves intensive fetal surveillance. The most widely accepted methods of monitoring the fetus are discussed in Chapter 8. In brief, serial ultrasound scans are performed to establish that some fetal growth is maintained; cessation of fetal growth may be an indication in itself for delivery. However, fetal biometry cannot give meaningful estimates of growth rate at intervals of less than 2 weeks, so dynamic tests of fetal well-being such as Doppler ultrasound and fetal cardiotocography are now the principal means of determining fetal well-being. Absence of blood flow in the umbilical artery during fetal cardiac diastole or reversed flow (i.e. back towards the heart) requires delivery in the near future, as it reflects high placental resistance and is usually a preterminal event. When this situation is seen at periviable gestations (24–28 weeks), more complicated fetal arterial and venous Doppler studies are used in some tertiary centres in an attempt to delay delivery. Unlike the umbilical artery Doppler, the role of other fetal Doppler studies has not yet been proven by large prospective trials.

No effective drug therapy for IUGR has yet been found. Small studies have suggested that aspirin, nitric oxide donors or anti-oxidants may be helpful in some cases. These drugs may act by reducing platelet activation in the uteroplacental circulation, or may be acting directly as vasodilators. Larger, prospective, placebo-controlled studies are awaited to assess the use of these agents in either the prevention or treatment of IUGR.

Prognosis

The main danger to the baby is intrauterine death, due either to failure in making the diagnosis or to excessive delay prior to delivery. Some babies will suffer morbidity, or die, as a result of premature delivery. The long-term prognosis for survivors is good, with low incidences of mental or physical handicap. Whilst height and weight curves for these infants remain slightly below the 50th centile, most infants with IUGR secondary to placental insufficiency show 'catch-up' growth after delivery, when feeding can be optimized. Where IUGR is related to a congenital infection, or chromosomal anomaly, subsequent development of the child will be determined by the precise abnormality present.

A link between IUGR and the adult incidence of both hypertension and diabetes has now been established. It remains to be seen whether other associations will be found in the future.

Placental abruption

Definition

This is uterine bleeding following premature separation of a normally sited placenta. It is concealed in approximately one-third of cases (i.e. no blood loss is seen per vagina) and revealed in two-thirds of cases.

Incidence

This has been documented as between 0.5 and 2.0 per cent of pregnancies, but varies depending on the criteria used for diagnosis. Where diagnosis is based on histological examination of the placenta, the incidence has been reported to be as high as 4 per cent.

Aetiology

This is unknown in the majority of cases, although there is evidence for an association with defective trophoblastic invasion, as with pre-eclampsia and growth restriction. Other associations include direct abdominal trauma (e.g. road traffic accidents, assault, external cephalic version), high parity, uterine over-distension (polyhydramnios and multiple gestation),

sudden decompression of the uterus (e.g. after delivery of the first twin or release of polyhydramnios) and smoking. The association with hypertension may reflect a direct cause, or may be a manifestation of poor trophoblastic invasion.

Risk factors for placental abruption

- Hypertension
- Smoking
- Trauma to abdomen
- Crack cocaine usage
- Anticoagulant therapy
- Polyhydramnios
- Low socio-economic group
- Intrauterine growth restriction

Clinical presentation

The classical presentation is that of abdominal pain, vaginal bleeding and uterine contractions. The vaginal bleeding is usually dark and non-clotting; however, as the bleeding may be concealed, its absence does not preclude the diagnosis. Abruptio placentae often occurs close to term and frequently during labour. Although abdominal pain is a common feature, and is probably due to extravasation of blood into the myometrium, 'silent' abruptions have also been described. Some patients present additionally with nausea, restlessness and faintness.

Clinical features of placental abruption

- Tender, tense uterus
- Tachycardia and hypotension out of proportion to vaginal bleeding
- Renal compromise
- Coagulation disorders: possibly disseminated intravascular coagulation

---

If blood loss is significant, there may be signs of hypovolaemic shock, with increased pulse rate, hypotension and signs of peripheral vasoconstriction. Abdominal palpation reveals a tender uterus that is often described as being 'woody hard'. The uterus may be larger than gestation suggests and the fetus is often difficult to palpate.

Depending on the size of the abruption, and the area of placental separation, the fetus may be dead, in distress or unaffected. Vaginal examination may reveal blood or cervical dilatation if the abruption has precipitated labour.

Diagnosis

This is usually made on clinical grounds. Where abruption has not been severe, the diagnosis may only be made by inspection of the placenta after the third stage of labour is complete. Ultrasound can be helpful in some cases, demonstrating retro-placental clot and excluding placenta praevia. Ultrasound examination is also important where abruption is managed conservatively (see 'Effects on the fetus', below). The differential diagnosis of placental abruption can be broadly divided into two groups: other causes of vaginal bleeding and other causes of abdominal pain in pregnancy.

Effects on the mother

Hypovolaemic shock
There is a tendency to underestimate the amount of blood loss. This is due to some haemorrhage being concealed behind the placenta and within the uterine wall. In addition, some patients will have been hypertensive prior to the abruption, masking the hypotensive effect of blood loss. Central venous pressure measurement is extremely helpful, both in assessing the degree of blood loss and in accurate fluid replacement.

Disseminated intravascular coagulation
DIC is always a secondary phenomenon following a trigger to generalized activation of coagulation systems. Consumption of fibrin, clotting factors and platelets occurs, resulting in continued bleeding and further depletion of these factors. The triggers known to precipitate DIC include tissue thromboplastin release, endothelial damage to small vessels and pro-coagulant phospholipid production secondary to intravascular coagulation. The incidence is very variable, but serious DIC probably affects about 0.1 per cent of pregnancies. Laboratory investigations include measuring

the thrombin time (estimating clottable fibrinogen in whole blood), fibrin degradation products (FDPs) and platelet count. These tests should be repeated at regular intervals as resuscitation takes place. In cases of significant DIC, it is vital to involve the haematologist in the early care of the woman.

Acute renal failure
This is a consequence of poor renal perfusion, secondary to hypovolaemia, hypotension and DIC (microthrombi in the kidneys). The patient initially becomes oliguric and may develop acute tubular necrosis if the reduced renal perfusion is prolonged. After adequate fluid replacement and treatment of the DIC, the patient may become polyuric, during which phase the plasma urea and creatinine concentrations may continue to rise. Fluid, acid–base and electrolyte balance must be carefully monitored. Dialysis may be required. In general, the prognosis for acute renal failure after placental abruption in women who are adequately resuscitated is excellent.

Feto-maternal haemorrhage
This can lead to sensitization of the mother to fetal blood group antigens. This is particularly important for the rhesus D blood group, and all mothers who are D negative should have a Kleihauer test to quantify the size of the feto-maternal haemorrhage and an appropriate dose of anti-D immunoglobulin.

Maternal mortality
Successive Confidential Enquiries into Maternal Deaths continue to record placental abruption as a significant cause of death, usually as a consequence of the complications listed above.

Recurrence
After a single episode of abruption, the recurrence rate is approximately 10 per cent, increasing to 25 per cent after two episodes.

Effects on the fetus

Perinatal mortality
Abruption is a significant cause of fetal and neonatal loss. Perinatal mortality rates are influenced by the size of abruption, interval to delivery, gestational age at which the abruption and delivery have occurred,

and other associated factors such as growth retardation related to poor placentation.

Intrauterine growth restriction

This probably has two main components. The first cause is probably inadequate trophoblast invasion of the maternal decidua and spiral arteries, as with the increased risk of pre-eclampsia. Where abruption is chronic, or recurrent, the area of placenta available for nutrient and waste exchange between the fetus and the mother is reduced. This may also contribute to fetal growth restriction.

Management

A large placental abruption is an obstetric emergency, as it is life threatening for both mother and fetus. The immediate management of a patient with a large antepartum haemorrhage due to placental abruption is discussed in detail in Chapter 18.

Where smaller degrees of abruption have occurred and there is no evidence of fetal distress, particularly where gestational age favours delaying the delivery to allow greater fetal maturity, conservative management may be instituted. This will require close monitoring of fetal well-being, using ultrasound scans of fetal growth, amniotic fluid volume, umbilical artery Doppler and cardiotocography. As with many complicated obstetric problems, the timing of delivery will be based on when the perceived risks of leaving the fetus undelivered outweigh the risks of premature delivery, and the decision is best taken in conjunction with either local paediatricians or the regional neonatal unit.

Key Points

- Abnormal trophoblast invasion in the first trimester of pregnancy will not enable a low-resistance uteroplacental circulation to develop.
- The mechanism for this is not known, but its presence can be detected non-invasively by uterine artery Doppler ultrasound in the second trimester: 'notched' uterine artery waveforms indicate high resistance to flow before any problem is manifest.
- The consequences of abnormal trophoblast invasion are pre-eclampsia, IUGR, placental abruption and intrauterine death.
- The search for effective prophylaxis of these conditions has to date been only partially successful, and remains a major aim of perinatal medicine for the future.

Additional reading

James DK, Steer PJ, Weiner CP, Gonik B. *High risk pregnancy*, 2nd edn. London: WB Saunders, 1999.
Lewis G (ed.) *Why mothers die 1997–1999. The Confidential Enquiries into Maternal Deaths in the United Kingdom*. London: RCOG Press, 2001. http://www.cemach.org.uk/publications/CEMDreports/cemdrpt.pdf

Preterm labour

OVERVIEW

Spontaneous preterm labour and preterm prelabour rupture of membranes account for approximately two-thirds of preterm births. They are the predominant causes of perinatal mortality and morbidity. To achieve significant reductions in this perinatal mortality and morbidity, efforts must focus on the earliest births, particularly those before 32 weeks' gestation. As well as the prognosis, the aetiology underlying spontaneous preterm delivery varies with gestational age.

Definition

In pregnancy, term refers to the gestational period from 37^{+0} to 41^{+6} weeks, with preterm births occurring between 24^{+0} and 36^{+6} weeks. Although earlier births are referred to as miscarriages, occasional survivors are seen after delivery at 23 weeks. Preterm births occur either because delivery is felt to be in the best interests of the mother or baby (indicated preterm deliveries) or because the mother goes into spontaneous labour earlier than normal (spontaneous preterm births). The latter group is the focus of this chapter and has two sub-divisions: spontaneous preterm labour and preterm prelabour rupture of membranes (PPROM). Each of these three groups accounts for one-third of early births (Fig. 14.1).

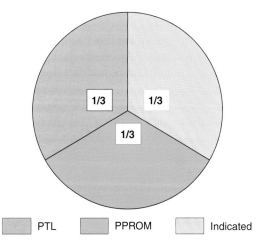

Figure 14.1 Origin of preterm births. (PTL, preterm labour; PPROM, preterm prelabour rupture of membranes.)

Prevalence

Gestationally based national data are difficult to obtain in the UK. In 1994–95, 6.6 per cent of all UK births were preterm, approximately 40 000 deliveries per annum. It is much easier to find current data based on birth weight. Of all babies born in the UK in 2002, 7.7 per cent weighed less than 2500 g. Although this roughly approximates to preterm births, it also includes intrauterine growth restriction (IUGR) in term births and macrosomia in preterm ones.

Significantly higher rates of preterm birth of 11 per cent are reported from the USA. Conversely, many Nordic countries with very reliable data quote rates below 5 per cent. This must reflect, at least in part, differing socio-economic and cultural factors.

There is no evidence that the incidence of preterm birth is declining. In fact, the rate appears to be slowly increasing, in part due to an increasing incidence of multiple pregnancy.

Preterm births contribute significantly to perinatal mortality and morbidity. Babies born before 32 weeks account for more than half of all perinatal mortality. Survival figures for the UK for each gestational age have been published (Fig. 14.2). Predicted survival can be modified if accurate information concerning fetal sex, weight and well-being is available. Parents are particularly anxious about the risks of later disability and handicap. These risks are especially significant below 28 weeks' gestation. Half the survivors at 23–25 weeks' gestation will have some functional impairment, often amounting to severe disability. There are other long-term worries after very preterm births, including subsequent growth, educational needs and social behaviour. There may also be influences on later adult health.

Classification

For reasons related to aetiology, outcome and recurrence risk, preterm births should be divided into three gestational periods: mildly preterm births at 32^{+0} to 36^{+6} weeks (incidence 5.5 per cent), very preterm births at 28^{+0} to 31^{+6} weeks (incidence 0.7 per cent), and extremely preterm births at 24^{+0} to 27^{+6} weeks (incidence 0.4 per cent).

Aetiology

Infection

Subclinical infection of the choriodecidual space and amniotic fluid is the most widely studied aetiological factor underlying spontaneous preterm births. In most cases, the bacteria are thought to ascend from the vagina. Vaginal colonization with a variety of genital tract micro-organisms, including bacterial vaginosis (BV), has been associated with an increased risk of spontaneous preterm delivery. Early-onset neonatal sepsis, maternal postpartum endometritis and histological chorioamnionitis are all significantly more common after preterm birth.

Over-distension

In pregnancy, there are two main causes of uterine over-distension: multiple pregnancy and polyhydramnios.

Vascular

Antepartum haemorrhage and abruption are commonly reported prior to spontaneous preterm deliveries. Blood is known to irritate the myometrium and weaken the membranes.

Intercurrent illness

Serious infective illnesses such as pyelonephritis, appendicitis and pneumonia are associated with

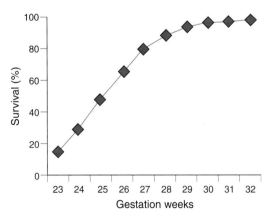

Figure 14.2 Median survival of infants alive at the onset of labour in the UK Trent Health Region for 1998–2001.

preterm labour. In these cases, preterm labour is presumed to be due either to direct blood-borne spread of infection to the uterine cavity or indirectly to chemical triggers, such as endotoxins or cytokines. Many other illnesses, such as cholestasis of pregnancy, and surgical procedures are associated with preterm labour, although the mechanisms for this remain obscure.

Cervical weakness

This remains a notoriously difficult diagnosis to make, either within or outside of pregnancy.

Idiopathic

In many cases, especially mildly preterm births, no cause will be found. In these cases, the physiological pathways to parturition may simply have been turned on too early.

Other physiology

Fetal fibronectin (fFN) is a 'glue-like' protein binding the choriodecidual membranes. It is rarely present in vaginal secretions between 23 and 34 weeks. Any disruption at the choriodecidual interface results in fFN release and possible detection in the cervico-vaginal secretions. Such a disruption commonly precedes preterm labour, often by many weeks. Two tests are available to detect fFN in the vaginal secretions: a slow, quantitative, laboratory-based assay gives precise concentrations, and a rapid, qualitative, bedside test has been designed to give a positive/negative result.

Risk factors

Risk factors for preterm labour/PPROM

Non-modifiable, major
- Last birth preterm: 20% risk
- Last two births preterm: 40% risk
- Twin pregnancy: 50% risk
- Uterine abnormalities
- Congenital anomalies:
  - cervical damage (cone biopsy, repeated dilatation)
  - fibroids (cervical)

- Factors in current pregnancy:
  - recurrent antepartum haemorrhage
  - intercurrent illness (e.g. sepsis)
  - any surgery

Non-modifiable, minor
- Teenagers having second or subsequent babies
- Parity (=0 or >5)
- Ethnicity (black women)
- Poor socio-economic status
- Education (not beyond secondary)

Modifiable
- Smoking: two-fold increase of PPROM
- Drugs of abuse: especially cocaine
- Body mass index (BMI) <20: underweight women
- Inter-pregnancy interval <1 year

Clinical features – preterm labour

History

The diagnosis of preterm labour remains notoriously difficult in the absence of advanced dilatation (>3 cm) or ruptured membranes. Less than 50 per cent of all women presenting with threatened preterm labour will deliver within 7 days. Symptoms such as low backache or cramping are often cyclical. Vague complaints such as pelvic pressure or increased discharge are also common. The co-existence of vaginal bleeding should always be taken seriously. Too much emphasis is often placed on the contraction frequency. In isolation, it correlates poorly with the risk of preterm birth. Markers of intensity, such as analgesic requirements or simple bedside clinical impression, may add refinement.

Examination

Abdominal examination may reveal the presence of uterine tenderness, suggesting abruption or chorioamnionitis. A careful speculum examination by an experienced clinician may yield valuable information; pooling of amniotic fluid, blood and/or abnormal discharge may be observed. A visual assessment of cervical dilatation is usually possible and has been shown to be as accurate as digital examination findings. Digital exams should be limited, as they are known to stimulate prostaglandin production and may introduce organisms into the cervical canal.

Differential diagnosis

- Urinary tract infection
- Red degeneration of fibroid
- Placental abruption
- Constipation
- Gastroenteritis

Investigations

Bedside fibronectin

Bedside fibronectin testing offers a rapid assessment of risk in symptomatic women with minimal cervical dilatation. If performed correctly, the test has a greater predictive value than digital examination. In one study, 30 per cent of women with a positive fibronectin test delivered within 7 days, compared with only 10 per cent of women who were 2–3 cm dilated.

Cervical length

Cervical length measurement by transvaginal ultrasound has also been shown to improve diagnostic accuracy. A normal cervix measures approximately 35 mm in length (Fig. 14.3a). Significant cervical shortening is often accompanied by dilatation and funnelling of the membranes down the cervical canal (Fig. 14.3b). Although measurements can be repeated frequently and with little expense, skilled ultrasonographers and suitable machines with transvaginal probes are required.

Repeat vaginal examination

Repeat vaginal examination in 1–4 hours should be considered essential in the absence of specialized tests. The interval between assessments should be guided by the severity of the symptoms.

Clinical features – preterm prelabour rupture of the membranes

History

The most reliable diagnostic feature of PPROM from the history is the report of a 'gush of fluid' vaginally, usually followed by a more-or-less continuous dribble. This must be distinguished from leaking urine (ask about frequency, urgency, leakage and dysuria), as incontinence or a urinary tract infection (UTI) may present in a similar way. The presence of any vaginal discharge should be ascertained. Fetal movements may be reduced in strength or frequency after PPROM, and occasionally uterine irritability or contractions may be reported.

Examination

Infection may lead to an increased pulse and temperature and a flushed appearance. Abdominal examination may reveal a clinical suspicion of oligohydramnios or uterine tenderness if chorioamnionitis is present. The definitive diagnosis of PPROM can only be made by performing a sterile speculum examination; a pool of amniotic fluid in the posterior vagina is diagnostic. It is also important at this point to visualize the cervix and establish whether dilatation is present. Digital vaginal examinations should be avoided if possible in

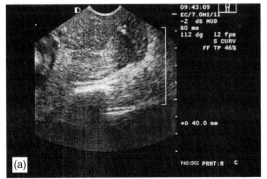
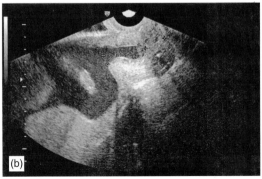

Figure 14.3 (a) Normal cervix. (b) Cervical length and funnelling on ultrasound.

PPROM, as they are associated with a significant reduction in the latent interval before labour. This reduction is most dramatic at the earliest gestations.

Investigations

Nitrazine testing

Amniotic fluid is alkaline, whereas the vaginal secretions are usually acidic. An elevated pH turns a nitrazine stick black. Some units use nitrazine sticks to define the presence of amniotic fluid. Unfortunately, false positives occur, with blood, semen and even urine limiting its usefulness. However, the predictive value of a negative test is very high.

Genital tract swabs

A high vaginal swab (HVS) may help to guide antibiotic therapy, if subsequently required. Screening for group B *Streptococcus* (GBS) can also be performed, as there is a substantial risk of labour in the next few days.

Maternal well-being

This should include regular assessment of the mother's blood pressure, pulse and temperature. Some advise serial white cell counts and C-reactive proteins, used as early markers of infection.

Fetal well-being

Serial antepartum cardiotocography is important after PPROM, as a gradually increasing baseline heart rate or fetal tachycardia is suggestive of intrauterine infection.

Ultrasound

Ultrasound can give valuable information about the amniotic fluid volume. The presence or absence of oligohydramnios provides further diagnostic support. In established PPROM, there is a direct correlation between the amount of amniotic fluid remaining and the latency period. Unlike preterm labour, cervical length measurements do not have predictive ability in PPROM.

Amniocentesis

A sample of amniotic fluid can be sent for Gram stain, microscopy and culture, to establish whether there is an intrauterine infection (chorioamnionitis). There is, however, a risk of stimulating preterm labour by performing an invasive test, and amniocentesis can be technically very difficult if there is virtually no amniotic fluid.

Treatment

Maternal steroids

Current evidence shows that a single course of maternal steroids (two injections 12–24 hours apart) given between 28 and 34 weeks' gestation and received within 7 days of delivery results in markedly improved neonatal outcomes. This is primarily due to a reduction in neonatal respiratory distress syndrome (RDS). Maximum benefit from the injection is seen after 48 hours. Courses received less than 48 hours or more than 7 days before delivery still lead to benefit, as may courses given below 28 weeks.

There is considerable reassuring evidence about the long-term safety of single courses of maternal steroids, with paediatric follow-up into the teenage years. However, there is growing concern about adverse consequences of repeat dosing. Like antibiotics, steroids have the potential for harm in pregnancy and should be used carefully.

Tocolytics

The Canadian Preterm Labor Trial remains the most influential tocolytic trial to date. It concluded that ritodrine had no significant benefit on perinatal mortality or the prolongation of pregnancy to term, although it was able to reduce the number of women delivering within 48 hours by 40 per cent. This window of opportunity is the sole reason for using tocolytics. If steroids have been given and special care baby unit cots are available, tocolytics are probably inappropriate. Beta-agonists have significant maternal side effects, and maternal deaths from acute cardiopulmonary compromise are described. There are now accepted guidelines for their use involving small-volume infusions. The oxytocin antagonist atosiban now has a UK product licence. Although side effects are less frequent, it has no greater clinical effectiveness than ritodrine and the cost is much higher. Other smooth muscle relaxants used to treat preterm labour include magnesium sulphate, nifedipine and glyceryl trinitrate. There is no evidence of increased efficacy or improved outcomes with any of them.

As prostaglandins appear to be one of the pivotal chemicals involved in parturition, non-steroidal anti-inflammatories such as indomethacin have attracted considerable interest as tocolytics. There are potential fetal side effects, but these can be limited by restricting use to less than 72 hours below 30 weeks' gestation.

Antibiotics

The Medical Research Council Oracle Study concluded that the routine use of antibiotics in uncomplicated preterm labour did not confer benefit. However, a 10-day course of erythromycin led to improved neonatal outcomes after PPROM. Most North American centres continue to give intrapartum antibiotics to women in preterm labour unless GBS status is known to be negative.

Fetal assessment

Maternal steroid therapy can suppress both fetal activity and heart rate variability. Doppler studies are not influenced. Whenever possible, the presentation in preterm labour should be confirmed by ultrasound, as clinical palpation is notoriously unreliable. An estimated fetal weight, particularly below 28 weeks, can be helpful. Preterm infants have less reserve to tolerate the stress of labour, particularly in the presence of oligohydramnios. Therefore, continuous fetal monitoring is required, although there may be considerable difficulties interpreting the fetal heart rate pattern in extremely preterm infants.

Mode of delivery

Many clinicians feel that fetal morbidity and mortality, the difficulty in diagnosing intrapartum hypoxia/acidosis and maternal risk do not justify Caesarean section for fetal indications below 26 weeks. As gestation advances, both neonatal outcomes and the ability to diagnose fetal compromise improve, and intervention for fetal reasons becomes appropriate. The safety of preterm breech vaginal delivery is often questioned and Caesarean section commonly performed.

Type of Caesarean section

At the earliest gestations and in the presence of oligohydramnios, the lower segment is often poorly formed. Vertical uterine incisions may be necessary. This 'classical' uterine incision carries an up to 5 per cent risk of uterine rupture in subsequent pregnancies, some of which will occur antenatally.

Analgesia

In terms of intrapartum analgesia, the use of epidural anaesthesia is frequently advocated. Postulated benefits include avoiding expulsive efforts before full dilatation or a precipitous delivery, a relaxed pelvic floor and perineum and the ability to proceed quickly to abdominal delivery.

Communication

There are two vital areas of communication in the management of threatened preterm labour or PPROM. Communication with the woman and her family ensures that they have a full understanding of the risks involved and enables a clear management plan to be discussed. Communication with the neonatal unit staff ensures that adequate and appropriate resources are available at the time of delivery. Parents often appreciate the opportunity to have discussed the care of their baby with the neonatology staff in advance of delivery.

In-utero transfer

If local resources are unable to care for the newborn, in-utero transfer to a unit with adequate neonatal facilities is recommended. It is generally accepted that this will improve the outcome for babies.

Management of high-risk asymptomatic women

Due to limited resources, most aspects of prematurity prevention are targeted at asymptomatic women with known risk factors for preterm birth. After a preterm birth, a postnatal visit should be organized to review the events leading to the delivery and any investigations taken at the time, such as placental apthology. Ideally, a management plan for any subsequent pregnancy should be made. If first seen in early pregnancy, a careful analysis of events surrounding the last birth must be undertaken.

Early dating scan

A first trimester dating scan ensures the precise assessment of gestational age in the current pregnancy.

Bacterial vaginosis

Bacterial vaginosis has been associated with an increased risk of preterm birth in many observational studies. Randomized studies have demonstrated that oral antibiotics such as clindamycin or metronidazole significantly lower the risk of preterm birth, by 60 per cent in high-risk women positive for BV. In contrast, no benefit has been found from treating low-risk BV-positive women.

Asymptomatic bacteriuria

This also carries an increased risk of preterm birth. Short courses of antibiotics based on culture sensitivities should be prescribed.

Group B streptococcal genital colonization

Preterm infants are more susceptible to early-onset GBS infection, acquired during passage through the birth canal. In women known to be at increased risk of early delivery, testing for GBS antenatally with a combined low vaginal/rectal swab allows appropriate intrapartum prophylaxis. Antenatal treatment has repeatedly been shown to be of no benefit.

Cervical ultrasound

Cervical length can be accurately and repeatedly measured by transvaginal ultrasound. In asymptomatic women with a short cervix, the risk of very preterm delivery rises to 4 per cent with lengths of 11–20 mm. At 10 mm, the risk is 15 per cent, and it increases dramatically with further decreases in length. When significant cervical shortening is found before 24 weeks' gestation, cervical cerclage is an option (see Chapter 10). At present, randomized trials are yielding conflicting results. In the presence of a normal cervical length, cerclage can usually be deferred.

Fetal fibronectin

Fetal fibronection testing can only be undertaken after 23 weeks, as high levels may be physiological before then. In high-risk asymptomatic women with a positive fibronectin test at 24 weeks' gestation, nearly half will deliver before 30 weeks' gestation. Conversely, the chance of such an early birth is less than 1 per cent with a negative test.

Tocolysis

Many studies, meta-analyses and reviews have shown no evidence of benefit from oral or maintenance tocolytics.

Lifestyle modification

Randomized trials of social support in the UK failed to improve pregnancy outcomes. In some studies, hospitalization for bed rest led to an increase in preterm birth. Roles for sexual abstinence and/or psychological support are no clearer.

Key Points

- Preterm delivery complicates about 7 per cent of UK pregnancies.
- Major risk factors are a previous early birth and multiple pregnancy.
- The diagnosis of spontaneous preterm labour is difficult before advanced cervical dilatation.
- Histological chorioamnionitis is much more common after spontaneous preterm birth than after either term birth or indicated preterm deliveries.
- Ninety per cent of histologically proven cases of chorioamnionitis are sub-clinical with no overt clinical signs of infection.
- The most beneficial treatment in preterm labour is with maternal steroids, which substantially improve neonatal outcomes.

New developments

- Epidemiological evidence suggests an increased chance of a positive thrombophilia screen after preterm deliveries associated with evidence of placental dysfunction such as abruption, recurrent bleeding or IUGR. Whether this translates into an increased recurrence risk is unclear, as is the role of treatment.

- Inflammatory cytokines are now thought to be involved in the aetiology of many neonatal injuries, such as bronchopulmonary dysplasia and cerebral palsy. High levels of these chemicals are found in preterm births complicated by chorioamnionitis.
- Recent studies suggest a possible role for progesterone supplementation in the prevention of preterm birth.

CASE HISTORY

Mrs A, a 28-year-old Nigerian, is a non-smoker and works as a catering manager in a school. She and her husband (a building society manager) live in their own home.

This is her third pregnancy. At the age of 18, she had a termination of pregnancy at 10 weeks' gestation. At the age of 27, she had a spontaneous vaginal delivery at 30 weeks' gestation. The baby was born in good condition, weighing 1.6 kg, and required 5 weeks in the neonatal unit. Mrs A had a knife cone biopsy 3 years ago and a normal cervical smear 2 years ago. She has no history of pelvic inflammatory disease. She had an appendicectomy at the age of 26.

She is now 8 weeks pregnant, fit and well, and is taking iron supplements. When seen in the antenatal booking clinic, concerns were raised about her risks of having a further episode of preterm labour.

What risk factors does Mrs A have for preterm labour?

Termination of pregnancy in the first trimester is unlikely to predispose towards preterm labour. However, having had a previous preterm labour and delivery at 30 + 5 weeks is a definite risk factor and puts her in the 'high-risk' category.

A knife cone biopsy is probably more traumatic to cervical competence than the more commonly performed LLETZ (long loop excision of the transformation zone) procedure and may have affected cervical function, leading to an increased risk of preterm labour. Mrs A is therefore at high risk of having a preterm delivery.

What care should Mrs A receive?

In view of her high risk of preterm delivery, she should receive consultant-led care in a hospital. It may be a good idea for her to meet a neonatologist, and to be shown around the neonatal unit. Some units, especially in the USA, utilize home monitoring of contractions (tocography) to assess the possible onset of preterm labour.

How can her risk be more accurately assessed?

Clinical risk factors for preterm labour, as described above, are only good enough to be a vague guide as to the likelihood of preterm delivery. Further measures that may allow not only greater predictive accuracy but also the chance of intervening to improve outcome include screening for BV, scanning for cervical length and fFN assay (see 'New developments' above).

Medical diseases complicating pregnancy

OVERVIEW

Pregnancy is a normal physiological event during which most women remain fit and well. However, it may cause specific medical conditions. There are few medical disorders that are associated with sterility, although some may reduce a woman's fertility. Therefore it is not uncommon to encounter pregnant women with pre-existing medical diseases. Both pregnancy-specific and pre-existing medical conditions may in some circumstances be associated with significant maternal and fetal morbidity and, more rarely, mortality.

A multidisciplinary approach is vital in helping to ensure appropriate levels of care for pregnant women with medical problems. Members of such a team include specialist midwives, obstetricians, physicians and obstetric anaesthetists, and dieticians and physiotherapists will often provide support. Ideally, assessment of medical conditions and discussion regarding any implications for pregnancy should be available and offered and a plan of care documented before pregnancy. Such pre-conception counselling does occur, but it is not universal and often takes place either once the woman becomes pregnant or after a first pregnancy has ended in failure. For example, women with insulin-dependent diabetes should only embark on pregnancy when their diabetic control is very tight; failure to do so is associated with a significantly increased risk of pregnancy failure, complications and fetal abnormality. Counselling prior to the pregnancy allows women with, for example, severe heart or renal disease to understand the possible risks in pregnancy and the level of antenatal care they will require.

Contraceptive advice

In women in whom pregnancy or further pregnancies are not advised, contraceptive advice is extremely important. Women with medical problems are often advised against using the combined oral contraceptive pill, because of real (hypertension, thromboembolism) or perceived (insignificant heart disease) contraindications. They are thus denied an effective form of contraception, and efforts should be taken to ensure appropriate advice is given regarding effective alternatives such as an intrauterine system (Mirena) or implantable progesterone-only contraceptive (Implanon). Barrier methods may be appropriate, but they have a higher failure rate so should not be recommended as the sole form of contraception in those for whom pregnancy would be dangerous. An intrauterine contraceptive device is associated with an increased risk of infection, not to be desired in a woman with diabetes, for example.

Heart disease

Prevalence and aetiology

Heart disease in pregnancy is rare, but potentially serious, and complicates approximately 1 per cent of all pregnancies. This prevalence varies from one community to another, principally because the incidence of rheumatic heart disease and undiagnosed or uncorrected congenital heart disease is higher in developing countries and in immigrants from such countries. In the UK 50 years ago, rheumatic heart disease accounted for 90 per cent of all heart disease in pregnancy, but since the widespread use of antibiotics in streptococcal infection, this figure has fallen dramatically. Rheumatic heart disease nonetheless remains an important cause of heart disease in ethnic minority immigrants. In contrast, advances in paediatric cardiac surgery since the mid-1960s have resulted in an increase in the number of women with congenital heart disease surviving to reach childbearing age. Congenital heart disease now accounts for approximately 50 per cent of the heart disease in pregnant women in the UK. Acquired ischaemic heart disease is becoming more common in pregnancy, related to a delay in the average age of childbearing and the epidemic of smoking amongst women.

Physiology

Irrespective of the underlying condition, pregnancy imposes a significant burden on the heart due to the normal physiological changes that occur. Both blood volume and cardiac output increase by 40 per cent. The increase in cardiac output is achieved by an increase in stroke volume and a rise in heart rate of 12–15 beats per minute (bpm). These changes are discussed in more detail in Chapter 5.

Maternal risks

Although maternal mortality is seen with all forms of heart disease, it is most likely in conditions that restrict an increase in pulmonary blood flow, typically pulmonary hypertension and mitral stenosis. In these circumstances, an obstruction exists either within the pulmonary vessels or at the mitral valve. There is a 40–50 per cent maternal mortality rate amongst women with pulmonary hypertension and Eisenmenger's syndrome. In other complex cardiac lesions, such as Fallot's tetralogy, the risk of maternal mortality is much lower (5 per cent in some series), because there is no pulmonary hypertension. Other common cardiac causes of maternal death are cardiomyopathy, rupture or dissection of the aorta or its branches and ischaemic heart disease. Infective endocarditis is rare since the use of antibiotics became routine, but fatal cases do occur when the underlying heart defect (often a bicuspid aortic valve) is not recognized. Prior episodes of arrhythmia, heart failure or stroke, severe impairment of left ventricular function or severe left heart obstruction from aortic stenosis or hypertrophic cardiomyopathy (HOCM) predict maternal morbidity in pregnancy.

Fetal risks

The fetus is at increased risk of growth restriction and preterm delivery in pregnancies complicated by cyanotic congenital heart disease, when total fetal loss rate may be as high as 40 per cent. Uncorrected coarctation of the aorta is associated with fetal growth restriction in more than 10 per cent of cases due to reduced placental perfusion.

The incidence of congenital heart disease in the general population is 8 per 1000 live-born babies. If a parent is affected, the risk is increased to 5 per cent. Therefore all pregnant women with congenital heart disease should be referred for expert fetal cardiology scanning.

Pre-pregnancy management

Most women with heart disease will be aware of their condition prior to becoming pregnant. Ideally, such women should be fully assessed before embarking on a pregnancy and the maternal and fetal risks carefully explained. A cardiologist should be involved in this assessment, which should include maternal echocardiography. Any concurrent medical problems should be aggressively treated and medical therapy optimized. If there is a possibility that the heart disease will require surgical correction, it is recommended that this should be undertaken before a pregnancy if at all possible.

Key points in pre-pregnancy counselling are shown in the box below.

Antenatal management

Pregnant women with significant heart disease should be managed in a joint obstetric/cardiac clinic by experienced physicians and obstetricians. Continuity of care makes the detection of subtle changes in maternal well-being more likely. This is important because many of the symptoms and signs of heart failure are common in normal pregnancy, such as breathlessness, tachycardia, ankle swelling, a third heart sound and an ejection systolic heart murmur. In trying to distinguish between these 'normal' symptoms and impending cardiac failure, it is important to ask the woman if she has noted any breathlessness, particularly at night, any change in her heart rate or rhythm, any increased tiredness or a reduction in exercise tolerance. Physical examination should include the points listed in the box below. In the majority of cases, women will remain well during the antenatal period and outpatient management is usually possible, although women should be advised to have a low threshold for reducing their normal physical activities.

Risk factors for the development of heart failure

- Respiratory or urinary infections
- Anaemia
- Obesity
- Corticosteroids
- Tocolytics
- Multiple gestation

- Hypertension
- Arrhythmias
- Pain-related stress
- Fluid overload

Any signs of deteriorating cardiac status should be carefully investigated and treated. Hospital admission for bed rest will reduce the workload of the heart. Admission should not be a blanket policy, but rather it should be assessed on an individual basis.

The use of anticoagulants during pregnancy is a complicated issue because warfarin is teratogenic if used in the first trimester. However, anticoagulation may be essential in patients with congenital heart disease who have pulmonary hypertension or artificial valve replacements and in those in or at risk of atrial fibrillation. There are three broad strategies for anticoagulation in pregnancy; which is chosen will depend on the perceived degree of thrombotic risk and the woman's choice once the risks and benefits have been carefully explained. The first option is to continue warfarin throughout pregnancy, replacing this with heparin for delivery only. As the fetus clears warfarin less rapidly than the mother, the changeover is usually performed 1–2 weeks prior to planned delivery. This is the safest option for the mother with an old-fashioned metal valve in the mitral position. However, warfarin increases the risk of maternal bleeding, teratogenesis, miscarriage and stillbirth and intracerebral bleeding in the fetus. The second option is as the first but replacing warfarin with heparin in the first trimester to avoid the teratogenic risk. The third option is to use heparin throughout pregnancy. Heparin is usually given as subcutaneous low-molecular-weight heparin, but for women with metal valves this may be insufficient, necessitating the use of intravenous unfractionated heparin. Should labour commence whilst the woman is receiving warfarin, fresh frozen plasma (FFP) and vitamin K should be given to reduce the risk of bleeding.

Treatment of heart failure in pregnancy

The development of heart failure in pregnancy is dangerous. The principles of treatment are the same as in the non-pregnant individual. The woman should be admitted and the diagnosis confirmed by clinical examination for signs of heart failure, and echocardiography. Drug therapy may include diuretics, vasodilators and digoxin. Oxygen and morphine may also be required. Dysrhythmias also require urgent correction and drug therapy, including adenosine for supraventricular tachycardias, and selective beta-adrenergic blockade may be required. In all cases, assessment of fetal well-being is essential and should include fetal ultrasound to assess fetal growth and regular cardiotocography (CTG). If there is evidence of fetal compromise, premature delivery may be considered. Similarly, in cases of intractable cardiac failure, the risks to the mother of continuing the pregnancy and the risks to the fetus of premature delivery must be carefully balanced.

> ### Essential points of examination in pregnant women with heart disease
>
> - Pulse rate and rhythm
> - Blood pressure
> - Jugular venous pressure
> - Presence of basal crepitations
> - Ankle and sacral oedema
> - Symphysis–fundal height measurement

Management of labour and delivery

In most cases the aim of management is to await the onset of spontaneous labour, as this will minimize the risk of intervention and maximize the chances of a normal delivery (see box below). Induction of labour should be considered for the normal obstetric indications and in very high-risk women to ensure that delivery occurs at a reasonably predictable time when all the relevant personnel are present or available. Epidural anaesthesia is often recommended, as this reduces the pain-related stress, and thereby some of the demand on cardiac function. Regional anaesthesia and analgesia are not without some risk to both the mother and baby in some cardiac conditions, principally because of the potential complication of maternal hypotension. The input of a senior anaesthetist to formulate and document an anaesthetic management plan and minimize the procedure-related risks is essential. Prophylactic antibiotics should be given to any woman with a structural heart defect to reduce the risk of bacterial endocarditis. Depending on the severity of the condition, other forms of monitoring may be appropriate during labour, including oxygen saturation and continuous arterial blood pressure monitoring.

Additional points in management

> ### Management of labour in women with heart disease
>
> - Avoid induction of labour if possible
> - Use prophylactic antibiotics
> - Ensure fluid balance
> - Avoid the supine position
> - Discuss regional/epidural anaesthesia/analgesia with senior anaesthetist
> - Keep second stage short
> - Use Syntocinon judiciously

Assuming normal progress in labour, the second stage may deliberately be kept short, with an elective forceps or ventouse delivery if normal delivery does not occur readily. This reduces maternal effort and the requirement for increased cardiac output. Caesarean section should only be performed for the normal obstetric indications. Liberal use of Caesarean delivery is associated with an increased risk of haemorrhage, thrombosis and infection, conditions that are likely to be much less well tolerated in women with cardiac disease. Ergometrine may be associated with intense vasoconstriction, hypertension and heart failure, and therefore active management of the third stage is usually with Syntocinon alone. Syntocinon is a vasodilator and therefore should be given slowly to patients with significant heart disease.

Specific heart conditions occurring during pregnancy

Mitral stenosis

Mitral stenosis is the commonest acquired cardiac lesion, accounting for 90 per cent of rheumatic valvular problems. The stenosis produces a left atrial obstruction with consequent elevated left atrial and pulmonary wedge pressures (Fig. 15.1). Eventually, pulmonary oedema and atrial fibrillation may occur. There is a fixed cardiac output, with limited ability to adapt to the increased demands placed on the heart during pregnancy by a raised intravascular volume and heart rate. The most useful investigation is echocardiography, which is able to assess the mitral valve area and left atrial size. Echocardiography performed early in pregnancy will act as a baseline against which subsequent investigations may be compared if there is deterioration in symptoms.

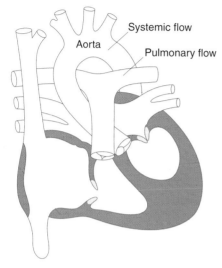

Figure 15.1 Mitral stenosis producing left atrial obstruction.

Significant problems may be anticipated if the valvular area falls below 2 cm². The woman is at particular risk as the cardiac output increases in early pregnancy and also at and immediately after delivery as the third stage leads to autotransfusion of blood from the uterus into the venous circulation. Surgical valvotomy in suitable cases can ideally be undertaken before the pregnancy, although it may be safely performed during pregnancy.

Eisenmenger's syndrome

Eisenmenger's syndrome is associated with a very high maternal mortality, up to 50 per cent. The syndrome develops when initially there is a left-to-right shunt across, for example, a ventricular-septal defect with consequent pulmonary hypertension. Eventually the shunt reverses and cyanosis occurs (Fig. 15.2). The major risk in pregnancy is during labour and delivery, when there may be sudden changes in systemic vascular resistance leading to increased right-to-left shunting and desaturation. Because of the very high maternal mortality, the option of terminating the pregnancy should be carefully discussed with the mother. In women who decide to continue with their pregnancy, miscarriage and fetal growth restriction are common because of the relative hypoxia and cyanosis.

Coarctation of the aorta and Marfan's syndrome

Although coarctation may be detected in childhood, and is therefore usually repaired when encountered in pregnancy, in less severe cases it may not present until the second and third decades when hypertension develops. The principal risk is of dissection of the aorta associated with the increased cardiac output of pregnancy and a possible increase in medial vessel degeneration. In addition, endocarditis, intracranial haemorrhage and death have been reported. There is a 2 per cent risk that the fetus will also develop coarctation. The risk of maternal death in unoperated coarctation is approximately 15 per cent, and the option of termination should be discussed. Antenatally, any hypertension should be aggressively treated.

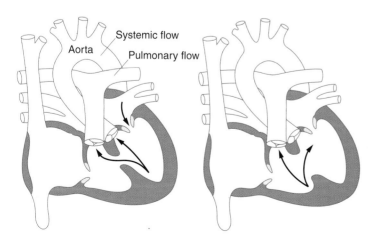

Figure 15.2 Eisenmenger's syndrome: initial left-to-right shunting is reversed, with consequent cyanosis.

Marfan's syndrome is an autosomal dominant connective tissue abnormality that may lead to mitral valve prolapse and aortic regurgitation, aortic root dilatation and aortic rupture or dissection. Pregnancy increases the risk of aortic rupture or dissection and has been associated with maternal mortality of up to 50 per cent with very marked aortic root dilatation.

Echocardiography is the principal investigation, as it is able to determine the size of the aortic root, and should be performed serially throughout pregnancy, especially in women who enter pregnancy with an aortic root that is already dilated.

Hypertensive disorders

Prevalence and aetiology

Hypertensive disease complicates 5–7 per cent of all pregnancies. It may be categorized into pre-existing hypertension, pregnancy-induced hypertension and pre-eclampsia. Pre-existing hypertension may be diagnosed before gestation or assumed when a woman is found to be hypertensive in early pregnancy. Pregnancy-induced hypertension occurs when new-onset hypertension develops in the second half of pregnancy but in the absence of significant proteinuria or any other features of pre-eclampsia (see Chapter 13).

> Hypertension is defined as changes of blood pressure recorded on at least two occasions of either:
> - diastolic blood pressure >90 mmHg, or
> - systolic blood pressure >140 mmHg, or
> - a rise (compared to booking) in diastolic blood pressure of at least 15 mmHg, or
> - a rise (compared to booking) in systolic blood pressure of at least 30 mmHg.

Physiology

Because the blood pressure falls in the first trimester, pregnancy may mask pre-existing hypertension. Blood pressure rises again in the third trimester and therefore, if hypertension is noted for the first time in the third trimester, this may be due to unrecognized pre-existing hypertension, pregnancy-induced hypertension or pre-eclampsia. Often a clear diagnosis is

only possible several months after delivery when the blood pressure does or does not revert to normal.

Significant proteinuria is defined as 300 mg or more in a 24-hour urine sample. Although reagent strips give an indication as to the degree of proteinuria, accurate quantification relies on a 24-hour collection. Other causes of proteinuria include renal disease, vaginal discharge or contamination and urinary tract infection. Oedema is a non-specific, generalized accumulation of fluid, which affects more than 50 per cent of the pregnant population and is therefore non-discriminatory. Pre-eclampsia and eclampsia (see Chapter 13) will typically relate to elevations in blood pressure after the 20th week of pregnancy. It is for this reason that it is useful to have a pre-pregnancy or early pregnancy recording of blood pressure with which to compare subsequent changes.

Chronic hypertension preceding pregnancy

Essential hypertension is the underlying cause in 90 per cent of cases. A list of causes is shown in the box below.

> ### Causes of chronic hypertension
>
> - Essential hypertension
> - Renal disease:
>   - glomerulonephritis
>   - polycystic disease
>   - diabetic nephropathy
>   - renal artery stenosis
> - Collagen vascular disease:
>   - systemic lupus erythematosus (SLE)
>   - scleroderma
> - Coarctation of the aorta
> - Endocrine causes:
>   - phaeochromocytoma
>   - Conn's syndrome

Before a diagnosis of essential hypertension is made, these other possibilities need to be excluded. Irrespective of the underlying cause, the principal concern for the obstetrician is that these women may develop superimposed pre-eclampsia. This may occur in up to one-third of women with pre-existing hypertension and is more likely in women with severe hypertension, defined as a diastolic blood pressure of 110 mmHg or higher before 20 weeks' gestation, and in those with renal disease. The risk factors for developing superimposed pre-eclampsia are listed in the box below. The maternal risks of pre-existing hypertension include pre-eclampsia, but also abruption, heart failure and intracerebral haemorrhage. Abruption is rare, but in severe hypertensive disease the risk is in the order of 10 per cent. Fetal risks include growth restriction from placental insufficiency. Morbidity and mortality are closely related to the degree of severity and the gestational age at delivery.

Risk factors for developing superimposed pre-eclampsia

- Renal disease
- Maternal age >40 years
- Diabetes
- Connective tissue disease, e.g. SLE and antiphospholipid syndrome (APS)
- Coarctation of the aorta
- Blood pressure >160/100 mmHg in early pregnancy

Management

If the blood pressure is elevated for the first time in pregnancy, appropriate investigations should be performed to exclude renal, cardiac and autoimmune disease (see box below). In mild cases (blood pressure <150/100 mmHg) there is no immediate indication to treat; however, the pregnancy should be monitored carefully to detect any rise in blood pressure or features of pre-eclampsia or fetal growth restriction. Women who are receiving antihypertensive medication before pregnancy are often able to discontinue this for the first part of pregnancy because of the physiological fall in blood pressure at this time. Some antihypertensives such as the angiotensin-converting enzyme (ACE) inhibitors should be discontinued because of the risk of fetal damage.

Investigation of hypertension

- Creatinine, electrolytes, urate
- Liver function tests
- 24-Hour urinary protein/creatinine clearance
- Renal scan
- Autoantibody screen
- Complement studies
- Cardiac investigations including electrocardiography (ECG) and echocardiography

The development of proteinuria may herald the development of superimposed pre-eclampsia. Pregnancies should be monitored for the development of fetal growth restriction, and serial ultrasound examination may be appropriate.

If the blood pressure is consistently noted to be >150/100 mmHg, antihypertensive medication will need to be introduced or recommended. This is to reduce the risk of severe hypertension and the attendant risks of intracerebral haemorrhage and heart failure.

Care should be taken not to lower the blood pressure excessively, as this may adversely affect the fetus by reducing placental blood flow. Preferred antihypertensive agents include methyldopa (centrally acting agent) – which is generally well tolerated, especially if women are forewarned about the common transient side effects of lethargy and postural hypotension – labetalol (alpha- and beta-blocker), and nifedipine (calcium-channel blocker). The aim of antihypertensive medication is to maintain the blood pressure below 160 mmHg systolic and 100–110 mmHg diastolic. The optimum target blood pressure to reduce the danger to the mother, without compromising the fetus, is disputed. This is currently the subject of clinical studies.

The obstetric management of pre-existing hypertension involves close monitoring for the development of superimposed pre-eclampsia. Each case must be individually assessed, but early delivery is rarely indicated unless pre-eclampsia ensues or the blood pressure is very difficult to control. In general, it is reasonable to await spontaneous labour or attempt vaginal delivery by induction of labour (at 38 weeks), ensuring the maternal blood pressure is well controlled. If delivery is contemplated before 34 weeks' gestation, the mother should be given steroids to increase fetal lung maturation. Continuous fetal monitoring is advocated in labour if the fetus is growth restricted.

The management of pre-eclampsia is discussed in Chapter 13.

Postnatally, the maternal blood pressure will often decrease, but careful observation is required in the first 48 hours because blood pressure tends to increase again on the third or fourth postpartum day. Breastfeeding is encouraged and although some antihypertensive medication may enter the breast milk, none of the standard antihypertensive medications is contraindicated in breastfeeding mothers.

Endocrine disorders

Diabetes

Physiology

Significant hormonal changes affect carbohydrate metabolism during pregnancy. In particular, there is an increase in human placental lactogen and cortisol, both of which are insulin antagonists and therefore the mother develops relative insulin resistance. These changes are most marked during the third trimester. To balance these changes during normal pregnancy, the maternal pancreas secretes increased amounts of insulin to maintain carbohydrate metabolism. Typically in pregnancy, this will result in a fall in the fasting level of glucose. In contrast, following a carbohydrate challenge, the levels of glucose are higher than in the non-pregnant state. Glucose crosses the placenta by facilitated diffusion and the fetal blood glucose level closely follows the maternal level. Fetal glucose levels are therefore normally maintained within narrow limits, as in the mother.

Diabetes may complicate a pregnancy either because a woman has pre-existing insulin-dependent (IDDM) or non-insulin dependent diabetes mellitus (NIDDM) before pregnancy or because she develops usually transient impaired glucose tolerance or diabetes during the course of her pregnancy. Approximately 1–2 per cent of pregnant women will develop gestational diabetes. Certain groups of women are more likely to develop diabetes at some time during their life and are labelled as potential diabetics. The risk factors that are important for the obstetrician to note are listed below.

Definition of diabetes

The World Health Organization (WHO) has defined diabetes mellitus as either a raised fasting blood glucose level of >7.8 mmol/L or a level of >11.1 mmol/L 2 hours following a 75 g oral glucose load. The significance of impaired glucose tolerance (2-hour value 7.8–11.1 mmol/L) in pregnancy has been much debated, but many now feel that it is unlikely to have any untoward effect on pregnancy outcome unless the WHO criteria for diabetes are reached.

> **Risk factors for the development of diabetes in pregnancy**
>
> - Obesity (body mass index >30)
> - Family history of diabetes
> - Previous baby >4.5 kg
> - Previous unexplained stillbirth
> - Previous congenital abnormality

The importance of good glycaemic control during pregnancy is reinforced by the direct relationship between blood glucose levels and the incidence of fetal and maternal complications. For this reason, women who plan to become pregnant should be advised to aim for optimal control of their diabetes prior to conception and throughout pregnancy. This may necessitate a change to insulin therapy prior to conception in women with NIDDM. Women should be advised of the risks of pregnancy and diabetes, and the importance of diet and exercise should be reiterated. Careful self-monitoring of glucose levels by women with diabetes is a critical aspect of care. This helps to highlight excessive swings in blood glucose levels. Women using a twice-daily insulin regime will often have to change to a four times daily insulin regimen. Women with diabetes require increased insulin doses during pregnancy.

Fetal and neonatal complications of diabetic pregnancy

There is an increased risk of miscarriage and congenital fetal abnormality. Good diabetic control, particularly prior to conception, reduces these risks substantially. Measurement of glycosylated haemoglobin gives a retrospective assessment of diabetic control; high levels in early pregnancy are associated with neural tube defects, congenital heart disease and other spinal anomalies, including a rare condition called caudal regression syndrome. Congenital abnormality is the most important cause of mortality and morbidity in diabetic pregnancies and is seen two to four times more often than in normal pregnancies. Malformations at present account for 40 per cent of the perinatal mortality associated with diabetic pregnancies. The mechanism that gives rise to these abnormalities is not fully understood, but it is thought that hyperglycaemia in the critical stages of organogenesis may be the underlying cause, and this has been demonstrated in animal models. Apart from structural malformations, fetal macrosomia is a major problem associated with traumatic birth, shoulder dystocia and therefore possible hypoxic damage (Fig. 15.3). Accelerated growth patterns are typically seen in the late second and third trimesters and are associated with poorly controlled diabetes (Fig. 15.4). Sudden, unexplained, late stillbirths occurred in 10–30 per cent of diabetic pregnancies, but are much less common now that the importance of good diabetic control and timely delivery is appreciated. However, this remains a risk in women whose diabetes is poorly controlled and in those who have vascular disease and in pregnancies complicated by macrosomia or polyhydramnios. The

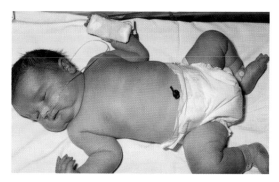

Figure 15.3 The 5.1 kg macrosomic infant of a diabetic mother.

mechanism of such losses is not fully understood, although several possible mechanisms may contribute to chronic hypoxia and fetal acidosis.

Maternal mortality and morbidity in diabetic pregnancy

There has been a marked reduction in maternal mortality in diabetic pregnancies and this is now a very rare event. Those at most risk are women with pre-existing coronary artery disease. In general, the maternal morbidity is related to the severity of diabetic-related disease preceding the pregnancy. The risk of pre-eclampsia is increased two–four-fold in women with diabetes. Women with co-existing microalbuminuria or frank nephropathy are at particular risk of developing pre-eclampsia. Although the renal condition may worsen during pregnancy, this is rarely permanent and tends to improve following delivery. In contrast, women with diabetic retinopathy are at risk of progression of the disease and they should be kept under careful surveillance. Other complications include an increased incidence of infection, severe hyperglycaemia or hypoglycaemia, diabetic ketoacidosis and the complications that may arise from the increased operative delivery rate, including thromboembolic disease (see box below).

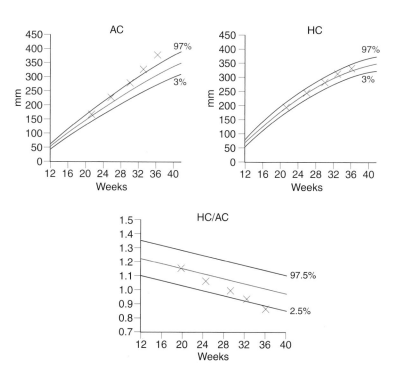

Figure 15.4 Growth patterns of the fetal abdominal circumference (AC) and head circumference (HC) and the HC/AC ratio in the fetus of a poorly controlled insulin-dependent diabetic mother. The increased growth mainly affects the abdominal organs, hence the accelerated growth rate of the AC.

Maternal complications of diabetic pregnancy

- Nephropathy (temporary worsening)
- Retinopathy (progression)
- Coronary artery disease
- Hyperglycaemia/hypoglycaemia/ketoacidosis
- Pre-eclampsia
- Infection
- Thromboembolic disease

Neonatal complications

Neonatal morbidity in diabetic pregnancy has fallen dramatically over the last three decades, with improvement of glycaemic control antenatally, but it remains significantly increased compared to non-diabetic pregnancies and is related to the degree of antenatal glucose control. Babies of mothers with diabetes should be monitored for possible complications, especially hypoglycaemia.

Causes of neonatal morbidity

- Congenital abnormalities:
  - cardiac
  - neural tube defects
- Macrosomia:
  - birth asphyxia
  - traumatic birth injury, e.g. brachial plexus injury
- Respiratory distress syndrome
- Hypoglycaemia
- Hypomagnesaemia
- Polycythaemia
- Hyperbilirubinaemia

Hypoglycaemia, particularly in the first 24 hours following delivery, is anticipated because the infant continues to produce large amounts of insulin in the immediate neonatal period due to recent fetal hyperglycaemia. However, once the umbilical cord is clamped, the neonate is no longer exposed to high levels of glucose from the mother. Mothers should be encouraged to breastfeed straight away; monitoring of the baby's blood glucose should be undertaken and, if necessary, a formula feed or glucose infusion commenced. Less common abnormalities include disturbances of hypocalcaemia and magnesium deficiency,

in extreme cases leading to apnoeic episodes and fits. Polycythaemia is often found and may need correction by a partial exchange transfusion. Finally, jaundice caused by hyperbilirubinaemia may result from the neonatal polycythaemia.

Screening for diabetes in pregnancy

This is an extremely controversial area, as there is no agreed definition for gestational diabetes in terms of specific blood glucose levels and it is disputed whether treatment of gestational diabetes, however defined, improves fetal and neonatal outcome. There is particular controversy regarding the significance of impaired glucose tolerance in pregnancy, where the diabetic 'label' may do more harm than good. Part of the problem relates to the fact that many confounding variables, especially maternal weight, increase the risk of both diabetes and macrosomia, thus making causality hard to prove. Screening for diabetes in pregnancy can be justified to diagnose previously unrecognized cases of pre-existing diabetes and to identify a group of women who are at risk of developing NIDDM later in life. No single screening test has been shown to be perfect in terms of high sensitivity and specificity for gestational diabetes. Urinary glucose is unreliable, and most screening tests now rely on blood glucose estimation. An oral glucose tolerance test is used by many units, but this is expensive, time consuming, and does not have good reproducibility in pregnancy. Other units use a random blood glucose test (interpreted according to the time since the last meal), or a blood glucose taken 1 hour following a 50 g glucose meal (sometimes called a mini glucose tolerance test).

Antenatal management

Pregnant women with diabetes should be managed in a joint clinic with an obstetrician and physician. Women with pre-existing diabetes should be referred directly to this clinic at booking, and those in whom a diagnosis of gestational diabetes is made at a later stage should also be referred. The aim of treatment is to maintain the blood glucose level as near normal as possible, with a combination of diet and insulin. In women with IDDM, this will usually require three or four daily doses of insulin or the newer rapidly acting insulin analogues. All women with diabetes should be instructed in self-monitoring with their own glucose meters. Long-term control may be checked using glycosylated haemoglobin or fructosamine measurements. Input from a dietician is also important and often a nurse or midwife specialist will act as an adviser to adjust the dose of insulin.

Obstetric management is aimed initially at ensuring that the appropriate screening tests are performed, including nuchal translucency scanning, detailed ultrasound assessment for fetal anomalies and fetal echocardiography. Serial growth scans are recommended to detect fetal macrosomia, although this is rarely a problem before the third trimester. As well as assessing the fetal size, ultrasound may also alert the team to developing polyhydramnios. Concern for fetal well-being should lead to increased surveillance with Doppler ultrasound and CTG. In principle, provided the pregnancy has gone well, management attempts to achieve a vaginal delivery between 38 and 40 weeks' gestation. The development of macrosomia or maternal complications such as pre-eclampsia together with the rate of failed induction is such that the Caesarean section rate amongst diabetic women often is as high as 50 per cent.

The management of preterm labour or polyhydramnios is particularly difficult in diabetic pregnancies. Tocolytics such as ritodrine or salbutamol are themselves diabetogenic and will tend to elevate blood glucose levels. In addition, the administration of intramuscular steroids to improve fetal lung maturation will also destabilize diabetic control. Under these circumstances, increasing doses of insulin are required and an intravenous insulin and glucose infusion may be appropriate to ensure normoglycaemia.

Intrapartum management

During either induced or spontaneous labour, normoglycaemia should be maintained using a sliding scale of insulin. Blood glucose levels should be tested at hourly intervals. Continuous fetal monitoring is advised and fetal scalp blood sampling should be undertaken in the presence of an abnormal CTG. Following delivery, the insulin requirements of established diabetics will rapidly fall and return to pre-pregnancy levels. Women with gestational diabetes should stop their insulin at delivery. A full glucose tolerance test is performed 6 weeks following delivery to ensure that the diabetes has resolved.

🔍 Key Points

Diabetes in pregnancy

- The incidence of large babies (macrosomia) can be reduced with good blood glucose control.
- Gestational diabetes has a very high recurrence rate in subsequent pregnancies.
- The commonest congenital abnormalities are cleft palate, sacral agenesis and cardiac defects.
- Reduced fetal movements at or near term in women with diabetes with a non-reassuring CTG should lead to delivery as a priority (especially if there are abnormal ultrasound findings, as in the case of Mrs K, below).

CASE HISTORY

Mrs K is a 38-year-old Asian woman who is pregnant for the third time. Her two previous pregnancies were complicated by gestational diabetes and both culminated in Caesarean sections at term, with birth weights of 3.9 and 4.2 kg. Her body mass index is 38.

Mrs K booked for a hospital delivery at 12 weeks. An ultrasound showed a singleton pregnancy with a normal nuchal scan giving a risk of Down's syndrome of 1:1400. An anomaly scan and fetal echocardiography at 20 weeks were normal.

In her previous pregnancy, Mrs K had required insulin in a four times daily regimen from 20 weeks' gestation. Unfortunately, she was poorly motivated to check her blood glucose and modify her diet. In this pregnancy, insulin was started at 14 weeks (HbA1c prior to commencing insulin was 8.6 per cent) with short-acting insulin before meals

and long-acting insulin at night. Despite advice from dieticians and weekly diabetic clinic attendance, blood glucose control was poor and serial ultrasound (see Fig. 15.4) showed fetal growth accelerating beyond the 95th centile from 32 weeks onwards. At 36 weeks and 3 days, Mrs K noticed reduced fetal movements. An ultrasound scan showed polyhydramnios (amniotic fluid index 26 cm) and an estimated fetal weight of 4.6 kg. CTG was reactive but variability was reduced (<5 bpm).

A semi-elective Caesarean section was performed the following day; a 5.1 kg female infant was delivered in good health. The baby was hypoglycaemic after delivery and required 4 days' care on the neonatal unit while blood glucose levels stabilized and feeding became established. She suffered no respiratory complications.

Thyroid disorders

Pregnancy has a significant impact on the normal maternal thyroid physiology. During pregnancy, the production of thyroid-binding globulin by the liver doubles as a result of oestrogenic stimulation. As a consequence, there is an increased amount of total thyroxine (T4) and tri-iodothyronine (T3), but importantly there is no significant change in the amount of circulating free thyroid hormone (FT4 and FT3) (see Chapter 5). The renal clearance of iodine increases in pregnancy.

Maternal hyperthyroidism

Hyperthyroidism in the mother occurs in 1 in every 500 pregnancies. In the majority of cases the condition has been diagnosed before pregnancy and 90 per cent of cases are secondary to Graves' disease. This autoimmune disorder is associated with the presence of circulating thyroid-stimulating antibodies. Less common causes of hyperthyroidism include:

- toxic nodules
- Hashimoto's thyroiditis
- multinodular goitre
- trophoblastic disease (extremely rare).

Clinically, the diagnosis may be difficult to make in pregnancy because mild maternal tachycardia, weight loss, heart murmurs and heat intolerance are all symptoms in early pregnancy. If there is a past history, or clinical suspicion of thyroid disease, thyroid function tests (including a free T4) should be performed. Hyperthyroidism is confirmed by high levels of FT4 and FT3, with reduced levels of thyroid-stimulating hormone (TSH). Uncontrolled maternal hyperthyroidism is associated with maternal cardiac arrhythmias, including atrial fibrillation, diarrhoea, vomiting, abdominal pains and psychosis. If the underlying aetiology is autoimmune disease, the thyroid-stimulating antibodies may cross the placenta and cause fetal thyrotoxicosis and goitre. The main complications for the fetus include fetal growth restriction, stillbirth, fetal tachycardia and premature delivery.

Following the diagnosis of hyperthyroidism, the treatment during pregnancy should be drug therapy aiming to maintain maternal FT3 and FT4 levels in the high/normal range. Radioactive iodine is contraindicated because it completely obliterates the fetal thyroid gland. Treatment is usually medical with carbimazole or propylthiouracil (PTU). Beta-blockers may be indicated initially before the antithyroid drugs take effect. Surgical treatment may be necessary in rare circumstances when the thyrotoxicosis does not respond to medical treatment. The lowest dose of carbimazole or PTU must be used, as high doses cross the placenta and may cause fetal hypothyroidism. However, in severe thyrotoxicosis it is important to control the disease as quickly as possible, if necessary with high doses of antithyroid drugs. Careful monitoring of maternal thyroid function is essential under these circumstances.

Maternal hypothyroidism

The commonest cause of hypothyroidism worldwide is iodine deficiency, but this is rarely seen in the UK. Maternal iodine deficiency is associated with the development of cretinism in the newborn as a result of congenital hypothyroidism. The commonest reason for maternal hypothyroidism in the UK is autoimmune Hashimoto's thyroiditis, followed by treated (with surgery, radioiodine or drugs) hyperthyroidism. Women treated with radioactive iodine frequently require T4 supplements, and the dose should be checked in early pregnancy to ensure appropriate levels of FT4 and FT3. Women diagnosed with hypothyroidism should continue full thyroid replacement during pregnancy. Thyroid function tests should be performed serially in each trimester, or more often if dose adjustments are required. Provided a woman is receiving an adequate dose of T4 prior to pregnancy, there is only rarely a need to increase this dose in pregnancy.

Postpartum thyroiditis may present with thyrotoxicosis or hypothyroidism, but most commonly with postnatal depression (in the hypothyroid phase), 4–6 months following delivery. Although this is often a self-limiting condition, many will suffer recurrence after a subsequent pregnancy and these women are at risk of permanent hypothyroidism.

Pituitary disorders

Hyperprolactinaemia is an important cause of infertility and amenorrhoea. It is most often due to a benign pituitary microadenoma. It may also be due to drugs that act as dopamine antagonists, such as methyldopa and the phenothiazines. The diagnosis is confirmed with a combination of measurement of the prolactin level and computerized tomography (CT) or magnetic resonance imaging (MRI) scanning of the pituitary fossa. In 80 per cent of cases it may be treated with the dopamine agonists bromocriptine or cabergoline, which cause the tumour to diminish in size. Larger tumours may require surgery or radiotherapy, which is best undertaken before pregnancy. Bromocriptine and cabergoline are usually stopped in pregnancy. The pituitary gland enlarges during pregnancy, but it is rare for microadenomas to cause problems. It is important to monitor the visual fields during pregnancy. If there is evidence of tumour growth during pregnancy, bromocriptine or cabergoline should be recommenced. In women with macroadenomas (>1 cm), it is best to continue with dopamine agonists because of the risk of the tumour enlarging under oestrogenic stimulation. There is no evidence that bromocriptine or cabergoline is teratogenic.

Adrenal disorders

Cushing's syndrome

All adrenal disease is rare in pregnancy. Cushing's syndrome is characterized by increased glucocorticoid production, usually due to hypersecretion of adrenocorticotrophic hormone (ACTH) from a pituitary tumour. However, in pregnancy, adrenal causes are more common. Most women with Cushing's syndrome are infertile and, in the few reported cases of pregnancy, a high incidence of preterm delivery and stillbirth is described. Diagnosis may be difficult because many of the symptoms mimic normal pregnancy changes such as striae, weight gain, weakness, glucose intolerance and hypertension. If suspected, plasma cortisol levels should be assayed (remembering that the levels increase in pregnancy) and adrenal imaging with ultrasound, CT or MRI should be used.

Addison's disease

Addison's disease (adrenal insufficiency) is usually an autoimmune process. The clinical picture is of exhaustion, nausea, hypotension, hypoglycaemia and weight loss. The diagnosis is difficult to make in pregnancy because the cortisol levels, instead of being characteristically decreased, may be in the low–normal range due to the physiological increase in cortisol-binding globulin in pregnancy. Occasionally, the disease may present as a crisis, and treatment consists of glucocorticoid and fluid replacement. In adequately treated patients, the pregnancy usually continues normally.

It is important to remember that replacement steroids should be continued in pregnancy and increased (and given parenterally) at times of stress such as hyperemesis and delivery.

Phaeochromocytoma

Phaeochromocytoma is a rare catecholamine-producing tumour. The tumours arise from the adrenal medulla in 90 per cent of cases. Its importance in pregnancy is that it may present as a hypertensive crisis and the symptoms may be similar to those of pre-eclampsia. A characteristic feature is paroxysmal hypertension, whilst the other symptoms of headaches, palpitations, blurred vision, anxiety and convulsions may occur in pre-eclampsia. The diagnosis is confirmed by measurement of catecholamines in a 24-hour urine collection and, if elevated, in plasma. Treatment is by alpha-blockade with phentolamine. Caesarean section is the preferred mode of delivery, as it minimizes the likelihood of sudden increases in catecholamines associated with vaginal delivery.

Respiratory disorders

Asthma

Asthma is reversible bronchial airway obstruction, and is commonly encountered in pregnancy (up to 5 per cent of pregnancies). In most cases the disease is well controlled with inhaled beta-2 agonists (salbutamol 'relievers') and corticosteroids (betamethasone 'preventers'). Pregnancy itself does not increase the frequency or severity of asthma in most women. Problems may occur in patients whose asthma is poorly controlled, in those who are not compliant with their medication or are told not to continue it, or from failure of clinicians to recognize the severity of the problem. In such cases there may be an increased incidence of fetal growth restriction. Care should be aimed at optimizing medical treatment to prevent exacerbations of asthma and the aggressive treatment of acute attacks. Patient inhalation techniques should be carefully reviewed, and regular respiratory peak flow assessment performed by the woman herself is the best way of monitoring the severity of the condition. In severe exacerbations, hospital admission for nebulized treatment with bronchodilators, oxygen and steroids is indicated.

Labour is rarely a problem for women with asthma, and epidural is the preferred analgesia. General anaesthesia should be avoided if possible, as it increases the risk of bronchospasm and chest infection. In the postnatal period, non-steroidal anti-inflammatory drugs (NSAIDs), often used for pain relief, should be avoided. Prostaglandin F2α (carboprost) may cause intense bronchoconstriction.

Sarcoid

Sarcoid is a non-caseating granulomatosis that may affect any organ, but principally affects the lung and skin. Complications include severe progressive lung problems with pulmonary fibrosis, hypoxaemia and pulmonary hypertension, and these features are associated with a poor prognosis. Women are best jointly managed with a chest physician. Treatment is with steroid therapy. Sarcoid is uncommonly diagnosed in pregnancy, since it usually improves, although erythema nodosum (which may occur in normal pregnancy and in sarcoidosis) may cause diagnostic confusion. Pregnancy does not influence the long-term natural history of the condition. If there is progressive lung involvement, anaesthetic input should be obtained prior to labour.

Cystic fibrosis

This is an autosomal recessive condition. The life expectancy of affected women is increasing all the time and many more women are surviving to an age at which pregnancy is possible. It is a multi-system disorder, principally affecting the lungs and liver. Malabsorption due to pancreatic insufficiency is often a major problem, and women are typically underweight. Many women develop diabetes and this risk is increased during pregnancy.

It is important to check the cystic fibrosis carrier status of the woman's partner, and the couple should be offered genetic counselling regarding the risks of the fetus having cystic fibrosis or being a carrier. The main risks to the fetus include growth restriction and preterm delivery, the latter usually being iatrogenic if there is evidence of deteriorating maternal respiratory function. Fetal growth and well-being are monitored by serial ultrasound scans. Mothers should be jointly managed between the obstetrician and a respiratory physician with expertise in cystic fibrosis. Most women will have a daily physiotherapy regime and will require prolonged antibiotic therapy and hospital admission during exacerbations. If delivery is contemplated before 34 weeks' gestation, steroid therapy should be given to improve fetal lung maturation. Ideally, a vaginal delivery should be the aim and epidural analgesia offered. The second stage can be shortened in the event of maternal exhaustion.

Haematological abnormalities

Anaemia

The WHO defines anaemia as a haemoglobin concentration of $<11.0\,g/dL$. During pregnancy, although the red cell mass increases, the plasma volume expansion is relatively greater and therefore the haemoglobin concentration falls. Anaemia in pregnancy is most commonly due to a lack of haemoglobin production because of low levels of essential precursors such as iron and folate. Less commonly, it may be secondary to chronic blood loss or haemolysis.

Microcytic anaemia
Iron demand in pregnancy increases from 2 mg to 4 mg daily. A healthy diet contains 10 mg. The diagnosis of iron deficiency is suspected if the mean corpuscular volume (MCV) is below 85 fL, assuming electrophoresis is normal. Low levels of serum iron and ferritin help to confirm the diagnosis. Treatment is with iron supplementation and a single 60 mg tablet daily should suffice. If the woman is unable to tolerate this because of common side effects, including nausea and constipation, different iron preparations are available, including liquid formulae. Other means of increasing haemoglobin concentration have their drawbacks: intramuscular iron is painful, intravenous iron may cause allergic reactions, and blood transfusions should be avoided, if possible, because of the small risk of antibody production and transfusion reactions.

Macrocytic anaemia
Folate deficiency is less common in the UK, as many foods include folate supplements, but may be suggested by an increased MCV. Folate requirements are increased in pregnancy, as all tissues require it for the manufacture of DNA. The normal values of folate concentrations fall in pregnancy due to the haemodilutional effect of plasma expansion. All women

considering pregnancy should be encouraged to use folate supplementation (0.4 mg daily), as it has been shown to reduce the incidence of neural tube defects. Additional supplements (5 g daily) are required in women receiving anticonvulsant medication.

Worldwide, the commonest cause of a raised MCV is alcohol consumption. Vitamin B12 deficiency (pernicious anaemia) is another cause of macrocytic anaemia, but is unlikely to present in pregnancy, as severe cases are associated with infertility. Diagnosed cases should continue vitamin B12 injections throughout gestation.

Haemolytic anaemia

Sickle-cell syndromes

These are autosomally inherited diseases. Abnormal haemoglobin (HbS) contains beta-globin chains with an amino acid substitution that results in it precipitating when in its reduced state. The red blood cells become sickle shaped and occlude small blood vessels – this is known as sickling.

Sickle-cell disease

Sickle-cell disease (HbSS) is a severe condition and in pregnancy women are at high risk of complications. Pregnancy is associated with an increased incidence of sickle-cell crises that may result in episodes of severe pain, typically affecting the bones or chest. These crises may be precipitated by hypoxia, stress, infection and haemorrhage. Mothers are at increased risk of miscarriage, pre-eclampsia, chest and urinary tract infections and premature labour. The fetal loss rate is higher than normal, as is the incidence of growth restriction. Ideally, these potential problems of pregnancy should be discussed with the woman before pregnancy.

Sickle-cell trait

Sickle-cell carriers have a 1:4 risk of having a baby with sickle-cell disease if their partner also has sickle-cell trait (HbAS). Carriers of the trait are usually fit and well, but are at increased risk of urinary tract infection. Very rarely, they may suffer from crises.

Sickle-cell haemoglobin C disease

Although sickle-cell haemoglobin C disease (HbSC) may cause only mild degrees of anaemia, it is associated with very severe crises that are more common throughout pregnancy. The danger of this condition relates to a false reassurance because women are not as anaemic as those with SS disease; thus the severity of crises may be underestimated.

Antenatal management

All women should be screened at booking to detect haemoglobinopathies. If a woman is found to be a heterozygote for a haemoglobinopathy, her partner should also be tested. Prenatal diagnosis can be offered to couples at risk of having an affected baby. No specific treatment exists to prevent sickle-cell crises; however, hypoxia, dehydration and infection should be avoided by aggressive treatment with adequate analgesia, antibiotics, oxygen and rehydration. Ideally, a haemoglobin concentration of at least 10.0 g/dL with 60 per cent normal HbA will minimize the risk of crises. In some cases, blood transfusion or exchange transfusion may be used to increase the percentage of circulating normal haemoglobin A; however, blood transfusion is not without risk and its role in sickle pregnancies is controversial.

Vaginal delivery should be the aim and epidural anaesthesia advised, to reduce the stress of labour. Care should also be taken to avoid dehydration, cooling, infection or hypoxia during labour. Continuous fetal monitoring is recommended. In the postnatal period, women with sickle-cell disease remain at increased risk of suffering a crisis, as this is a stressful time. Contraception should be carefully discussed and both the combined contraceptive and progesterone-only pills may be safely used.

Thalassaemia

The thalassaemia syndromes are the commonest genetic blood disorders. The defect is a reduced production of normal haemoglobin. The syndromes are divided into the alpha and beta types, depending on which globin chain is affected. In alpha-thalassaemia minor, there is a deletion of one of the two normal alpha genes required for haemoglobin production. Although the affected individual is chronically anaemic, this condition rarely produces obstetric complications except in cases of severe blood loss. It is important to screen the woman's partner for thalassaemia and to consider prenatal diagnosis (see Chapter 9); if he is also affected, there is a 1:4 chance of the fetus having alpha-thalassaemia major.

In alpha-thalassaemia major, there are no functional alpha chains, no normal haemoglobin is synthesized and the condition is incompatible with life. The fetus develops marked hydrops, and pregnancies are complicated by polyhydramnios and preterm delivery. If affected, the baby will only survive a few hours following delivery. These pregnancies may also be complicated by severe pre-eclampsia related to the enlarged and hydropic placenta. There is no treatment, but individuals can be offered the option of antenatal diagnosis in subsequent pregnancies.

The beta-thalassaemias result from defects in the normal production of the beta chains. Normal haemoglobin contains mostly HbA1, with a small percentage of HbA2. If the gene for HbA1 is missing, the individual has beta-thalassaemia minor. These abnormalities are more commonly found in people from the East Mediterranean, but may also occur sporadically in other communities. Consequently, all pregnant women should be offered electrophoresis as part of the antenatal screening process. Beta-thalassaemia minor/trait is not a problem antenatally, although women will tend to be mildly anaemic and have a low MCV. Iron and folate supplements should be given and partners should also be screened. However, if both partners have beta-thalassaemia minor, there is a 1:4 chance the fetus could have no gene for the production of HbA1, and this is termed beta-thalassaemia major. The fetus produces HbF in utero and this is not a problem; however, in postnatal life, normal HbA1 cannot be produced and severe anaemia develops, requiring serial blood transfusion. Eventually this leads to the problems of iron overload and death.

Thrombocytopenia

Thrombocytopenia is a reduction in platelet number below 150×10^9/L. There are many causes and these are classified in the box below.

Classification of thrombocytopenia

- Incidental thrombocytopenia of pregnancy
- Increased consumption
- Autoimmune thrombocytopenia
- SLE/APS
- Activated clotting mechanism:
  - pre-eclampsia
  - HELLP (haemolysis, elevated liver enzymes, low platelets) syndrome
  - disseminated intravascular coagulation
- Thrombotic thrombocytopenic purpura
- Hypersplenism
- Decreased platelet production/bone marrow suppression:
  - sepsis
  - human immunodeficiency virus (HIV)
- Malignant marrow infiltration

Incidental thrombocytopenia

Incidental thrombocytopenia is common and may be present in 7–8 per cent of the pregnant population. Mild falls in platelet counts to between 100 and 150×10^9/L are only very rarely associated with poor maternal outcome. Bleeding is rarely a complication unless the count is $<50 \times 10^9$/L. The diagnosis of incidental thrombocytopenia is a diagnosis of exclusion and can only be made when autoimmune and other causes have been excluded.

Autoimmune thrombocytopenic purpura

Autoimmune thrombocytopenic purpura (ITP) may present acutely, typically in children after a viral illness. In adults, the presentation is more chronic. The incidence in pregnancy is 1:5000. Autoantibodies are produced against platelet surface antigens, leading to platelet destruction by the reticulo-endothelial system. In pregnancy, the condition may present with bruising or be suspected for the first time following a routine blood count. The count is typically 30–80 $\times 10^9$/L and it is rare for it to fall to extremely low levels. Other associated autoimmune conditions should be considered, including SLE and APS.

Management in pregnancy should include serial platelet counts and, provided the count remains above 80×10^9/L, no bleeding complications are likely. Regional epidural/spinal anaesthesia and analgesia may be used. If the count falls below 80×10^9/L, other forms of pain relief for labour, or general anaesthesia for Caesarean section, may be indicated. If the platelet count falls below 50×10^9/L approaching term, treatment should be considered. Corticosteroids act by suppressing platelet autoantibodies; however, high doses are often required to improve the platelet count, and long-term use is associated with weight gain, hypertension, diabetes and osteoporosis. Corticosteroids also take 2–3 weeks to have an effect. Although much more expensive, the use of intravenous immunoglobulin G (IgG) has been a major advance in the treatment of autoimmune thrombocytopenia. The precise mechanism of its action is not known, but it is thought that the administration of human IgG prolongs the clearance time of IgG-coated platelets by the reticulo-endothelial system. The platelet response is usually rapid. Because of cost implications, this treatment is usually reserved for cases that do not respond to steroids, or when a rapid response is required prior to delivery, or if there is bleeding in the postpartum period. The resulting increase in platelets will normally allow delivery in the next 2–3 weeks with adequate platelet cover, and therefore the option of an epidural in labour can be considered. A final treatment is splenectomy, but this is very rarely undertaken in pregnancy as it is associated with significant maternal and perinatal mortality.

In pregnancy, antiplatelet antibodies may cross the placenta and destroy the fetal platelets; however, severe fetal thrombocytopenia is unusual and occurs in less than 5 per cent of the fetuses of women with maternal ITP.

Thrombophilia
See Chapter 11.

Neurological disease

Epilepsy

Epilepsy is a relatively common disorder, occurring in 0.15–1 per cent of women of childbearing age. Pregnancy has no consistent effect on epilepsy: some women will have an increased frequency of fits, others a decrease, and some no difference. In the majority of cases, women will have been commenced on anticonvulsant medication prior to pregnancy. Many factors contribute to altered drug metabolism in pregnancy and result in a net decrease in anticonvulsant drug levels. These include reduced compliance because of fears of teratogenicity, an increase in plasma volume, an increase in extracellular fluid volume, a reduced albumin concentration and increased renal and hepatic clearance of the drug.

The principal concern related to epilepsy in pregnancy is the increased risk of congenital abnormality caused by anti-epileptic medications. All anti-epileptic drugs (AEDs) are associated with an approximate doubling of the risk of fetal abnormality. The major

fetal abnormalities associated with AEDs (including sodium valproate, carbamazepine, phenytoin, phenobarbitone) are neural tube defects, facial clefts and cardiac defects. Many of these abnormalities are detectable by ultrasound and therefore all women should be offered detailed anomaly scanning. In addition, each AED has been associated with a specific syndrome that includes developmental delay, nail hypoplasia, growth restriction and mid-face abnormalities. Despite the risks of continuing AEDs in pregnancy (6–7 per cent risk of fetal abnormality), failure to do so may lead to an increased frequency of epileptic seizures that may result in both maternal and fetal hypoxia. Women with epilepsy require careful pre-pregnancy counselling. Those on multiple drug therapy should, wherever possible, be converted to monotherapy, and all women receiving AEDs should be advised to start taking a 5 mg daily folic acid supplement prior to conception. Women should be reminded that uncontrolled seizures are more harmful to the fetus than the potential risks of drug therapy. In women who have been free of seizures for 2 years, consideration may be given pre-pregnancy to discontinuing AEDs. In general, the risk of recurrent seizures is about 25 per cent within 1 year of starting to taper the medication. The risk is higher in women with adolescent-onset or adult-onset epilepsy, in those requiring more than one AED to control their epilepsy, in those who had seizures while on medication, and in those with an abnormal electroencephalogram in the last year.

Monitoring of drug levels in pregnancy is difficult. The measured drug level (usually total, not free) falls, but in a majority of cases this is not associated with an increased frequency of fits. An increase in dosage to combat the anticipated fall may lead to an increased fetal risk. In the majority of cases, provided there is no increase in frequency of seizures, the prenatal drug dosage can be continued. However, an increase in seizure frequency or a recurrence of seizures, especially in the context of sub-therapeutic drug levels, should prompt an increase in dosage. In the event of a first tonic–clonic seizure in pregnancy, it is important to exclude other possible causes, particularly eclampsia.

Causes of seizures in pregnancy

- Eclampsia
- Epilepsy
- Encephalitis/meningitis

- Space-occupying lesion:
  - tuberculoma
  - toxoplasmosis
  - cerebral tumour
- Cerebral vascular accident
- Thrombotic thrombocytopenic purpura
- Drug withdrawal
- Toxic overdose
- Metabolic disturbance (hypoglycaemia)

In the fetus and neonate, many of the AEDs have been shown to be competitive inhibitors of the prothrombin precursors, resulting in deficiency of vitamin K-dependent clotting factors. It is essential that the neonate receives prophylactic vitamin K at delivery. Mothers may suffer from a marked loss of sleep in the postnatal period, which can predispose to seizures. It is important to ensure good compliance with drug therapy at this time and therefore to reassure women that breastfeeding is safe.

Migraine

Up to one-fifth of pregnant women will experience migraine, many of whom do not get migraines outwith pregnancy. Seventy per cent of migraine sufferers feel that their migraine improves during pregnancy. Obstetric complications are not increased in migraine sufferers. Migraine during pregnancy should be treated with analgesics, anti-emetics and, where possible, avoidance of factors thought to trigger the attack. Low-dose aspirin or beta-blockers may be used to prevent attacks.

Bell's palsy

This is a unilateral neuropathy of the VIIth cranial nerve leading to paralysis of the forehead and lower face; loss of taste on the ipsilateral anterior tongue may also occur. The incidence of this palsy is increased ten-fold during the third trimester of pregnancy. The outcome is generally good and complete recovery may be anticipated if the time of onset is within 2 weeks of delivery. The role of corticosteroids and antiviral agents for Bell's palsy is controversial, but they may hasten recovery if given within the first 24 hours of the onset of symptoms. A reducing dose regime of steroids is used over a 10-day period. Bell's palsy does not affect pregnancy outcome.

Autoimmune disease

Systemic lupus erythematosus is a multi-system chronic autoimmune inflammatory disease. It is five to ten times more common in women, particularly in black and Asian populations. It may cause disease in any system, but principally it affects the joints, skin, lungs, nervous system, kidneys and heart. SLE may be diagnosed prenatally or may be suspected for the first time during pregnancy or the postpartum period, usually as a result of complications. The diagnosis is suggested by the finding of a positive assay for antinuclear antibodies. The presence of antibodies to double-stranded DNA is the most specific for SLE.

Systemic lupus erythematosus is a relapsing condition, and pregnancy increases the risk of disease flare. Approximately one-third of mothers with SLE will experience an exacerbation during pregnancy. The term APS is used to describe the association of anti-cardiolipin antibodies and/or lupus anticoagulant with the typical clinical features of arterial or venous thrombosis, fetal loss after 10 weeks' gestation, three or more miscarriages at less than 10 weeks' gestation, or delivery before 34 weeks due to intrauterine growth restriction (IUGR) or pre-eclampsia. APS may be primary or found in association with SLE.

Maternal and fetal risks of SLE and APS

Maternal
- Lupus flare
- Worsening nephropathy/proteinuria
- Pre-eclampsia
- Thrombosis
- Thrombocytopenia

Fetal
- Miscarriage
- Fetal death
- Growth restriction
- Preterm delivery
- Neonatal lupus due to transplacental passage of anti-Ro/anti-La antibodies

Because of these significant risks, pregnant women with SLE and APS require intensive monitoring for both maternal and fetal indications. The mother should be seen frequently, and baseline renal studies, including a 24-hour urine collection for protein, should be performed. Blood pressure should be monitored closely because of the increased risk of pre-eclampsia. Serial ultrasonography is performed to assess fetal growth. If antenatal treatment is required for SLE, steroids and azathioprine may be given safely, for example in women with lupus nephritis. NSAIDs should be avoided in pregnancy because of adverse effects on the fetus. In women with APS who have suffered repeated pregnancy loss or severe obstetric complications, the use of aspirin ± heparin has been shown to reduce the pregnancy loss rate.

Liver disorders

Acute fatty liver of pregnancy

This is a rare but very serious disorder of liver function occurring in approximately 1 in 10 000 pregnancies. The condition typically develops in the third trimester or within a few days of a stillbirth. The presenting complaints are of abdominal pain, headache, nausea and vomiting. Progressive jaundice, encephalopathy, hypoglycaemia, coagulopathy and renal failure may develop. The aetiology of the condition is unknown, but histologically a perilobular fatty infiltration of the liver cells is noted. There is a significant risk of maternal or fetal death. Following the onset of the condition, there may be a rapidly worsening cascade of problems, and the situation is frequently complicated by hypertension and disseminated intravascular coagulation. Maternal death results from encephalopathy or overwhelming haemorrhage associated with the clotting defect. Fetal death is not uncommon and is thought to be related to maternal liver failure and the metabolic disturbance.

Management relies on early diagnosis. Liver function tests are markedly deranged and there may be renal impairment. There is no place for liver biopsy in view of the bleeding risks. Treatment is to deliver the baby as soon as possible. This will frequently be by Caesarean section under general anaesthesia if clotting disorders preclude the use of regional techniques. Supportive therapy with blood transfusion, fresh frozen plasma, vitamin K, platelets, 50 per cent glucose, acetyl cysteine

and dialysis may be required prior to delivery and in the immediate postnatal period. The management in severe cases should include liaison with a regional liver unit. Postnatally, the liver function usually returns to normal over a few weeks and there is no long-term liver dysfunction.

Obstetric cholestasis

Obstetric cholestasis is an uncommon condition of pregnancy occurring in approximately 0.5–1 per cent of pregnancies. Its incidence varies widely geographically, and it is especially common in certain South American countries, particularly Chile. It presents most commonly in the third trimester (usually 32–36 weeks), with generalized itching, worst on the palms and soles. Anorexia, pale stools, dark urine and steatorrhoea may develop. There is no rash except marks resulting from skin scratching. Jaundice is unusual.

The importance of the condition is that it is associated with sudden intrauterine death. Most reported deaths occur at term. The mechanism for this is not clear, but it is often associated with meconium-stained liquor and premature labour. Cholestasis is not associated with major maternal complications.

Maternal liver function is often only mildly deranged, with raised transaminases and bile acids being the most sensitive finding. Cholestasis must be differentiated from other causes of liver dysfunction in pregnancy, including viral hepatitis, extrahepatic obstruction from gallstones, autoimmune hepatitis, pre-eclampsia, HELLP syndrome or acute fatty liver of pregnancy, sepsis and drug-induced hepatitis.

Investigation of cholestasis

Maternal
- Liver function tests
- Bile acids (may be first/only abnormality)
- Full blood count
- Clotting profile
- Renal function
- Hepatitis serology
- Autoimmune antibodies
- Liver ultrasound

Fetal
- Ultrasound for growth, amniotic fluid
- CTG

Management includes the symptomatic relief of pruritus with emollients and antihistamines, for instance oral chlorpheniramine (chlorphenamine). Ursodeoxycholic acid reduces maternal itching and improves liver function in most women. Because the risk of intrauterine death increases beyond 38 weeks, delivery is normally induced before this gestation. Maternal oral vitamin K given antenatally may reduce the risk of postpartum haemorrhage associated with reduced clotting factors. After delivery, the itching normally abates and maternal liver function returns to normal within days to weeks. In subsequent pregnancies, the recurrence risk of cholestasis is very high.

Complications of obstetric cholestasis

Maternal
- Haemorrhage
- Premature labour
- Steatorrhoea

Fetal
- Stillbirth
- Intrapartum fetal distress
- Meconium staining of amniotic fluid

Skin diseases

There are extensive physiological changes to the skin during pregnancy. Increased pigmentation, especially on the face (melasma), areolae, axillae and abdominal midline (linea nigra), is common. Spider naevi affect the face, arms and upper torso, and broad pink linear striae (striae gravidarum) frequently appear over the lower abdomen and thighs. Striae gravidarum fade and become white and atretic after pregnancy, but never disappear. Their appearance may be related to the increased levels of free cortisol during pregnancy. Pruritus without rash affects up to 20 per cent of normal pregnancies, but liver function tests should always be performed to exclude obstetric cholestasis (see above).

Pre-existing skin conditions such as eczema or acne may worsen in pregnancy.

There are dermatoses specific to pregnancy.

Polymorphic eruption of pregnancy

Polymorphic eruption of pregnancy (PEP), the commonest pregnancy-specific dermatosis, is a pruritic eruption that appears late in the third trimester and affects about 1 in 200 pregnancies. The lesions occur mainly over the abdomen and upper thighs. Usually, the lesions run linearly along vertical striae. No side effects to the fetus are described, and the rash resolves rapidly after delivery. Management is symptomatic, with emollients such as aqueous cream and antihistamines. Topical or, rarely, systemic steroids may be required.

Pemphigoid gestationis

Pemphigoid gestationis (PG) was previously called herpes gestationis and is a very rare but serious condition that is associated with an increased perinatal mortality. The eruption causes intense pruritus and begins in the peri-umbilical region, spreading to the limbs, palms and soles. The eruption begins with papules and plaques, but these develop into vesicles and tense bullae after 2 or more weeks. The condition usually begins in the third trimester, and although it may improve towards the end of pregnancy, there is typically flare postpartum, with persistence for several months. The diagnosis is by skin biopsy and direct immunofluorescence, which shows complement (C3) deposition in the basement membrane and confirms the nature of the lesion as an autoimmune condition, possibly related to fetal antigens. The presence of complement distinguishes PG from PEP. This distinction is important because PG is associated with low birth weight, preterm labour and intrauterine death, so intensive fetal monitoring is required. Treatment is with potent topical or systemic (e.g. prednisolone 40 mg daily) steroids and sedative antihistamines.

Prurigo of pregnancy

This pruritic condition consists of groups of red or brown papules that cover the abdomen and extensor surfaces of limbs. It develops in late pregnancy and improves after delivery. No effects on the fetus are known and the condition usually responds to topical steroids. It should be distinguished from pruritic folliculitis, which is an acneiform eruption occasionally complicating pregnancy.

Key Points

- Women with medical conditions that may adversely affect pregnancy outcome should be offered pre-pregnancy counselling by appropriately experienced healthcare professionals.
- Women with medical problems that preclude safe pregnancy should be offered safe, effective and appropriate contraception.
- Pregnant women with significant heart disease should be treated in joint obstetric/cardiac clinics by experienced physicians and obstetricians.
- Eisenmenger's syndrome and any pulmonary hypertension is associated in a risk of maternal morbidity of up to 50 per cent in pregnancy.
- Women found to be hypertensive in the first half of pregnancy require investigation for possible underlying causes of their hypertension.
- Women with pre-existing hypertension are at increased risk of superimposed pre-eclampsia, fetal growth restriction and placental abruption.
- Pre-existing diabetes increases maternal and fetal obstetric morbidity.
- Iron deficiency is the commonest cause of anaemia, but all forms of iron supplements commonly cause side effects.
- The risk of perinatal and maternal morbidity is increased in pregnancies complicated by sickle-cell disease.
- The main issue for pregnant women with epilepsy relates to the teratogenic risk of anti-epileptic drugs.
- Obstetric cholestasis is associated with an increased risk of term stillbirth.

Additional reading

Department of Health, Welsh Office, Scottish Home and Health Department and Department of Health and Social Services, Northern Ireland. *Why mothers die: Confidential Enquiries into Maternal Deaths in the United Kingdom 1997–99*. London: RCOG Press, 2001.

Nelson-Piercy C. *Handbook of obstetric medicine*, 2nd edn. London: Martin Dunitz, 2002.

Perry KG Jr, Morrison JC. The diagnosis and management of hemoglobinopathies during pregnancy. *Seminars in Perinatology* 1990; **14**:90–102.

Tomlinson MW, Cotton DB. Cardiac disease. In: James DK, Steer PJ, Weiner CP, Gonik B (eds). *High-risk pregnancy*, 2nd edn. London: WB Saunders, 1999.

Perinatal infections

OVERVIEW

Infection presents a major challenge to the obstetrician in both developed and developing countries. The extremely high rates of maternal mortality due to puerperal sepsis during the nineteenth and early twentieth centuries were mainly due to transmission of infection within the hospital. Group A *Streptococcus* was the commonest pathogen. Semmelweis, working in mid-nineteenth-century Vienna, was the first to demonstrate the value of aseptic technique and handwashing between patients. With improved infection control measures and the availability of intravenous antibiotics, maternal death from sepsis in hospital is now rare. Unfortunately, neonatal death still occurs from infections such as group B streptococcal meningitis, septicaemia and viral infections such as herpes encephalitis.

Altered maternal physiology during pregnancy places the mother at additional risk of certain infections. Decreased smooth muscle tone leads to increased vulnerability to pyelonephritis developing as a complication of cystitis. Subtle shifts in immunity due to T-helper cells may lead to increased susceptibility to intracellular infections such as tuberculosis, chickenpox (varicella zoster infection), listeria and *Chlamydia psittaci*.

Infections associated with congenital abnormality

The infections that cause congenital abnormality have been traditionally summarized by the acronym TORCH (toxoplasmosis, rubella, cytomegalovirus, herpes). It is clear that many other infections may adversely affect a fetus or neonate and these have been re-summarized as STORCH[5] (Table 16.1). However, pregnancy loss may occur in the first trimester in association with any acute infections in the mother, e.g. influenza.

Syphilis

Syphilis is a sexually transmitted infection caused by the sphirochaete *Treponema pallidum*. It is common in many developing countries, where up to 10 per cent of pregnant women may have positive serological tests. There was an explosive epidemic in Russia and Eastern Europe during the 1990s, but in Western Europe and the USA the incidence fell progressively over the course of the second half of the twentieth century.

Primary syphilis presents as a painless genital ulcer (Fig. 16.1) 3–6 weeks after the infection is acquired, with local lymphadenopathy. In women the ulcer is

Table 16.1 – STORCH[5]: specific infections that adversely affect a fetus, neonate or pregnant woman

S	Syphilis
T	Toxoplasmosis
O	Other
	Bacterial vaginosis
	Trichomoniasis vaginalis
	Group B *Streptococcus*
	Escherichia coli
	Ureaplasma urealyticum
	Haemophilus influenzae
	Varicella
	Listeria monocytogenes
R	Rubella
C	Cytomegalovirus
H[5]	Herpes
	Human immunodeficiency virus (HIV)
	Hepatitis B
	Human papillomavirus
	Human parvovirus

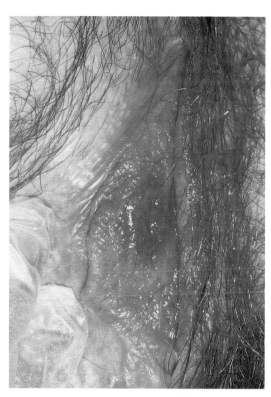

Figure 16.1 Primary syphilitic chancre. A painless rubbery ulcer is seen on the vulva. In many women the chancre is sited on the cervix, in which case the infection may pass asymptomatically. (Courtesy of Dr Raymond Maw, Royal Victoria Hospital, Belfast.)

most often on the cervix and may therefore pass unnoticed. At this stage the infection is highly contagious. Secondary manifestations of syphilis occur 6 weeks to 6 months after infection, often just as the primary chancre is regressing, and present as a non-itchy maculopapular rash affecting the palms of the hands and soles of the feet. Lesions affecting the mucous membranes are warty growths called condylomata lata. Other manifestations include alopecia, uveitis and sensorineural deafness. If no specific treatment is administered, the lesions regress after 2–4 weeks, but the infected patient may suffer relapses during the following 2 years, when lesions may reappear. At this stage the infection is called early latent, as it may be transmitted during relapses. Late infection ensues and syphilis cannot be transmitted sexually. Ultimately, 20 per cent of untreated patients will develop symptomatic cardiovascular tertiary syphilis and 5–10 per cent will develop symptomatic neurosyphilis.

Up to 70 per cent (the highest risk) of fetuses become infected if the mother has primary or secondary syphilis during pregnancy. With later stages of syphilis, the risk is smaller, being approximately 14 per cent 5 years after the mother has acquired infection. The spectrum of congenital syphilis varies from a severe fetal infection causing intrauterine death, to a neonate with symptomatic disease (early congenital syphilis), a child who subsequently develops the stigmata of congenital syphilis (late congenital syphilis), and a child who is asymptomatically infected. The key features are summarized in Table 16.2.

Any woman presenting during pregnancy with small genital ulcers should be screened for syphilis and herpes. A dark ground examination should be performed to look for *T. pallidum* and blood should be taken for serology. A fluorescent treponemal antibody absorption (FTA) test is the first serological test to become positive in early syphilis. The *Treponema pallidum* haemagglutination assay (TPHA) and FTA are specific tests for treponemal antibody, confirming exposure to infection at some stage of life; these remain positive even after treatment. The Venereal Diseases Research Laboratory (VDRL) test is measured quantitatively: a high titre of 1:64 or greater is found in secondary or early latent syphilis. After treatment, the

---

Table 16.2 – Features of congenital syphilis

Severe intrauterine infection leading to miscarriage

Early congenital syphilis:
  maculopapular rash
  hepatitis splenomegaly
  mucous patches, lymphadenopathy
  bone abnormalities, anaemia
  active neurosyphilis

Late congenital syphilis:
  Stigmata: Hutchinson's signs
    interstitial keratitis
    sensorineural deafness
    Hutchinson's teeth
    Clutton's joints
  Active disease: general paresis of the insane,
  gummata

VDRL titre falls progressively and will be unreactive in most individuals after 2 years.

The majority of pregnant women with syphilis are detected during routine screening at their booking visit. Biological false-positive VDRL tests may occur in women with systemic lupus erythematosus (SLE) or the antiphospholipid syndrome, usually at a titre of 1:8 or less. Thus, if the VDRL is positive but the FTA and TPHA are negative, an autoantibody screen should be performed and lupus antibody sought. People originating from tropical countries may have one of the tropical treponematoses that are not sexually transmitted or transmissible to a fetus, such as pinta and yaws.

Treatment

Penicillin is the treatment of choice for syphilis. For early syphilis (primary, secondary or early latent), protein penicillin should be prescribed, 1.2 MU daily, intramuscularly, for 12 days. Later stages of syphilis require 21 days of treatment. A Jarish–Herxheimer reaction may occur with treatment as a result of release of pro-inflammatory cytokines in response to dying organisms. This presents as a worsening of symptoms, and fever for 12–24 hours after starting treatment, and may be associated with uterine contractions and the onset of preterm labour. Some clinicians therefore advocate admitting women to initiate treatment with intravenous penicillin (1.2 MU per day in divided doses).

Women who are allergic to penicillin represent a problem. Tetracycline is the usual second-line treatment, but is contraindicated in pregnancy. Erythromycin is less reliable and resistance has been reported; it is best administered intravenously. It is essential that current and recent sex partners of women with syphilis are screened. Older children may also need to be screened.

Toxoplasmosis

Toxoplasma gondii is a protozoan parasite that may be acquired from exposure to cat faeces or from eating uncooked meat. The prevalence varies widely according to eating habits. In France, more than 70 per cent of pregnant women have been infected and have acquired immunity before pregnancy, whereas in the UK only 10–20 per cent of women are immune. Despite this, it is estimated that approximately 1 in 140 pregnant women in France acquire the infection during pregnancy, compared to 1 in 400 in the UK. Primary infection often passes asymptomatically. It may cause a glandular fever-like illness with atypical lymphocytes seen on a blood film, but, rarely, it causes fulminating pneumonitis or fatal encephalomyelitis. Eye infections, presenting as chorioretinitis, can occur from either congenital or acquired infection. In acquired immunodeficiency syndrome (AIDS), as immunity deteriorates, previously quiescent toxoplasmosis may recur, causing multiple brain abscesses.

Most infections are, however, asymptomatic. Infection during the first trimester of pregnancy is most likely to cause severe fetal damage, but only 10–25 per cent of infections are transmitted to the fetus. In the third trimester, 75–90 per cent of infections are transmitted, but the risk of fetal damage decreases from 65 per cent in the first trimester to almost zero for those infected near to the time of delivery. Severely infected infants may have the classic tetrad of hydrocephalus or microcephaly, chorioretinitis, convulsions and cerebral calcifications. In such cases extensive neurological damage occurs and the neonate may die. The majority of infected infants are asymptomatic at birth but develop sequelae several years later.

Only about ten severely affected babies are diagnosed per year in the UK. Routine screening in pregnancy is therefore not undertaken. A variety of serological tests are available. The Sabin–Feldman dye test is performed in reference laboratories. Enzyme-linked immunosorbent assays (ELISA) are available and immunoglobulin M (IgM) antibody can also be measured. The most definitive test is demonstration of the parasite in lymph node tissue or cerebral spinal fluid (CSF). It can be isolated by inoculation into mice. A high titre of antibody on the dye test (1–500 or higher) is suggestive but not diagnostic of current infection, as titres may fall for several years. Similarly, IgM antibody may persist for several months in adults. A presumptive clinical diagnosis can be made for congenital infection if the full spectrum of clinical features is present and the infant has an elevated *Toxoplasma* antibody titre. If the titre remains high for at least 6 months, the diagnosis becomes definite. The presence of IgM antibody in cord blood is suggestive, but can occur from a placental leak, and repeat testing should be performed. A negative IgM test does not exclude congenital toxoplasmosis.

Treatment

A combination of sulphadiazine and pyrimethamine is used in symptomatic adults. Pyrimethamine is, however, potentially teratogenic and should not be used during the first trimester. Spiramycin, a macrolide antibiotic, is less toxic and is devoid of teratogenic effects. A 3-week course of 2–3 g per day is administered during pregnancy. Whilst this reduces the incidence of transplacental infection, it has not been shown definitively to reduce the incidence of clinical congenital disease. In France, where many more women acquire infection during pregnancy, women are screened antenatally, but again the benefits of such a programme appear to be limited. Congenital toxoplasmosis should always be treated with pyrimethamine and sulphonamide.

Prevention

Pregnant women should be informed of the mode of spread of toxoplasmosis from meat and cat faeces. They should avoid eating rare steaks or hamburgers and take care when handling raw meat in the kitchen. Handwashing with soap and water is essential. Pregnant women should avoid handling cats and particularly cat litter. Children's sandpits should be covered to prevent cats from defaecating in them.

Cytomegalovirus

Cytomegalovirus (CMV) is a herpes virus and therefore has the ability to establish latency. In the UK, approximately 40 per cent of women are susceptible when they become pregnant. It is spread through the respiratory and genitourinary tracts and high levels of virus may be present in the urine. Primary infection often produces no symptoms or mild non-specific symptoms. The incidence of infection in pregnancy is therefore not known precisely but is estimated to be as high as 1 in 200 pregnancies, of which around 40 per cent will result in fetal infection. It is possible that infection later in pregnancy is more likely to result in fetal morbidity. Ninety per cent of infected infants are asymptomatic. Thus, of an estimated 1000 infected babies born per year in the UK, approximately 100 are damaged by the virus.

The principal features are microcephaly, blindness and deafness. Other manifestations include pneumonitis, chorioretinitis, cerebral calcification and developmental delay. Because the primary infection in the mother is usually asymptomatic, the diagnosis is rarely made before birth. Probably about another 100 children are born each year with sensorineural hearing loss as the only sign of congenital CMV infection.

After infection, the virus is excreted for weeks or months by adults and for years by infants. It persists in the lymphocytes throughout life and can therefore be transmitted by blood transfusion or transplantation. Reactivation occurs intermittently, with shedding in the genital, urinary or respiratory tract. In temperate countries, infection is usually transmitted by close contact, kissing or sexual contact; approximately 1–2 per cent of the population becomes infected each year. In tropical countries, most infections take place in childhood and 60–70 per cent of individuals are infected within 6 months of birth. The remainder are mostly infected by the age of 5 years and therefore there are few susceptible pregnant women. Clinical features in infected infants include hepato-splenomegaly, jaundice and purpura.

Diagnosis

A definitive diagnosis of congenital infection can be made by isolating the virus in cell culture from throat swabs, urine, blood or CSF in the first 3 weeks of life. Infants may secrete the virus for a prolonged period and therefore isolation of virus in the postnatal period does not confirm recent infection. Serological diagnosis is made by demonstrating a rising titre of IgG antibody or specific CMV IgM antibody. Specific IgM antibodies persist for a few weeks to a few months, and specific IgA antibodies from a few months to a year.

The diagnosis may be made in utero by amniocentesis and polymerase chain reaction (PCR), as the virus is concentrated in the urine. The congenital manifestations need to be differentiated from other congenital infections such as toxoplasmosis, rubella, herpes simplex and syphilis.

Treatment

Specific antiviral agents are available for CMV such as ganciclovir and foscarnet. These are not used in pregnancy, and have to be given by intravenous infusion. These agents are used in immunosuppressed individuals with AIDS or after transplantation, but are not indicated for infected infants with congenital defects. Assistance with rehabilitation for congenital abnormalities may be required.

Rubella

This togavirus causes a usually insignificant infection in adults or adolescents but can cause devastating congenital infection. In most countries between 70 and 90 per cent of young adults are immune to rubella, but in some parts of Asia only 50 per cent are immune. In temperate climates, acquired disease is most common in the spring and early summer, with an increase in local incidence every 3–5 years.

The incubation period is 2–3 weeks and clinical manifestations include mild fever, sore throat, enlarged cervical glands and a rash that may be discreet or give a general pink flush to the trunk. Painful joints are common in adults, and symptoms persist for 3–7 days. However, infection in children often passes unnoticed. Any symptoms suggestive of rubella during pregnancy should lead to investigation. Similar clinical pictures (except those of congenital infection) are produced by many other viral infections.

Gregg's triad of cardiovascular defects, eye defects and deafness summarizes congenital infection. In addition, hepatitis, thrombocytopenia, bone involvement, microcephaly, behavioural change and mental retardation have been reported. Abortions and stillbirths can occur, as can preterm birth. The diagnosis should be suspected in any small for gestational age baby with congenital abnormalities. The congenital syndrome occurs most commonly in early pregnancy; the incidence is 50 per cent following infection in the first month, dropping to 10 per cent if infection occurs in the fourth month of pregnancy. The virus can be isolated from more than 90 per cent of embryos of infected pregnancies and it appears that approximately half the cases are able to clear the infection, as only 50 per cent of proven maternal infections result in infants with persistent IgG or IgM antibodies.

Diagnosis is based on serological tests. At booking, maternal antibody levels are measured and if the antibody titre is low (<15 iu/mL), a booster vaccination should be given after delivery. A very high IgG antibody titre is suggestive of recent infection, but specific IgM is only detectable for 4–6 weeks in most cases. Non-immune women should be advised to stay away from known cases of rubella, as there is no specific treatment available. Congenital rubella can be diagnosed by detecting the virus in secretions from the throat, urine and faeces. It can also be found in CSF, blood, eyes and ears. Excretion diminishes slowly and has ceased by the age of 6 months in 70 per cent of cases. The presence of IgG antibody after 6 months of age is confirmatory. Rubella-specific IgM may be found for 3–9 months.

Many children are so handicapped by deafness or blindness that they are unable to attend normal schools. If rubella is diagnosed during the first trimester, the risk of congenital infection is so high that many women elect to have a termination of pregnancy. In the past, adolescent girls were vaccinated against rubella; vaccination has now been incorporated within the measles, mumps, rubella (MMR) vaccine given in infancy. Following scares related to the measles vaccine, uptake has dropped below 90 per cent in the UK, which means that a cohort of women susceptible to rubella will continue to present in pregnancy. However, a vaccination programme has led to a significant reduction in the incidence of congenital rubella to two cases per year for the UK.

Varicella zoster

Varicella zoster virus is another herpes virus. It is transmitted easily from adults with chickenpox or shingles (herpes zoster), and 90 per cent of adults in the UK are immune to chickenpox. Shingles is a reactivation that can occur during pregnancy but does not pose any threat to the fetus. Transmission occurs through droplet spread, with an incubation period of about 2 weeks. In children, the illness is often mild and there may be only a handful of lesions. In adults, there is usually a prodrome with headache, general aches and pains and malaise. Clusters of vesicles emerge at different stages; most are usually densely grouped centrally. If there is any doubt, the diagnosis can be confirmed by electron microscopy and culture of vesicle fluid. Once the infection clears, latent infection of both sensory and motor nerve cells is established. This infection can reactivate with dissemination of the virus into a dermatome causing the eruption recognized as shingles. Pregnant women are more vulnerable to chickenpox and may develop pneumonitis (to which smokers are particularly prone), which can be fatal. Early administration of intravenous aciclovir may ameliorate the severity, but intensive care support may be needed.

1. Varicella zoster can affect the fetus in two ways. If infection occurs prior to 20 weeks' gestation, there is a small risk (approximately 1 per cent) of a congenital varicella syndrome. This consists of hypoplastic limbs, scarring and central nervous system (CNS) anomalies. If a pregnant woman is exposed to chickenpox or shingles, she should be tested for varicella zoster antibody. If she is not immune, varicella zoster immune globulin (VZIG) should be administered. The possible role of antiviral agents has not yet been evaluated.

2. Neonatal chickenpox can also occur if the mother presents with infection from 2 days before to 5 days after delivery, as the fetus is exposed to virus in the absence of maternal antibody. Neonatal varicella may be very severe, although early reports of a mortality rate of up to 30 per cent were overestimated. VZIG should be administered to the neonate immediately if the mother develops chickenpox. If chickenpox develops during the first month of life, intravenous aciclovir should be administered.

The diagnosis of chickenpox is usually clinical but can be confirmed by electron microscopy or culture of scrapings taken from vesicles. Serological tests are negative during the acute presentation, but the absence of antibody confirms that the mother is susceptible to infection. Chickenpox should be differentiated from other acute viral exanthems: smallpox has now been eradicated, but eczema herpeticum might be mistaken for chickenpox.

Other infections associated with pregnancy loss and preterm birth

Parvovirus B19

Infection with human parvovirus has been recognized to cause acute aplastic crises in individuals with reduced red cell survival, such as those with sickle-cell anaemia. In children it causes the viral exanthem known as 'fifth disease', erythema infectiosum or slapped cheek syndrome.

The infection is asymptomatic in 25 per cent of adults and in more than 50 per cent of children. It may be associated with only mild symptoms of malaise or may present with a macular rash and it can be associated with severe arthralgia. In approximately 15 per cent of infections occurring during pregnancy, the fetus becomes chronically infected. This leads to persistent anaemia in utero, which may develop into non-immune hydrops fetalis, which may resolve spontaneously or may require intrauterine blood transfusion.

The diagnosis of parvovirus infection is confirmed by demonstrating either virus-specific IgM in maternal serum or seroconversion with a specimen that previously proved negative. It should be sought in mothers who have the clinical features, or when hydrops fetalis develops. There is no specific treatment for parvovirus infection, but the baby should be monitored carefully, with repeated ultrasound examinations. The virus is not teratogenic.

Listeria monocytogenes

This bacterium has been isolated from more than 50 species of domestic and wild animals, including birds, fish, insects and crustaceans. It is found in sewage, water and mud and can grow in refrigerated food, including meat, eggs and dairy products, particularly soft cheeses. Asymptomatic carriage in humans as well as animals is common, with up to 29 per cent of healthy people having detectable organisms in the faeces. Such carriage is often transient. Cooking destroys the bacterium and therefore the risk of infection is greatest with uncooked food. Most infections are probably subclinical, but pregnant women are more vulnerable. In the UK, the incidence of *Listeria* infection is approximately 1 in 37 000 births.

In adults, the anginose type of listeriosis may be confused with glandular fever, and in pregnancy, an episode of malaise, headache, fever, backache, conjunctivitis and diarrhoea associated with abdominal or loin pain may occur. In 40 per cent of cases fever is not marked at any time and the disease presents as a mild, flu-like illness. In animals, recurrent or persistent genital *Listeria* infection causes habitual abortion and it may do the same in humans.

Listeria infection of the newborn occurs in two forms. The early-onset type results from in-utero infection that manifests as septicaemia within 2 days of birth. Usually the infant is born prematurely with signs of respiratory distress and there may be a rash. The late form presents predominantly as meningo-encephalitis after the fifth day. Approximately 30 per cent of babies with early-onset disease are stillborn. In France, *Listeria monocytogenes* ranks third, after *Escherichia coli* and group B *Streptococcus*, as a cause of neonatal sepsis. The organism has a predilection for infecting the CNS in the newborn and also in immunosuppressed adults. There may be only a low-grade fever and focal neurological signs may develop.

Diagnosis in the neonate requires a high index of suspicion. Specimens from affected sites, including the throat, liver, CSF, vagina, placenta, and urine, faeces and blood can be used for culture. Isolation is enhanced by cold passage at 4 °C. Serological diagnosis is unsatisfactory, although finding a rising titre of *Listeria*-specific IgM can be helpful.

The organism is susceptible to penicillins, macrolides and tetracyclines; ampicillin is the treatment of choice. Without recognition of the diagnosis, the mortality from infantile listeriosis is as high as 90 per cent and the prognosis is worse in preterm babies. Early diagnosis and prompt treatment have reduced this figure to only 50 per cent.

Malaria

Malaria is prevalent throughout the tropics and is a major cause of mortality in both children and adults. Major polymorphisms such as thalassaemia and sickle-cell trait provide a selection advantage in these areas because affected individuals are more resistant to severe manifestations of malaria. *Plasmodium falciparum* causes the most severe type of malaria, which can present with hepatic and cerebral forms of infection. It is transmitted between human hosts by the female *Anopheles* mosquito. Attempts to eradicate this intermediate host during the 1960s and 1970s with spraying of toxins such as dichlorodiphenyl-trichloroethane (DDT) have now been abandoned. *P. falciparum* has been able to develop resistance to most antimicrobials, creating a need for new agents to be developed. The other strains of malarial parasites (*P. ovale* and *P. vivax*) seldom cause fatal disease and have not so far developed chloroquine resistance

but cause considerable morbidity. The development of the parasite in the mosquito only occurs at warm temperatures, therefore infection is rarely transmitted at altitudes above 2200 m.

The principal feature of malaria is episodes of high body temperature and rigors followed by sweating as the temperature falls. There is headache, nausea and vomiting and, with *P. falciparum* malaria, the pyrexia may be continuous. The incubation period is approximately 2 weeks. In severe infections, 20 per cent or more of the red cells may be infected and haemolysis occurs, leading to anaemia. This may result in haemoglobinuria (blackwater fever), associated with acute renal failure. Hyponatraemia and disseminated intravascular coagulation may also occur. Cerebral malaria presents with disturbances in consciousness due to obstruction of the cerebral capillaries by infected red cells that have reduced deformability. Pregnant women are at increased risk of severe manifestations of malaria; infection may trigger a miscarriage or premature labour. Even non-*falciparum* malaria has been associated with intrauterine growth restriction. Congenital malaria has been described.

The diagnosis should be suspected in anyone who has been to the tropics and presents with a febrile illness. A history of taking prophylaxis does not exclude the diagnosis, as no prophylaxis is 100 per cent effective. A blood film should be requested and stained for malaria parasites. Repeated blood films should be taken during episodes of fever if the initial test is negative. As well as anaemia, there may be thrombocytopenia and elevation of liver enzymes. Fever in the tropics or in those recently returned from the tropics may be caused by many other infections, including typhoid, food poisoning organisms, and viral infections such as dengue fever.

Malaria is usually treated with quinine sulphate, initially administered intravenously. Individuals with *P. falciparum* malaria should be admitted to hospital and monitored closely, as sudden deterioration requiring intensive care may occur. Non-*falciparum* malaria establishes chronic infection of the liver. If the individual is not returning to an endemic area, acute treatment should be followed by a course of Fansidar to eradicate infection. Individuals living in endemic areas acquire immunity to malaria, but this is lost within a few months of moving away; therefore anyone travelling from the UK to an endemic area should consider taking prophylaxis. A combination of chloroquine and proguanil taken weekly provides protection against non-*falciparum* malaria and *falciparum* malaria in some areas. Malaria resistant to many antimicrobials is present in sub-Saharan Africa and South East Asia, where even mefloquine resistance has been reported. The choice of prophylactic agent should therefore be made after consulting current recommendations that give details of resistance patterns. Chloroquine is probably the least toxic prophylactic agent for pregnant women, and those travelling to areas of chloroquine resistance must balance the risk of malaria against the potential toxicity of prophylactic agents. It is safest to avoid travel to such areas when pregnant, but if the mother cannot be persuaded to delay travel, the potential risks and benefits of chemoprophylaxis must be discussed.

Chlamydia psittaci

This organism causes epidemic abortion in ewes and an atypical pneumonia in humans. Exposure to lambing ewes and the products of conception can lead to infection in pregnant women, which results in intrauterine infection and abortion. This has occurred most commonly in vets and farm workers, and all pregnant women should be advised to avoid sheep during the lambing season.

Urinary tract infection (see p. 128)

Bacterial vaginosis

Bacterial vaginosis is the commonest cause of vaginal discharge in women of childbearing age. The principal symptom is an offensive, fishy-smelling vaginal discharge that is often more apparent during menstruation or following unprotected intercourse. In some populations its prevalence is greater than 50 per cent, although in the UK it is found in 10–15 per cent of women. It is thought to represent a disturbance of the vaginal ecosystem in which the usually dominant lactobacilli are overwhelmed by an over-growth of predominantly anaerobic organisms, including *Gardnerella vaginalis*, *Bacteroides* spp., *Mycoplasma hominis* and *Mobiluncus* spp. Some of these organisms produce polyamines and trimethylamine, which are responsible for the fishy smell. There is also a rise in the vaginal pH from the normal level (below 4.5) to levels as high as 6 or 7.

It is not a sexually transmitted infection and there is no benefit from treating male partners.

Bacterial vaginosis is not usually associated with vaginal soreness. However, it may co-exist with either candidiasis or trichomoniasis, both of which cause irritation and soreness. On examination, a white or yellow, thin, homogenous discharge is seen. Examination of a 'wet mount' of vaginal fluid microscopically shows the presence of many small bacteria, which adhere to the epithelial cells giving them a fuzzy border, the so-called 'clue cell'. Similar features are seen on a Gram-stained smear. Vaginal pH can be measured simply by placing a small amount of vaginal fluid onto pH paper. A further criterion is the potassium hydroxide test, for which a sample of vaginal fluid is mixed with potassium hydroxide on a microscope slide. A strong fishy smell is produced if the woman has bacterial vaginosis. The condition may also be recognized on Papanicolaou-stained cervical smears. Culture of vaginal fluid is not useful for making the diagnosis, as the organisms can be found in more than 50 per cent of normal women.

Trichomoniasis or candidiasis can both produce discharges they produce can look similar to those of bacterial vaginosis. Microscopy and culture of vaginal fluid can confirm both of these alternatives. Discharge due to cervicitis is usually more mucoid or mucopurulent and there should be signs of clinical cervicitis on examination. Many observational studies have confirmed that women with bacterial vaginosis have an increased risk of second trimester loss and preterm birth; indeed, it may be the most important cause of idiopathic preterm birth. It is associated with chorioamnionitis, which can progress to deciduitis or amniotic fluid infection, which may result in fetal pneumonitis and ultimately fetal death may follow this from sepsis. Chorioamnionitis is associated with elevated levels of pro-inflammatory cytokines such as tumour necrosis factor-alpha (TNF-α), interleukin 6 (IL6) and IL12. These can stimulate the metabolism of arachidonic acid to prostaglandins, which is the final pathway for cervical ripening and the onset of labour. At present, studies are evaluating the use of antibiotics to treat pregnant women with bacterial vaginosis. Studies of selected women at high risk of preterm birth have shown a benefit from treatment with metronidazole. However, it is less clear whether women without high-risk factors for preterm birth should be screened and treated. Symptomatic women should, of course, be treated.

The standard treatment for bacterial vaginosis in the UK is metronidazole 400 mg twice a day for 5 days. This produces resolution within a few days, but relapse can occur, and as many as 30 per cent of women have bacterial vaginosis again within 1 month. Alternative treatments include intravaginal 0.75 per cent metronidazole gel, 2 per cent clindamycin cream, and oral clindamycin 300 mg twice a day for 5 days. Physicians have been wary of prescribing metronidazole during pregnancy because of reputed teratogenicity. Several meta-analyses have reviewed its use during pregnancy and have shown no excess of birth defects. If a woman requires treatment, it is sensible to discuss the potential risks and weigh them against the benefits. Both oral and intravaginal clindamycin have been associated with pseudomembranous colitis, a potentially fatal condition. Women who develop diarrhoea following such treatment, particularly with blood, should cease treatment and seek medical advice.

Infections affecting the neonate at birth

Herpes simplex virus

Herpes simplex is a virus that is well adapted to its human host. Primary infection usually presents within 7 days of exposure and may be accompanied by widespread lesions around the mouth and oropharynx and, in the case of genital herpes, around the vulva, vagina and cervix. If inoculation occurs on the skin, such as with occupational exposure for a healthcare worker, a herpetic whitlow may result. In many populations, more than 70–80 per cent are exposed to oral herpes, herpes simplex virus type 1 (HSV1), during childhood. This gives some degree of cross-protection against HSV2, traditionally the causative agent of genital herpes, and primary infection may be mild. With less exposure to childhood infections in Western societies, fewer young adults have been exposed to HSV1, and 50 per cent of cases of genital herpes are now due to this strain of virus. Primary infection may therefore follow oro-genital contact. Seroprevalence studies suggest that 15–70 per cent of the population have antibodies to HSV1 and approximately 20 per cent to HSV2.

Primary genital herpes presents with soreness and irritation of the affected part (Fig. 16.2). It may, however, pass completely unnoticed or be manifest with a

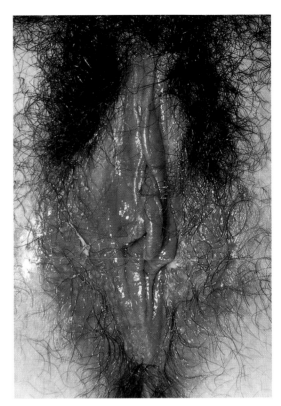

Figure 16.2 Primary genital herpes in a woman. Multiple ulcers are seen with a wide distribution and confluent in some areas. In pregnancy, recurrent herpes can resemble a primary episode. (Courtesy of Dr Richard Lau, St George's Hospital, London.)

widespread eruption of painful ulcers preceded by vesicles. Severe dysuria and peripheral nerve involvement may lead to urinary retention in women requiring admission for analgesia and a temporary suprapubic catheter. In pregnancy with altered T-helper cell immunity, recurrent herpes may be more severe than usual and mimic primary herpes. In primary herpes, the lesions heal during the course of 2–3 weeks. Recurrences (Fig. 16.3) usually last 3–7 days and are more localized, in a manner similar to an oral cold sore.

Vesicles and ulcers are seen on examination. The cervix may be severely inflamed and haemorrhagic. Cases of severe herpes mimicking pelvic inflammatory disease (PID) have been described, particularly in postnatal human immunodeficiency virus (HIV)-infected women.

More than half the men and women infected with genital herpes are unaware of its presence. Close and careful questioning may reveal a history of transient, almost trivial, sores occurring sporadically, usually in

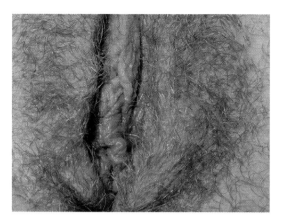

Figure 16.3 Recurrent genital herpes. There is a localized area of erythema and oedema on the left side of the labia majora, with early vesicle formation.

the same site. HSV2 is more likely than HSV1 to cause symptomatic recurrences. The frequency of recurrences varies from person to person and a small minority will have more than six recurrences per year; some are incapacitated due to neurological symptoms such as pains going down the legs.

The initial diagnosis is clinical but should always be confirmed by taking a swab from a vesicle or ulcer for culture or electron microscopy. Specific viral transport medium is essential. Serological tests have not been useful, as assays have not been able to distinguish between antibodies to HSV1 and HSV2.

Herpes simplex needs to be differentiated from other causes of genital ulcers. These include infections such as syphilis and tropical genital ulcer disease (see below). Genital ulcers can occur in association with systemic diseases such as sarcoidosis or SLE. Behçet's syndrome classically presents with oral and genital ulceration and may be accompanied by uveitis and CNS manifestations. The diagnosis is made by exclusion.

In the non-pregnant woman, a first presentation of herpes should be treated with a 5-day course of aciclovir 200 mg five times a day. This will stop further lesions developing and allow those that are present to heal. In many cases it will be a recurrent rather than a true primary infection that is being treated, but it is not possible to differentiate reliably unless there is a history of herpes infection. There are insufficient data to confirm that aciclovir is safe during pregnancy. However, to date, there is no excess of birth defects associated with its use. Topical aciclovir cream is not effective in the treatment of genital herpes.

It is important to diagnose herpes in pregnancy because a devastating neonatal infection can occur with involvement of the skin, liver and CNS. Neonatal mortality is 75 per cent. However, if aciclovir is administered rapidly, this can be reduced to 40 per cent. This syndrome is more common in the USA than in the UK, where the rates are 1 in 33 000 and 1 in 5000 live births respectively. The vast majority of these cases are associated with a primary herpes infection in the mother in the weeks prior to delivery. The baby then has no protective antibody and is vulnerable to disseminated infection, or localized hepes encephalitis. If primary herpes presents around the time of delivery, the case should be discussed with the paediatrician. Caesarean section will provide protection to the infant as long as no more than 4 hours have elapsed since rupture of the membranes. Genital swabs should be cultured from the mother and throat swabs from the baby, and intravenous acyclovir should be administered to the neonate. Women known to have recurrent herpes have also been offered Caesarean section if a recurrence occurs at the time of delivery. It has been found that the risk of infection to the neonate from a maternal recurrence of herpes is very small and many units have now abandoned Caesarean section for this indication. The potential role of aciclovir administration for the last 2–4 weeks of pregnancy in women with recurrent herpes has not been fully evaluated because neonatal herpes in such cases is so rare.

Infection during the first trimester may cause miscarriage. A congenital syndrome has also been described, associated with micro-ophthalmia, chorioretinitis and microcephaly.

Group B *Streptococcus*

This organism is a commensal in the gut and genital tract and is found in 20–40 per cent of women. It may cause severe neonatal infection leading to neonatal death and can cause upper genital tract infection progressing to septicaemia and occasionally maternal death.

Carriage of the organism is asymptomatic. It colonizes the vagina from the gut and then ascends into the uterus. It can be detected on culture of vaginal swabs, but colonization of the vagina can occur at any stage of pregnancy. Attempts have been made to screen for infection in early pregnancy and to eradicate the organism with penicillin; however, re-colonization frequently occurs and this approach has not been shown to reduce the incidence of neonatal infection. The current recommendation is therefore that the organism should be sought by culture of vaginal swabs in complicated pregnancies or when they has been a prior preterm birth. If the organism is present, penicillin should be administered intravenously at the time of delivery. The infants most at risk are premature, have undergone delivery after prolonged rupture of membranes, are growth restricted or have birth asphyxia. Early disease presents as overwhelming septicaemia and pneumonia. Occasionally an infant colonized in the perinatal period may develop secondary disease between 1 and 4 weeks of age, presenting as meningitis. Hospitals in which there is a high incidence of neonatal infection have developed protocols to screen mothers whose pregnancies are considered high risk and to treat them at about 28 weeks' gestation with penicillin if the organism is detected on a vaginal swab. The case for such screening is weaker in units with a low prevalence of neonatal infection.

Chlamydia trachomatis

Chlamydia trachomatis is an obligate intracellular parasite. Genital infection with serotypes D–K is the commonest bacterial sexually transmitted infection in developed countries. It is also very common in developing countries. In many tropical countries, trachoma (caused by serotypes A–C) is endemic, and transmission is thought to occur amongst household contacts; it leads to blindness in the most severe cases. *Chlamydia trachomatis* is important in pregnancy because it causes neonatal eye infection (ophthalmia neonatorum) and neonatal pneumonitis.

Estimates of the prevalence of genital *Chlamydia trachomatis* infection vary between 2 per cent and 10 per cent of women in the UK. The organism is detected much more commonly in young sexually active women and women under the age of 25. The spectrum of disease varies from chronic asymptomatic infection to cervicitis, endometritis, salpingitis (PID) and intraperitoneal spread leading to perihepatitis (Fitz-Hugh Curtis syndrome). In men it causes non-gonococcal urethritis, which may present with urethral discharge and dysuria. Many male partners of women with *Chlamydia trachomatis* are, however, asymptomatic.

Pelvic inflammatory disease is uncommon during pregnancy and many pregnant women carrying *Chlamydia trachomatis* are only diagnosed after the neonate develops clinical disease. Where screening is undertaken, in communities with a high prevalence of *Chlamydia trachomatis*, asymptomatic infection will be detected. An infected cervix is friable and bleeds easily on contact, with an associated purulent discharge from the cervical os, termed mucopurulent cervicitis. The changes induced by pregnancy may be similar, so that the specificity of such findings is lower than in the non-pregnant woman. Tubal damage associated with previous chlamydial infection is an important predisposing factor for ectopic pregnancy.

Approximately 50 per cent of babies born to women with chlamydial infection develop ophthalmia neonatorum. This usually presents about a week after birth with a red sticky eye, which may be bilateral. Chloramphenicol drops, which are commonly prescribed, will only produce partial resolution. A swab for *Chlamydia trachomatis* should be taken from the baby's eye. The organism can also be sought in nasopharyngeal aspirates. Diagnosis of chlamydial infection is made by detecting the organism. ELISA tests are easily used to screen large numbers of samples, but unfortunately the sensitivity is only 60 per cent. For this reason, culture, DNA detection-based tests or direct immunofluorescence must be used. Tests that rely on amplification of DNA provide greater sensitivity and specificity and will become increasingly routine. The organism can be detected with such tests in endocervical swabs, first-pass urine samples, and even self-administered vaginal swabs. The most important differential diagnosis for cervicitis is gonorrhoea, which is described below.

The treatment of choice for *Chlamydia trachomatis* is tetracycline, usually doxycycline. However, tetracycline should be avoided in the second and third trimesters of pregnancy because it binds to developing bones and teeth in the fetus, causing brown staining of the teeth and dysplastic bones. Erythromycin 500 mg twice a day for 2 weeks is therefore prescribed. This causes nausea, and the pharmacokinetics are not reliable in pregnancy, so a test of cure 2 weeks after completing treatment is obligatory. It is essential that male partners are screened and treated before sexual intercourse is resumed. Azithromycin as a single 1 g dose is licensed for the treatment of *Chlamydia trachomatis* and may be useful if the woman is unable to tolerate erythromycin. Although penicillins are not considered adequate treatment to eradicate *Chlamydia trachomatis*, co-amoxiclav has been shown to be effective in preventing neonatal infection and may be used if macrolides are contraindicated. Definitive treatment with a tetracycline should be administered after delivery and breastfeeding. Neonates with ophthalmia neonatorum should be treated with tetracycline eye ointment. Because there is a risk of subsequent chlamydial pneumonitis, they should also be treated with a 2-week course of erythromycin syrup.

Many women with *Chlamydia trachomatis* have subclinical endometritis, which may predispose to early pregnancy loss, chorioamnionitis and preterm birth, and clinical postpartum endometritis. It has been associated with failure of implantation in women undergoing in-vitro fertilization (IVF). Such women and their partners should therefore be screened.

CASE HISTORY

A 21-year-old primigravida is admitted in labour at 26 weeks' gestation with a twin pregnancy. The membranes ruptured spontaneously 2 hours earlier. An emergency Caesarean section is performed. The first child is stillborn, and the second survives for only 12 hours in the neonatal intensive care unit. At post mortem, the first child was found to have had a *Gardnerella* pneumonitis. The mother develops pyrexia of 39° C and is commenced on intravenous co-amoxiclav. Cultures of blood and urine are sterile. A vaginal swab grows mixed anaerobes. The fever settles and she is discharged from hospital 5 days later.

Six months later, she presents with amenorrhoea of 7 weeks and right-sided pelvic pain. An ectopic pregnancy is confirmed and removed laparoscopically.

At this point, she is screened for sexually transmitted infections and found to have chlamydial cervicitis. Her partner is also infected. Both are treated with doxycycline 100 mg twice daily for 2 weeks. After a further 6 months, she becomes pregnant again with a singleton fetus. A screen for bacterial vaginosis, chlamydia, gonorrhoea and

trichomoniasis is negative. She has an uneventful pregnancy, delivering a healthy boy at 38 weeks' gestation.

Discussion points

- Infection is a major factor in the aetiology of idiopathic preterm birth. Bacterial vaginosis is associated with chorioamnionitis, fetal sepsis and postpartum endometritis. *Gardnerella* pneumonitis is suggestive of bacterial vaginosis in the mother.
- Preterm birth is more common in twin pregnancies than in singleton pregnancies.
- *Chlamydia trachomatis* is an important cause of ectopic pregnancy. It should be sought in women with an ectopic pregnancy, and their sex partners must also be screened and treated before intercourse is resumed.
- Forty per cent of women with a prior preterm birth have preterm delivery in the next pregnancy. It is possible that by eradicating infections the risk of preterm birth is reduced.

Gonorrhoea

Neisseria gonorrhoeae is a sexually transmissible agent causing cervicitis, urethritis, endometritis, salpingitis (PID) and perihepatitis in women. In men it causes urethritis and epididymitis, and in both men and women it causes proctitis and pharyngitis. It is common worldwide, although the incidence has decreased in developed countries since the Second World War. Infection in both sexes is often asymptomatic.

Like chlamydia, gonorrhoea is commonest in young sexually active women, with the incidence declining over the age of 25. Its importance in obstetrics is due to a neonatal eye infection that, if untreated, can progress to blindness due to corneal scarring. The

introduction of silver nitrate drops as prophylaxis produced a dramatic decline in the incidence of this complication.

The diagnosis of gonorrhoea is established by microscopy and culture. Gram-stained microscopy of cervical, urethral and rectal swabs is performed, although the sensitivity of Gram stain is only 50 per cent compared to culture in women. The organism prefers a high carbon dioxide environment and is cultured on selective media such as blood agar. Even with optimal conditions, however, a single set of cultures has a sensitivity of only 60–70 per cent for detecting infection. If clinical suspicion is high, a second set of cultures should be taken. It is routine practice to perform two sets of cultures as a test of cure following treatment. DNA detection-based tests are now available and these offer superior sensitivity to culture; however, at present they do not allow the opportunity for antibiotic resistance testing, for which culture remains necessary.

Neisseria gonorrhoeae has demonstrated a great ability to acquire resistance to antibiotics. It readily exchanges plasmids with other bacterial species, and plasmid-mediated resistance to penicillin and tetracycline appears rapidly under selection pressure with such antibiotics. In many developing countries, the price of antibiotics is prohibitive for most individuals, so that suboptimal doses are used. This encourages the development of resistant strains, which are then exported worldwide. Chromosomal mutation has also produced moderate levels of penicillin resistance and is responsible for resistance to quinolones. Quinolones are contraindicated in pregnancy and therefore in a penicillin-allergic woman, or a woman with penicillin-resistant infection, a cephalosporin, such as cefotaxime 2 g in a single intramuscular dose, should be administered. Table 16.3 details antibiotics and their use in pregnancy.

Table 16.3 – Commonly used antibiotics in pregnancy

Thought to be safe
Penicillins, e.g. amoxycillin
Cephalosporins, e.g. cefotaxime
Erythromycin
Nitrofurantoin in first and second trimesters

Probably safe but limited experience
Co-amoxiclav
Azithromycin

Significant caution required
Quinolones, e.g. ciprofloxacin
Folate reductase inhibitors, e.g. co-trimoxazole

Contraindicated
Tetracyclines

Neonates may present with ophthalmia neonatorum due to gonorrhoea a few days after birth. If *Neisseria gonorrhoeae* is cultured, topical and systemic treatment should be administered according to antibiotic sensitivities. In a similar way to *Chlamydia* *trachomatis* infection, gonorrhoea is associated with chorioamnionitis and preterm birth.

Trichomoniasis

Trichomonas vaginalis causes severe vulvo-vaginitis in susceptible women. It is generally sexually transmitted, although infection may persist asymptomatically for many months in women and in some men. In men it may cause urethritis, but is often asymptomatic. Transient infection can be transmitted to female infants, who will present with purulent vaginal discharge.

The incidence of trichomoniasis has fallen in developed countries. It remains highly prevalent in many developing countries, where as many as 20–30 per cent of pregnant women carry the infection. It presents with a purulent vaginal discharge and may be associated with severe inflammation causing soreness and itching with a 'tidemark' extending on to the thighs. The diagnosis is made by detecting the organism on wet mount microscopy, with a sensitivity of approximately 50–60 per cent.

Newborn girls have stratified squamous epithelium in the vagina, similar to that of an adult, due to the influence of high levels of maternal oestrogen in utero. They are therefore susceptible to infection and may develop asymptomatic discharge. As the influence of maternal oestrogen wanes over the first few weeks of life, such infection usually resolves spontaneously and specific treatment is rarely necessary.

Trichomoniasis often co-exists with disturbed vaginal flora that develops into bacterial vaginosis. The only established treatments for trichomoniasis are metronidazole or tinidazole, but these have been considered to carry a risk of teratogenicity. There are extremely limited animal data to support such a claim, although there is some evidence of mutagenesis. Retrospective studies of women who have taken metronidazole during pregnancy have shown no excess of fetal abnormalities and it is therefore reasonable to treat symptomatic women with a 5-day course of metronidazole 400 mg twice a day. It is sensible, however, to discuss the potential risks of any treatment with the mother so that she can make an informed decision. Clotrimazole has some activity against trichomoniasis, and the application of intravaginal clotrimazole pessaries may control symptoms until the end of the first trimester if a woman is particularly concerned about systemic treatment.

Other infections

Ureaplasma urealyticum is an organism in the *Mycoplasma* genus, which is a common commensal organism in the vagina. It has been detected in the membranes of women delivering preterm and has also been associated with neonatal pneumonitis. Its importance in inducing preterm birth and neonatal lung disease is not yet established. *Mycoplasma genitalium* appears to cause a spectrum of disease similar to *Chlamydia trachomatis*, with cervicitis, PID and non-gonococcal urethritis. It has not yet been studied extensively in pregnancy.

Infections affecting the mother

Vaginal candidiasis

More than three-quarters of women have at least one episode of vaginal candidiasis during their lifetime. A few women get frequent recurrences. The organism is carried in the gut, under the nails, in the vagina and on the skin. The yeast *Candida albicans* is implicated in more than 80 per cent of cases; *C. glabrata*, *C. krusei* and *C. tropicalis* account for most of the rest. Sexual acquisition is rarely important, although the physical trauma of intercourse may be sufficient to trigger an attack in a predisposed individual. *Candida* is an opportunistic organism, growing under favourable conditions. Symptomatic episodes are common in pregnancy; growth of the organism is favoured by the high levels of oestrogen, increased availability of sugars and subtle alterations in immunity.

The classical presentation is itching and soreness of the vagina and vulva with a curdy white discharge that may smell yeasty but not unpleasant. Not all candidiasis presents in the same way; in some cases there may be itching and redness with a thin, watery discharge.

The pH of vaginal fluid is usually normal, between 3.5 and 4.5. The diagnosis can be confirmed by microscopy and culture of the vaginal fluid. Asymptomatic women from whom *Candida* is grown on culture do not require treatment.

Recurrent candidiasis, or resistance to treatment, is relatively uncommon. If there appears to be a recurrence, it is important to consider other diagnoses, particularly herpes simplex, which causes localized ulceration and soreness, and dermatological conditions such as eczema and lichen sclerosis.

In general, it is better to use a topical rather than a systemic treatment. This minimizes the risk of systemic side effects and exposure of the fetus. Vaginal creams and pessaries can be prescribed at a variety of doses and duration of treatment. For uncomplicated candidiasis, a single-dose treatment, such as clotrimazole 500 mg, is adequate. If oral therapy has to be used, a single 150 mg tablet of fluconazole is usually effective, but its activity is limited to *Candida albicans* strains and its role in pregnancy is not yet defined.

Genital warts

Warts are caused by human papillomavirus (HPV) infections. More than 100 strains have so far been identified and certain strains are generally transmitted sexually, producing genital warts on the mucosa of the genital tract. Most symptomatic infections develop within 8 months of starting a sexual relationship with a new partner, but the incubation period may be a few years in some cases. It is thought that cell-mediated immunity is important for suppressing wart virus infections. With the alterations in maternal immunity that occur during pregnancy, a previously asymptomatic infection may start to produce genital warts or established infections may become more florid (Fig. 16.4). Topical application of podophyllin or podophyllotoxin is often used as first-line treatment,

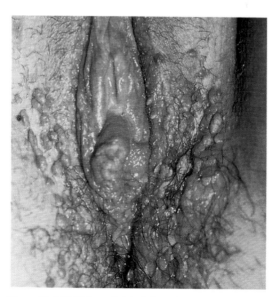

Figure 16.4 Multiple genital warts in a pregnant woman. Warts often increase in size and number during pregnancy. (Courtesy of Dr Richard Lau, St George's Hospital, London.)

but is contraindicated in pregnancy. The risk of fetal damage from the administration of a small amount of such chemicals to genital warts in a woman who does not realize she is pregnant is so low that it is not an indication for termination of pregnancy, unless applied to a very large area ($>10\,cm^2$). Surgical methods such as cryotherapy or excision are therefore the only treatments available for pregnant women. Even so, the warts may not fully resolve until the woman has delivered. Male partners should be advised to attend a genitourinary medicine clinic for screening and treatment of any warts that they may have, and condoms should be used during sexual intercourse. In an established relationship it is likely that wart virus transmission has already occurred, and therefore it is not necessary to give such advice unless a new relationship has started. HPV types 6 and 11 are the ones found most often in symptomatic lesions. These have a low association with malignant change in the cervix. The oncogenic strains 16 and 18 may be found alongside the other types, but do not often produce typical lesions on their own.

Any baby born to a mother harbouring wart virus will be exposed to the virus during delivery. It appears, however, that few neonates acquire infection from their mothers. Rarely, infants may present with laryngeal warts due to a genital strain of wart virus, but transmission appears to occur from less than 1 per cent of infected mothers. It is unlikely that maternal transmission leads to established infection in the genital tract of boys or girls.

Tropical genital ulcer disease

In many tropical areas, infections causing genital ulcers are common. Herpes simplex remains an important cause of genital ulcers worldwide, but lymphogranuloma venereum (LGV) caused by the LGV strains of *Chlamydia trachomatis*, donovanosis caused by *Calymmatobacterium donovanii* and chancroid caused by *Haemophilus ducreyi* are common. Specific diagnostic tests are expensive and such infections are usually managed according to protocols for syndromic management. The specific antibiotics prescribed depend on local availability and sensitivity patterns established in reference laboratories. In some areas of sub-Saharan Africa, up to 30 per cent of pregnant women are infected with HIV; therefore, altered immunity may lead to atypical presentation of any of

these infections, making diagnosis and treatment more difficult.

Other infections

With the altered immune state of pregnancy, chronic infections requiring cell-mediated immunity may flare up. These include wart virus infections, as discussed above. With the rising incidence of tuberculosis worldwide and recent increases in the UK and the USA, more pregnant women may present with severe manifestations of disease such as miliary tuberculosis. Pregnancy produces a transient fall in the CD4 lymphocyte count of HIV-infected women. (This is discussed more fully below.) Most of the UK now has effective screening programmes (Table 16.4).

Other vertically transmissible viral infections

Human T-cell leukaemia virus-1

Human T-cell leukaemia virus (HTLV-1) is a retrovirus that establishes life-long infection in affected individuals. The majority of such individuals remain asymptomatic, but a small proportion may develop T-cell leukaemia in adult life. It also causes tropical spastic paraparesis, which presents with demyelination of the spinal cord causing spastic weakness in the legs. Its prevalence is greatest in Japan, the Caribbean, the Indian sub-continent and parts of Africa. It is transmitted sexually or through breast milk, therefore if infection is identified, the mother should be advised not to breastfeed. There is no specific treatment, but barrier methods of contraception should be advised if the sex partner is uninfected.

Hepatitis A

This is caused by an RNA virus, which is spread through the oral–faecal route. Approximately 50 per cent of the UK population has antibodies from childhood infection but the prevalence is falling. The majority of individuals in developing countries acquire infection during childhood. Hepatitis A is usually a benign illness, but occasionally fulminating hepatitis has been described in pregnant women, although it has not been associated with congenital abnormalities.

Table 16.4 – Infection screening during pregnancy

Infection	Test	Action
Syphilis	VDRL/TPHA	Refer to specialist if reactive. If no history of prior treatment, will need parenteral penicillin for 12 days
Rubella	IgG	If negative, advise to avoid contact. Vaccinate after delivery
Hepatitis B	Surface antigen test	Immunoglobulin and vaccination for neonates. Check maternal liver function tests, and refer to hepatitis clinic
HIV	HIV antibody	Discuss ways to reduce risk of vertical transmission. Manage with multi-disciplinary team
UTI	Urinalysis/M,C&S	Prescribe antibiotics and check again after treatment

May be indicated in some cases/routine in some countries:
   group B *Streptococcus*
   herpes simplex
   toxoplasmosis
   bacterial vaginosis
   Chlamydia trachomatis
   gonorrhoea
   hepatitis C

VDRL, Venereal Diseases Research Laboratory test; TPHA, *Treponema pallidum* haemagglutination assay; IgG, immunoglobulin G; HIV, human immunodeficiency virus; UTI, urinary tract infection; M,C&S, microscopy, culture and sensitivities.

Individuals are most infectious before they develop jaundice. Some degree of protection may be provided through vaccination or the administration of human immune globulin during the incubation period.

Hepatitis B

Hepatitis B is a more severe infection that may be followed by chronic carriage and disease ending in cirrhosis. It is transmitted sexually, through blood products and through vertical transmission from an infected mother. Most acute infections are not clinically recognized, as only 20 per cent of individuals develop jaundice. The earlier in life the infection occurs, the more likely the person is to become a carrier; 80 per cent of infants infected perinatally become carriers. Infection is particularly common in China and South East Asia but it is prevalent in most tropical countries.

Pregnant women are screened for hepatitis B at booking. During acute infection, hepatitis B surface antigen (HBsAg) and e antigen (HBeAg) are detectable in serum. Hepatitis B core antibody appears after approximately 6 weeks and remains detectable thereafter as a marker of exposure. As immunity develops, anti-e antibody develops and the e antigen becomes undetectable. With clearance of the virus, surface antigen disappears and surface antibody is detectable. When HBeAg is present, the individual is highly infectious. Only a small proportion of individuals who are sAg positive but eAg negative have replicating virus and are infectious. Thus, to screen for chronic infection, anti-core antibody is sought. If this is positive, the other markers are tested to establish the degree of infectivity.

A proportion of individuals do not clear the acute infection and go on to develop chronic hepatitis. Treatment is available with interferon under the guidance of a liver specialist, and antiviral drugs with specific activity against hepatitis B are being introduced. Vertical transmission can be prevented by the vaccination of neonates born to mothers with hepatitis B. Hepatitis B immune globulin is given at birth additionally if the mother is eAg positive. Countries with a higher prevalence of hepatitis B infection than the UK have a policy of universal vaccination of all infants.

Hepatitis C

This is another RNA virus that causes chronic hepatitis. Again, acute infection often passes asymptomatically, but more than 50 per cent of infected individuals have active hepatitis that will progress to cirrhosis and possibly hepatocellular carcinoma. The prevalence varies widely across the world, with the highest incidence in Egypt, possibly associated with the use of contaminated needles for mass treatment for schistosomiasis. In the UK, infection is highly prevalent in those with a history of intravenous drug use. It may be transmitted sexually, but transmission is not very efficient, with only 1–2 per cent of long-term partners becoming infected. Vertical transmission again occurs uncommonly, although the risk is increased in those co-infected with HIV.

Hepatitis D

This is a defective virus that can only replicate in the presence of hepatitis B. Individuals who have this super-infection are more likely to develop severe hepatitis.

Hepatitis E

This virus is spread through the oral–faecal route and causes acute hepatitis. It can, like hepatitis A, be fulminating in pregnant women, with up to 20 per cent mortality. It is found mainly in tropical countries, where epidemics have occurred after natural disasters have allowed contamination of water with sewage. It is not thought to cause chronic hepatitis.

HIV infection

Human immunodeficiency virus infection is a major challenge for the obstetric team. There is a need to reduce the risk of vertical transmission to the fetus, and to maintain optimal health of the mother. This, however, usually involves the use of interventions such as drugs of known or unknown fetal toxicity, performing Caesarean section and advice not to breastfeed. It is best managed through a multi-disciplinary team incorporating obstetricians, midwives, paediatricians and HIV specialists.

Acquired immunodeficiency syndrome was first described in San Francisco in 1983. It is caused by infection with HIV. More than 20 million individuals are now infected worldwide and in countries with a high prevalence it is the leading cause of death in young adults. It is a particularly devastating disease because of the stigma of sexual transmission, the risk of vertical transmission to children, and the likelihood that other family members are infected. Even if a child is not infected, the death of one or both parents threatens their development and survival in many parts of the world. At present, HIV is increasing in prevalence in most parts of the world. In sub-Saharan Africa there are several cities in which as many as a third of pregnant women are infected. The epidemic in South East Asia is a few years behind that of Africa. By contrast, in London the prevalence in pregnant women is less than 1 per cent, and is considerably lower in most other parts of the UK. A resurgence of tuberculosis has occurred hand-in-hand with the AIDS epidemic.

The onset of immunodeficiency can be manifest in any organ system, so that a high index of suspicion is required to recognize the way in which other disease processes are altered.

Natural history and principles of treatment of HIV infection

Twenty per cent of those infected with HIV experience an acute seroconversion illness a few weeks after acquisition. Clinical features include fever, generalized lymphadenopathy, a macular erythematous rash, pharyngitis and conjunctivitis. A steady decline in immune function over the first few years may be manifest by non-life-threatening opportunistic conditions, such as recurrent oral and vaginal candidiasis, single dermatome herpes zoster (shingles), frequent and prolonged episodes of oral or genital herpes, persistent warts and genital ulcers (Fig. 16.5). Furry white patches on the sides of the tongue, termed oral hairy leuko-plakia (OHL), may come and go. This clinical sign is pathognomonic of immunodeficiency. Skin prob-lems include seborrhoeic dermatitis, folliculitis, dry skin, tinea pedis and a high frequency of allergic reactions.

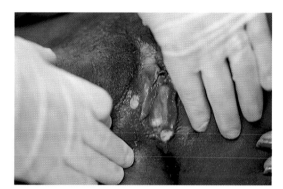

Figure 16.5 Genital ulcers in a woman with HIV infection. These persistent, painful ulcers were due to herpes simplex. Persistence for more than 1 month is AIDS defining. In the tropics, the differential diagnosis includes chancroid and donovanosis.

Without antiretroviral treatment, the average time for the development of AIDS is 10 years. Essentially, AIDS is defined by the onset of life-threatening opportunistic infections or malignancies associated with immunodeficiency. The commonest presenta-tions are listed in Table 16.5. There are two strategies used in treatment. Combinations of antiretroviral drugs are prescribed – the acronym HAART has been adopted for highly active antiretroviral therapy. Combinations may include two or more nucleoside analogues reverse transcriptase inhibitors, such as zidovudine or didanosine, a non-nucleoside reverse transcriptase inhibitor such as nevirapine, or one or more protease inhibitors such as nelfinavir. If suc-cessful, the immune system improves after a few months. These drugs, particularly some of the pro-tease inhibitors, have many potential interactions with other drugs through effects on the cytochrome P-450 enzymes. These include increasing the rate of breakdown of both the natural and synthetic oestro-gens used in oral contraceptive pills.

If immunodeficiency has already occurred, treat-ment and prevention of opportunistic infections are needed. These may include co-trimoxazole to prevent *Pneumocystis carinii* pneumonia and, in severely

Table 16.5 – Common AIDS-presenting illnesses

Pulmonary
Pneumocystis carinii pneumonia
Tuberculosis – pulmonary or extrapulmonary

Neurological
Cerebral toxoplasmosis
Cryptococcal meningitis
AIDS dementia

Gastrointestinal
Diarrhoea and wasting syndrome, which may be due
  to infection with *Cryptosporidium*, *Microsporidium*,
  Isospora
Oesophageal candidiasis

Ophthalmic
Cytomegalovirus retinitis
Malignancy
Kaposi's sarcoma
Non-Hodgkin's lymphoma

Systemic
Mycobacterium avium intracellulare complex (MAC)
  infection

immunosuppressed individuals with CD4 counts <0.05/L, azithromycin to prevent disseminated *Myco-bacterium avium intracellulare* complex (MAC) infec-tion, and ganciclovir to prevent CMV infection. Regular administration of antifungal agents may be necessary to control oral and vaginal candidiasis.

Virology

Human immunodeficiency virus is a retrovirus, with its genetic code in a single strand of RNA. Reverse transcriptase is carried within the core to enable pro-viral DNA to be produced in an infected cell. The outer membrane protein, gp-120, binds to CD4 receptors, which are present on T-helper lympho-cytes, macrophages, dendritic cells and microglia. Co-receptors, such as the CCR-5 chemokine receptor, are also used to enhance viral entry. Approximately 1 per cent of Caucasians have a homozygous mutation in the receptor, which is associated with resistance to acquiring infection. Another viral protein, p24, sur-rounds the RNA and enzymes present within the core of the virus, which enters the cytoplasm of an infected cell. Once pro-viral DNA has been integrated into the host, genome viral peptides are transcribed. Specific viral protease enzymes cleave these before the daughter virus particles are assembled.

Current antiretroviral drugs target reverse transcriptase or viral proteases. The aim of therapy is to reduce the level of virus in the plasma to zero with a combination of antiretroviral agents. If total suppression of viral replication is not achieved, resistant strains of virus will inevitably arise within the patient over the course of a few months. This is because reverse transcription is inherently inaccurate, leading to a high rate of mutation. With each cycle of replication of virus, which takes 48 hours, single point mutations arise, which will confer reduced sensitivity to antiviral agents. If therapy is effective, the CD4 lymphocyte count rises progressively, and at least partial immune restoration occurs. Unfortunately, HIV infects long-lived memory cells from which virus can rapidly reseed the body on the cessation of therapy. Eradication (and thus cure) is unlikely, even after several years of treatment.

Diagnosis

Human immunodeficiency virus infection is diagnosed by finding antibodies to gp-120. During seroconversion, p24 antigen is detectable in the serum before antibodies are produced. The disease is monitored by measuring the level of CD4 lymphocytes in peripheral blood. A normal level is >0.5/L. There is a 10 per cent risk of AIDS developing within 1 year when the CD4 lymphocyte count drops to 0.2/L. This is the level at which primary prophylaxis against *Pneumocystis carinii* pneumonia is recommended. Using PCR technology, it is also possible to measure the concentration of viral RNA in the plasma. A high level (>100 000 particles/mL) predicts rapid disease development, whilst a low level (<10 000 HIV viral load copies/mL) is associated with a low risk of disease progression.

Because the consequences of receiving a diagnosis of HIV are serious, a test should only be performed with informed consent from the patient, who may wish to discuss it with a partner, for whom the test may have major implications. To avoid the serious consequences of incorrect labelling or other human errors occurring, it is good practice to confirm correct labelling of the sample and request form with another healthcare worker.

If you suspect an individual has HIV, look for HOL (hairy oral leukoplakia), generalized lymphadenopathy and skin rashes. Kaposi's sarcoma may be evident,

with multiple red or purple tumours anywhere on the body. There is often lymphopenia or thrombocytopenia on a full blood count. Polyclonal IgG production produces a raised total protein level.

Transmission

In most developing countries, HIV is principally spread through vaginal intercourse, with approximately equal numbers of men and women infected. In developed countries, the majority of infections have been acquired through homosexual sex or intravenous drug use, although the incidence of heterosexual transmission is increasing. Genital infections are risk factors for HIV transmission and acquisition, including genital ulcer disease, *Chlamydia* and gonorrhoea. Bacterial vaginosis may also be a risk factor, and is very common in some African countries, with a prevalence of 50 per cent or more. Good control of sexually transmitted infections should reduce the incidence of HIV infection.

Vertical transmission

Vertical transmission occurs in 25–40 per cent of pregnancies if there are no interventions to reduce the risk. It is thought that a minority of infections occur during gestation. These babies can present with AIDS in the neonatal period. The majority of infections occur during parturition. Breastfeeding accounts for transmission in up to 15 per cent of pregnancies, corresponding to 37 per cent of infected infants. Transmission by this route may occur even after several months. The risk of vertical transmission is increased if there is a high HIV viral load or a preterm delivery. The role of genital infections in vertical transmission is still being assessed. Many children infected with HIV will survive into adolescence.

Three interventions have been shown to reduce the risk of vertical transmission of HIV:
- avoiding breastfeeding,
- elective Caesarean section,
- antiviral medication prescribed during the latter half of pregnancy, and to the neonate for 6 weeks.

If all three interventions are undertaken, the risk of transmission is less than 1 per cent. Zidovudine monotherapy has been studied most extensively in this context in randomized controlled trials. Since maternal HIV plasma viral load is predictive of vertical transmission, it is likely that combination therapies will be more effective. This approach has to be balanced against unknown potential toxicities for the neonate.

CASE HISTORY

A 25-year-old primigravida attends a booking clinic at 18 weeks' gestation. She has a history of intravenous drug use. After discussion with the midwife, she agrees to be screened for hepatitis viruses and HIV. She tests positive for syphilis: TPHA and FTA both reactive, VDRL negative. She also has evidence of past infection with hepatitis B: core antibody positive, surface antigen and e antigen negative. She is hepatitis C and HIV antibody positive.

She gives a history of treatment for syphilis 5 years earlier, with a 14-day course of penicillin injections. The HIV and hepatitis C tests are confirmed on a second sample. Her CD4 lymphocyte count is 0.35 cells/L and her HIV viral load is 15 000 copies/mL. She has vaginal candidiasis.

She is seen by the multi-disciplinary HIV team and agrees to a three-pronged approach to reduce the risk of vertical transmission: taking zidovudine 250 mg twice daily starting at 28 weeks' gestation, an elective Caesarean section at 38 weeks' gestation and not to breastfeed.

The pregnancy progresses uneventfully, and the child has negative HIV PCR tests at 3 months, 6 months and 9 months of age, confirming that HIV has not been transmitted. He is also hepatitis C negative.

Discussion points

- Tests for HIV and hepatitis B and C should be encouraged in all women with a history of intravenous drug use. Pre-test discussion is essential, and positive results should be confirmed on a second sample.
- If the history of prior syphilis treatment is confirmed, she does not need further treatment. Her serological test results are compatible with treated infection.
- There are no interventions to reduce vertical transmission of hepatitis C, which is more common in mothers co-infected with HIV.
- With the measures to prevent HIV vertical transmission, the risk of infection for the fetus is less than 3 per cent.
- The CD4 and viral load results suggest a low risk of developing AIDS in the next 3 years for the mother. She does not require aggressive triple therapy for HIV or prophylaxis against opportunistic infections at this stage.
- In developing countries, the risks of gastroenteritis from bottle-feeding have to be balanced against the risk of infection through breast milk. With prolonged breastfeeding (more than 1 year), 15–20 per cent of infants might acquire infection through this route.

Key Points

HIV and pregnancy

As a minimum, the following information needs to be discussed before a test is performed.

- The antibody test may take 3 months to become reactive after exposure.
- If there has been a recent high-risk exposure, the test should be repeated 3 months and 6 months after the event.
- A confirmatory sample should always be taken if the first test is reactive.
- Without specific treatment, the average time to develop AIDS is 10 years. It is possible to remain healthy even 15 years after initial infection.

- In countries with adequate healthcare resources, the prognosis is greatly improved by treatment.
- In pregnancy, the risk of vertical transmission is about 1 in 4 if no interventions are undertaken.
- A combination of antiretroviral medication, Caesarean section and avoidance of breastfeeding reduces the risk to <1 per cent.
- Who, if anyone, does the individual plan to tell about the test and its result?

Additional reading

Barton S, Hay P (eds). *Handbook of genitourinary medicine.* London: Arnold, 1999.

Labour

OVERVIEW

Labour can be defined as the process by which regular painful contractions bring about effacement and dilatation of the cervix and descent of the presenting part, ultimately leading to expulsion of the fetus and the placenta from the mother. Medical, social and ethical aspects combine together in a complex interplay which makes the obstetric management of labour a significant challenge. A doctor or midwife who manages labour must be aware of the normal anatomy and physiology of the mother and fetus, what distinguishes an abnormal from a normal labour, and when it is appropriate to intervene.

Introduction

Labour and delivery are the focus and climax of the reproductive process. They are both a physical and emotional challenge for the mother and a hazardous journey for the fetus. There is an interplay between the 'powers' of the uterus (the contractions), the 'passages' of the birth canal (the bony pelvis and the soft tissues of the pelvic floor and perineum) and the 'passenger' (the fetus). Each contraction necessary to promote dilatation of the uterine cervix and descent of the fetus transiently deprives the placenta of blood flow and consequently the fetus of oxygen. The duty of the midwife and obstetrician is to ensure this process is achieved with all parties healthy and satisfied.

Labour brings great joy and happiness to the majority of families, but occasionally death and catastrophe to others. Maternal death is rare in the West,

but remains frequent in many countries that have less developed healthcare systems. Complications of labour account for a significant proportion of maternal deaths in these countries, where childbirth is often unattended. This must not be confused with natural childbirth, a term used to describe a form of care in labour that utilizes minimal technology and natural methods of pain relief. Natural childbirth may be sought by women who perceive that birth in the West has been 'hijacked' by modern medicine and modern doctors. Conversely, there is now a small but significant minority of women who have the opposite philosophy: they have opted to avoid labour altogether and to elect for planned Caesarean section. Although this remains a contentious issue, many women have an increasing expectation that mode of delivery should be a matter of choice. The average Caesarean section rate in the UK is approximately 21 per cent, including both emergency and elective Caesarean sections. Although this is recognized by most as being too high, the reason for the steady rise in Caesarean births and the ideal rate are unclear. Undoubtedly, maternal choice is an important factor.

Before exploring the process of labour in detail, an understanding of the anatomy of the female pelvis and the fetus is crucial if the mechanisms of labour are to be understood.

Anatomy of the female pelvis and the fetus relevant to labour

The pelvis

The pelvic brim or inlet
The pelvic brim is the inlet of the pelvis and is bounded in front by the symphysis pubis (the joint separating the two pubic bones), on each side by the upper margin of the pubic bone, the ileopectineal line and the ala of the sacrum, and posteriorly by the promontory of the sacrum (Fig. 17.1). The normal

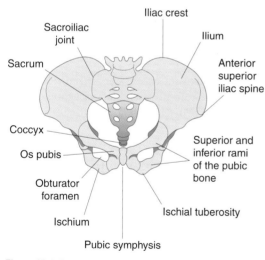

Figure 17.1 The bony pelvis.

transverse diameter in this plane is 13.5 cm and is wider than the anterior–posterior (AP) diameter, which is normally 11 cm (Fig. 17.2). The angle of the inlet is normally 60° to the horizontal in the erect position, but in Afro-Caribbean women this angle may be as much as 90° (Fig. 17.3). This increased angle may delay the head entering the pelvis in labour.

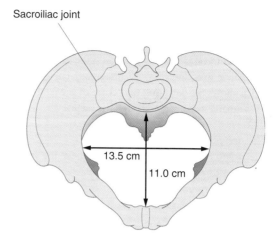

Figure 17.2 The pelvic brim.

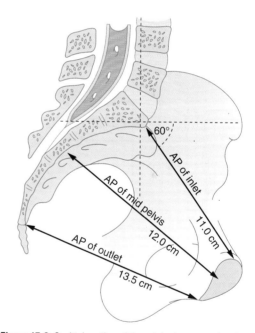

Figure 17.3 Sagittal section of the pelvis demonstrating the anterior–posterior (AP) diameters of the inlet and outlet.

The pelvic mid-cavity
The pelvic mid-cavity can be described as an area bounded in front by the middle of the symphysis pubis, on each side by the pubic bone, the obturator fascia and the inner aspect of the ischial bone and spines, and posteriorly by the junction of the second and third sections of the sacrum. The cavity is almost round, as the transverse and anterior diameters are similar at 12 cm. The ischial spines are palpable vaginally and are used as landmarks to assess the descent

of the head on vaginal examination (station). They are also used as landmarks for providing an anaesthetic block to the pudendal nerve. The pudendal nerve passes behind and below the ischial spine on each side. The pelvic axis describes an imaginary curved line, which shows the path that the centre of the fetal head takes during its passage through the pelvis.

The pelvic outlet
The pelvic outlet is bounded in front by the lower margin of the symphysis pubis, on each side by the descending ramus of the pubic bone, the ischial tuberosity and the sacrotuberous ligament, and posteriorly by the last piece of the sacrum. The AP diameter of the pelvic outlet is 13.5 cm and the transverse diameter is 11 cm (Fig. 17.4). Therefore, the transverse

is the widest diameter at the inlet, but at the outlet it is the AP. Recognizing this is crucial to the understanding of the mechanism of labour.

The pelvic measurements given here are obviously average values and relate to bony points. Maternal stature, previous pelvic fractures and metabolic bone disease such as rickets may all be associated with measurements less than these population means. Furthermore, as the pelvic ligaments at the pubic ramus and the sacroiliac joints loosen towards the end of the third trimester, the pelvis often becomes more flexible and these diameters may increase during labour. It is now uncommon to perform X-rays or computerized tomography (CT) scans of the pelvis to measure the pelvis because they have, on the whole, proven to be of minimal clinical use in predicting the outcome of labour.

A variety of pelvic shapes has been described, and these may contribute to difficulties encountered in labour. The gynaecoid pelvis is the most favourable for labour, and the most common (Fig. 17.5). Other pelvic shapes are shown in Figures 17.6 to 17.8. An android-type pelvis is said to predispose to deep transverse arrest (see Fig. 17.24, p. 240) and the anthropoid shape encourages an occipito-posterior (OP) position (see below). A platypelloid pelvis also is associated with an increased risk of obstructed labour.

The pelvic floor
This is formed by the two levator ani muscles which, with their fascia, form a musculofascial gutter during the second stage of labour (Fig. 17.9).

The perineum
The final obstacle to be negotiated by the fetus during labour is the perineum. The perineal body is a condensation of fibrous and muscular tissue lying between the

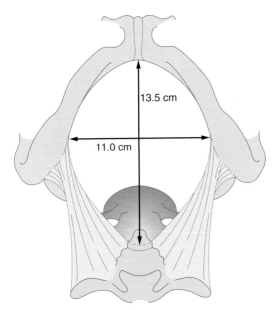

Figure 17.4 The pelvic outlet.

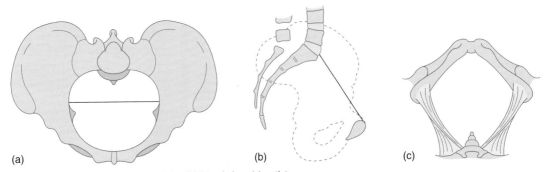

(a)   (b)   (c)

Figure 17.5 The gynaecoid pelvis: (a) brim, (b) lateral view, (c) outlet.

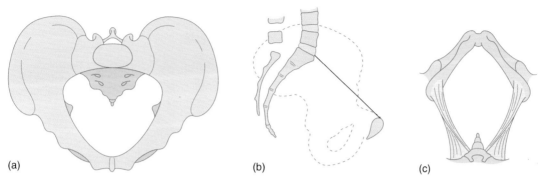

(a) (b) (c)

Figure 17.6 The android pelvis: (a) brim, (b) lateral view, (c) outlet.

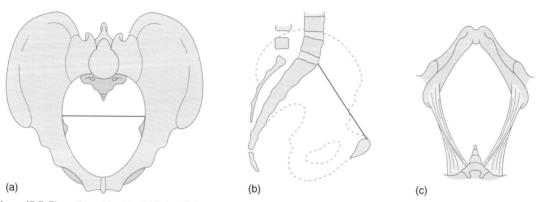

(a) (b) (c)

Figure 17.7 The anthropoid pelvis: (a) brim, (b) lateral view, (c) outlet.

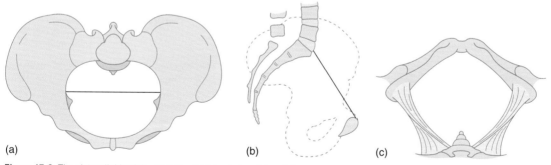

(a) (b) (c)

Figure 17.8 The platypelloid pelvis: (a) brim, (b) lateral view, (c) outlet.

vagina and the anus (Fig. 17.10). It receives attachments of the posterior ends of the bulbo-cavernous muscles, the medial ends of the superficial and deep transverse perineal muscles, and the anterior fibres of the external anal sphincter. It is always involved in a second-degree perineal tear and an episiotomy (see p. 256).

The fetal skull

The bones, sutures and fontanelles
The fetal skull is made up of the vault, the face and the base. The sutures are the lines formed where the individual bony plates of the skull meet one another.

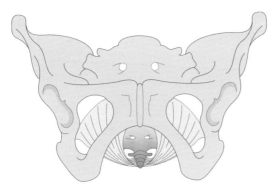

Figure 17.9 The musculofascial gutter of the levator sling.

At the time of labour, the sutures joining the bones of the vault are soft, unossified membranes, whereas the sutures of the face and the skull base are firmly united (Fig. 17.11).

The vault of the skull is formed by the parietal bones and parts of the occipital, frontal and temporal bones. Between these bones there are four membranous sutures: the sagittal, frontal, coronal and lambdoidal sutures.

Fontanelles are the junctions of the various sutures. The anterior fontanelle, or bregma (diamond shaped), is at the junction of the sagittal, frontal and coronal sutures. The posterior fontanelle (triangular shaped) lies at the junction of the sagittal suture and the lambdoidal sutures between the two parietal bones and the occipital bone. The fact that these sutures are not united is important for labour. It allows these bones to move together and even to overlap. The parietal bones usually tend to slide over the frontal and occipital bones. Furthermore, the bones themselves are compressible. Together, these characteristics of the fetal skull allow a process called moulding to occur, which effectively reduces the diameters of the fetal skull and encourages progress through the bony pelvis, without harming the underlying brain (Fig. 17.12). However, severe moulding can be a sign of cephalopelvic disproportion (CPD – see p. 238).

The area of the fetal skull bounded by the two parietal eminences and the anterior and posterior fontanelles is termed the vertex.

The diameters of the skull

The fetal head is ovoid in shape. The attitude of the fetal head refers to the degree of flexion and extension at the upper cervical spine. Different longitudinal diameters are presented to the pelvis in labour depending on the attitude of the fetal head (Figs 17.13 and 17.14).

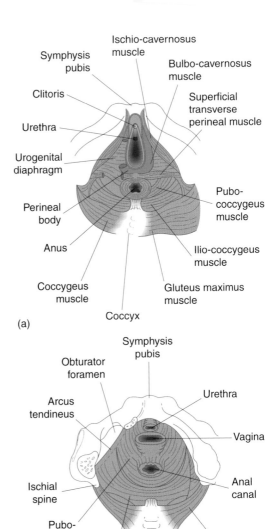

Figure 17.10 The perineum, perineal body and pelvic floor from below, showing superficial (a) and deeper (b) views. The pelvic floor muscles are made up of the levator ani (pubo-coccygeus and ilio-coccygeus).

The longitudinal diameter that presents in a well-flexed fetal head (vertex presentation) is the suboccipito-bregmatic diameter. This is usually 9.5 cm and is measured from the suboccipital region to the centre of the anterior fontanelle (bregma). The longitudinal diameter that presents in a less well-flexed head, such as is found in the OP position, is the suboccipito-frontal diameter, and is measured from the suboccipital region to the prominence of the forehead. It measures 10 cm.

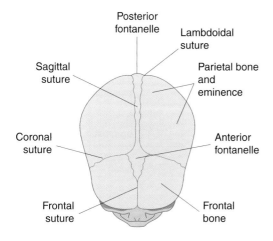

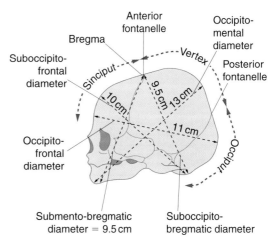

Figure 17.13 The diameters of the fetal skull.

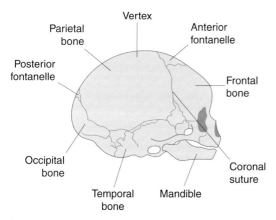

Figure 17.11 The fetal skull from superior and lateral views.

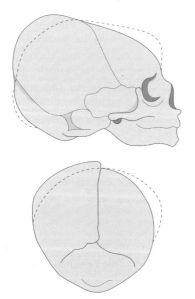

Figure 17.12 A schematic representation of moulding of the fetal skull.

With further extension of the head, the occipito-frontal diameter presents. This is measured from the root of the nose to the posterior fontanelle and is 11.5 cm. The greatest longitudinal diameter that may present is the mento-vertical, which is taken from the chin to the furthest point of the vertex and measures 13 cm. This is known as a brow presentation and it is usually too large to pass through the normal pelvis.

Extension of the fetal head beyond this point results in a smaller diameter. The submento-bregmatic diameter is measured from below the chin to the anterior fontanelle and is 9.5 cm. This is clinically a face presentation.

🔑 Key Points

The female pelvis
- The pelvic inlet is wider in the transverse than in the AP diameter.
- The pelvic outlet is wider in the AP than in the transverse diameter.
- Pelvic measurements may widen during labour due to pelvic ligament laxity.
- The soft tissues of the pelvic floor and perineum have a vital role to play in labour.
- Moulding may reduce the absolute measurements of the fetal skull during labour.
- The degree of flexion of the fetal skull at the neck (the attitude) determines the diameter of the fetal skull presenting to the pelvis.

	Flexed ➡️ Extended			
Attitude	Well flexed	Less well flexed (partially extended) or deflexed	Extended 'brow presentation'	Hyperextended 'face presentation'
Diameter	Suboccipito-bregmatic	Occipito-frontal	Occipito-mental	Submento-bregmatic
Measurement	9.5 cm	11.5 cm	13.0 cm	9.5 cm

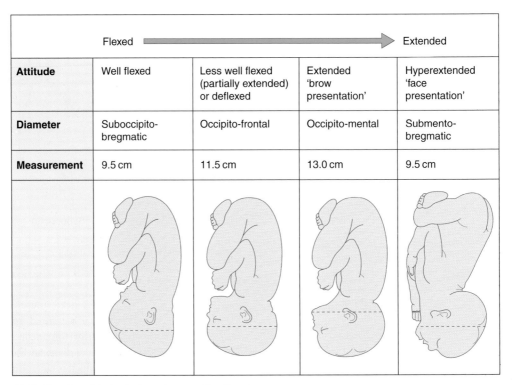

Figure 17.14 The effect of fetal attitude on the presenting diameter.

The process of labour

The onset of labour

The onset of labour can be defined as regular contractions bringing about progressive cervical change. Therefore, a diagnosis of labour is usually made in retrospect. Loss of a 'show' (a bloodstained plug of mucus passed from the cervix) or spontaneous rupture of the membranes (SROM) does not define the onset of labour, although they may occur at the same time. Labour can be well established before either of these events occurs, and both may precede labour by many days. Although much is understood about the physiology of labour in humans, the initiating biological event is still unclear (see 'Understanding the pathophysiology', below).

The stages of labour

Labour can be divided into three stages. The definitions of these stages rely predominantly on anatomical criteria, and in certain situations this may be a disadvantage, as labour is essentially a physiological process. In normal labour, the division into three stages is of little clinical significance. The important events in normal labour are the diagnosis of labour and the maternal urge to push, which usually corresponds with full dilatation of the cervix and the baby's head resting on the perineum. Defining the three stages of labour becomes more relevant if the labour does not progress normally. Because the definition of a normal labour can only be made retrospectively, there is difficulty in defining exactly when a normal labour becomes abnormal. Indeed, this definition will be different depending on the gestation, the previous obstetric record and the onset of labour.

The stages of labour are as follows.

First stage
This describes the time from the diagnosis of labour to full dilatation of the cervix (10 cm).

The first stage of labour can be divided into two phases. The latent phase is the time between the onset of labour and 3–4 cm dilatation. During this time, the cervix becomes 'fully effaced'. Effacement is a process by which the cervix shortens in length as it becomes included into the lower segment of the uterus. The process of effacement may begin during the weeks preceding the onset of labour but will be complete by the end of the latent phase. The cervical os cannot usually begin to dilate until effacement is complete. Effacement and dilatation should be thought of as consecutive events in the nulliparous woman, but may occur simultaneously in the multiparous woman. Dilatation is expressed in centimetres between 0 and 10. The duration of the latent phase is variable, and time limits are arbitrary. However, it usually lasts between 3 and 8 hours, being shorter in multiparous women.

The second phase of the first stage of labour is called the active phase and describes the time between the end of the latent phase (3–4 cm dilatation) and full dilatation (10 cm) (Fig. 17.15). It is also variable

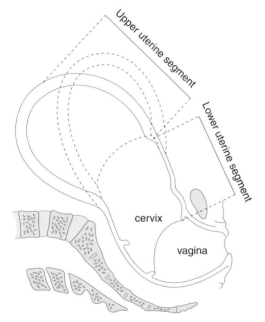

Figure 17.15 The thick upper segment and the thin lower segment of the uterus at the end of the first stage of labour. The dotted lines indicate the position assumed by the uterus during contraction.

in length, usually lasting between 2 and 6 hours. Again it is usually shorter in multiparous women. Cervical dilatation during the active phase usually occurs at 1 cm/hour or more in a normal labour (again, an arbitrary value).

Second stage
This describes the time from full dilatation of the cervix to delivery of the fetus or fetuses. The second stage of labour may also be subdivided into two phases. The passive phase is where there is no maternal urge to push and the fetal head is still relatively high in the pelvis. The second phase is rather confusingly called the active second stage. There is a maternal urge to push because the fetal head is low, causing a reflex need to 'bear down'. In a normal labour, second stage is often diagnosed at this point because the maternal urge to push prompts the midwife to perform a vaginal examination. Conventionally, a normal second stage should last no longer than 2 hours in a primiparous woman and 1 hour in a multipara. Again these definitions are largely arbitrary, but there is evidence that a second stage of labour lasting more than 3 hours is associated with increased maternal and fetal morbidity.

Use of epidural anaesthesia may influence the length and the management of the second stage of labour.

Third stage
This is the time from delivery of the fetus or fetuses until delivery of the placenta(s). The placenta is usually delivered within a few minutes of the birth of the baby. A third stage lasting more than 30 minutes should be considered abnormal.

The duration of labour

More than any other objective measurement, the duration of labour determines the impact of childbirth, particularly on mothers but also on babies, and also on those who care for both of them. The morale of most women starts to deteriorate after 6 hours in labour, and after 12 hours the rate of deterioration significantly accelerates. There is a greater incidence of fetal hypoxia and need for operative delivery associated with longer labours. Shorter labours will also mean that personal attention for each woman in labour is a realistic possibility. An early artificial rupture of membranes (ARM) does shorten the length of labour, but does not necessarily alter the outcome.

It is difficult to define prolonged labour, but it would be reasonable to suggest that labour lasting longer than 12 hours in nulliparous women and 8 hours in multiparous women should be regarded as prolonged.

The mechanism of labour

This refers to the series of changes in position and attitude that the fetus undergoes during its passage through the birth canal. It is described here for the vertex presentation and the gynaecoid pelvis. The relation of the fetal head and body to the maternal pelvis changes as the fetus descends through the pelvis. This is essential so that the optimal diameters of the fetal skull are present at each stage of the descent.

Engagement

The head normally enters the pelvis in the transverse position or some minor variant of this, so taking advantage of the widest diameter. Engagement is said to have occurred when the widest part of the presenting part has passed successfully through the inlet. Engagement has occurred in the vast majority of nulliparous women prior to labour, but not so for the majority of multiparous women.

The number of fifths of the fetal head palpable abdominally is often used to describe whether engagement has taken place. If more than two-fifths of the fetal head is palpable abdominally, the head is not yet engaged.

Descent

Descent of the fetal head is needed before flexion, internal rotation and extension can occur (Fig. 17.16). During the first stage and first phase of the second

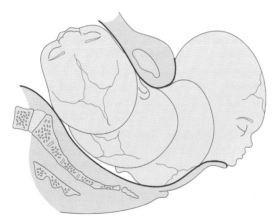

Figure 17.16 Descent and flexion of the head followed by internal rotation and ending in birth of the head by extension.

stage of labour, descent of the fetus is secondary to uterine action. In the active phase of the second stage of labour, descent of the fetus is helped by voluntary use of abdominal musculature and the Valsalva manoeuvre ('pushing').

Flexion

The fetal head may not always be completely flexed when it enters the pelvis. As the head descends into the narrower mid-cavity, flexion should occur. This passive movement occurs, in part, due to the surrounding structures and is important in minimizing the presenting diameter of the fetal head.

Internal rotation

If the head is well flexed, the occiput will be the leading point and on reaching the sloping gutter of the levator ani muscles, it will be encouraged to rotate anteriorly so that the sagittal suture now lies in the AP diameter of the pelvic outlet (i.e. the widest diameter). If the fetus has engaged in the OP position, internal rotation can occur from an OP position to an occipito-anterior (OA) position. This long internal rotation may explain the increased duration of labour associated with this malposition. Alternatively, an OP position may persist, resulting in a 'face to pubes' delivery. More often, the persistent OP position is associated with extension of the fetal head and a resulting increase in the diameter presented to the pelvic outlet. This may lead to obstructed labour and the need for instrumental delivery or even Caesarean section.

Extension

Following completion of internal rotation, the occiput is underneath the symphysis pubis and the bregma is near the lower border of the sacrum. The soft tissues of the perineum still offer resistance, and may be traumatized in the process. The well-flexed head now extends and the occiput escapes from underneath the symphysis pubis and distends the vulva. This is known as 'crowning' of the head. The head extends further and the occiput underneath the symphysis pubis acts as a fulcrum point as the bregma, face and chin appear in succession over the posterior vaginal opening and perineal body. This extension and movement minimize soft-tissue trauma by utilizing the smallest diameters of the head for the birth.

Restitution

When the head is delivering, the occiput is directly anterior. As soon as it escapes from the vulva, the head aligns itself with the shoulders, which have entered the pelvis in the oblique position. The slight rotation of the occiput through one-eighth of a circle is called restitution.

External rotation

In order to be delivered, the shoulders have to rotate into the direct AP plane (remember the widest diameter at the outlet). When this occurs, the occiput rotates through a further one-eighth of a circle to the transverse position. This is called external rotation (Fig. 17.17).

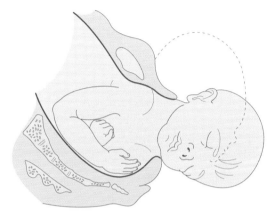

Figure 17.17 External rotation of the head after delivery as the anterior shoulder rotates forward to pass under the subpubic arch.

Delivery of the shoulders and fetal body

When restitution and external rotation have occurred, the shoulders will be in the AP position. The anterior shoulder is under the symphysis pubis and delivers first, and the posterior shoulder delivers subsequently. Although this process may occur without assistance, lateral traction is often exerted by gently pulling the fetal head in a downward direction to help release the anterior shoulder from beneath the pubic symphysis.

Normally the rest of the fetal body is delivered easily, with the posterior shoulder guided over the perineum by traction in the opposite direction, so sweeping the baby onto the maternal abdomen.

P Understanding the pathophysiology

The mechanism responsible for initiating human parturition is still unknown and is different from that in all other animal models that have been studied. There are, however, certain processes that seem to be of particular importance.

The onset of labour occurs when those factors which inhibit contractions and maintain a closed cervix diminish and are succeeded by the actions of factors which do the opposite. Both mother and fetus make contributions toward this.

Hormonal factors

Progesterone maintains uterine quiescence by suppressing prostaglandin production, inhibiting communication between myometrial cells and preventing oxytocin release. Oestrogen opposes the action of progesterone. Prior to labour, there is a reduction in progesterone receptors and an increase in the concentration of oestrogen relative to the progesterone. Oxytocin release from the pituitary and prostaglandin synthesis by the chorion and the decidua increase, leading to an increase in calcium influx into the myometrial cells. This change in the hormonal milieu also increases gap junction formation between individual myometrial cells, creating a functional syncytium, which is necessary for co-ordinated uterine activity. Maternal corticotrophin-releasing hormone (CRH) increases in concentration towards term and potentiates the action of prostaglandins and oxytocin on myometrial contractility.

Fetally produced cortisol may contribute to the conversion of progesterone to oestrogen. Which of these hormonal steps initiates labour is unclear. As labour becomes established, the output of oxytocin increases through the Fergusson reflex. Pressure from the fetal presenting part against the cervix is relayed via a reflex arc involving the spinal cord and results in increased oxytocin release form the posterior pituitary.

The myometrium

Myometrial cells contain filaments of actin and myosin which interact and bring about contraction, while their separation brings about relaxation. An increase in intracellular free calcium ions results in the formation of the contractile entity of actin-phosphorylated myosin. Beta-adrenergic compounds and calcium-channel blockers decrease intracellular calcium. Prostaglandins and oxytocin increase intracellular free calcium ions.

Individual myometrial cells are laid down in a mesh of collagen. There is cell-to-cell communication by means of gap junctions, which facilitate the passage of various products of metabolism and electrical current between cells. These gap junctions are absent for most of the pregnancy but appear in significant numbers at term. Gap junctions increase in size and number with the progress of labour and tend to disappear afterwards. Prostaglandins stimulate their formation, while beta-adrenergic compounds possibly do the opposite. A uterine pacemaker from which contractions originate probably does exist but has not been demonstrated histologically.

Retraction is a major feature of uterine contractility during labour. This is the progressive shortening of the uterine smooth muscle cells in the upper portion of the uterus as labour progresses. After the cells contract, they relax, but they do not return to their original length. The result of this retraction process is the development of the thicker, active, contracting segment in the upper portion of the uterus. At the same time, the lower segment of the uterus becomes thinner and more stretched. Eventually this results in the cervix being taken up into the lower segment of the uterus so forming a continuum with the lower uterine segment (see Fig. 17.15).

Uterine contractions are involuntary in nature and there is relatively minimal extrauterine neuronal control. The frequency of contractions may vary during labour and with parity. Throughout the majority of labour, they occur at intervals of 2 to 4 minutes. Their duration also varies during labour, from 30 to 60 seconds, or occasionally longer. The intensity or amplitude of the intrauterine pressure generated with each contraction averages between 30 and 60 mmHg.

The cervix

The cervix contains muscle cells and fibroblasts separated by a 'ground substance' made up of extracellular matrix molecules. Interactions between collagen, fibronectin and dermatan sulphate (a proteoglycan) during the earlier stages of pregnancy keep the cervix rigid and closed. Contractions at this point do not bring about effacement or dilatation. Under the influence of prostaglandins, and other humoral mediators, there is an increase in proteolytic activity and collagen turnover. Dermatan sulphate is replaced by the more hydrophilic hyaluronic acid, which results in an increase in water content of the cervix. This causes cervical softening or 'ripening', so that contractions, when they begin, can bring about the processes of effacement and dilatation.

Management of normal labour

At term, women are told to contact their local labour suite or their community midwife either when they have SROM or when their contractions are occurring every 5 minutes or more frequently. The need for pain relief may result in admission to hospital before either of these two criteria is reached. Whether at home or in hospital, the attending midwife will then make an assessment of the situation based on the history and on clinical examination.

History

The following are important points to note in the admission history.

- Details of previous births and the size of previous babies (the uneventful birth of normal or large babies is encouraging). A previous Caesarean section, for example, is an adverse feature, especially if it was performed because of a mechanical problem.
- The frequency, duration and perception of strength of the contractions and when they began.
- Whether the membranes have ruptured and, if so, the colour and amount of amniotic fluid lost.
- The presence of abnormal vaginal discharge or bleeding;
- The recent activity of the fetus.
- Any medical issues of note that may influence the labour and delivery, e.g. pregnancy-induced hypertension, fetal growth restriction.

General examination

It is important to recognize women who have a raised body mass index, as this may complicate the management of labour. The temperature, pulse and blood pressure must be recorded and a sample of urine tested for protein, blood, ketones, glucose and nitrates.

Abdominal examination

After the initial inspection for scars indicating previous surgery, it is important to determine the lie of the fetus (longitudinal, transverse or oblique?) and the nature of the presenting part (cephalic or breech?). If it is a cephalic presentation, the degree of engagement must be determined. A head that remains high and unengaged is a poor prognostic sign for successful delivery. If there is any doubt as to the presentation or if the head is high (five-fifths palpable), an ultrasound scan will determine the presenting part or the reason for the high head (e.g. OP position, deflexed head, placenta praevia, fibroid, etc.) An attempt to estimate the size of the fetus should be made.

Abdominal examination also includes an assessment of the contractions; this takes time (at least 10 minutes) and is done by palpating the uterus directly, not by looking at the tocograph, which provides information only on the frequency and duration of contractions, not the strength.

Vaginal examination

A full explanation of the purpose and technique of vaginal examination is given to the woman and her consent is obtained. The index and middle fingers are passed to the top of the vagina and the cervix. The cervix is examined for dilatation, effacement and application to the presenting part. The dilatation is estimated digitally in centimetres. When no cervix can be felt, this means the cervix is fully dilated (10 cm). The length of the cervix should be recorded. The cervix at 36 weeks is about 3 cm long. It gradually shortens by the process of effacement. In early labour it may still be uneffaced. At about 3 cm of dilatation, the cervix should be fully effaced. Providing the cervix is at least 3 cm dilated, it should be possible to determine both the position and the station of the presenting part.

In a normal labour, the vertex will be presenting and the position can be determined by locating the occiput. The occiput is identified by feeling for the triangular posterior fontanelle. Failure to feel the posterior fontanelle may be because the head is deflexed, the occiput is posterior or there is so much caput that the sutures cannot be felt. All of these indicate the possibility of a prolonged labour. Normally, the occiput will be transverse (OT position) or anterior (OA). Relating the lowest part of the head to the ischial spines will give an estimation of the station. This vaginal assessment of station should always be taken together with assessment of the degree of engagement by abdominal palpation. If the head is at or below the ischial spines (0 to +1 or more) and the occiput is anterior (OA), the outlook is favourable for vaginal delivery.

The condition of the membranes should also be noted. If they have ruptured, the colour and amount of fluid draining should be noted. Copious amounts of clear fluid are a good prognostic feature; scanty, heavily bloodstained or meconium-stained fluid is a warning sign for fetal compromise.

The admission history and examination act as an initial screen for abnormal labour and increased maternal/fetal risk. If all features are normal and reassuring, the woman will remain under midwifery care. If there are risk factors identified, medical involvement in the form of the on-call obstetric team may be appropriate. A flow chart of this process is shown in Figure 17.18.

Fetal assessment in labour

Fetal assessment in labour takes four forms:
- observation of the colour of the liquor – fresh meconium staining and heavy bleeding are markers of potential fetal compromise (Fig. 17.19),
- intermittent auscultation of the fetal heart using a Pinard stethoscope or a hand-held Doppler ultrasound,
- continuous external fetal monitoring (EFM) using cardiotocography (CTG),
- fetal scalp blood sampling (FBS).

Meconium is often passed by a healthy fetus at or after term as a result of maturation of gastrointestinal physiology; in this scenario it is usually thin and a very dark green or brown colour. However, it may also be expelled from a fetus exposed to marked intrauterine hypoxia or acidosis; in this scenario it is often thicker and much brighter green in colour.

In many hospitals, a CTG will be recommended for all women on admission to the labour suite. If the history, examination and admission CTG are all found to be reassuring, the woman can be considered low risk and continuous monitoring with the CTG is not indicated. Regular record of the colour of the amniotic fluid draining should be made and the fetal heart rate should be listened to every 15 minutes during and after a contraction. Detection of either an abnormal fetal heart baseline rate or decelerations by intermittent auscultation is an indication for continuous EFM. In second stage, the fetal heart rate should be listened to during and after every contraction. Only if there are pre-existing risk factors or if new risk factors are identified (such as meconium, prolonged labour, siting of an epidural, use of Syntocinon, abnormal intermittent auscultation) is there a need for continuous

ADMISSION MANAGEMENT FLOW CHART

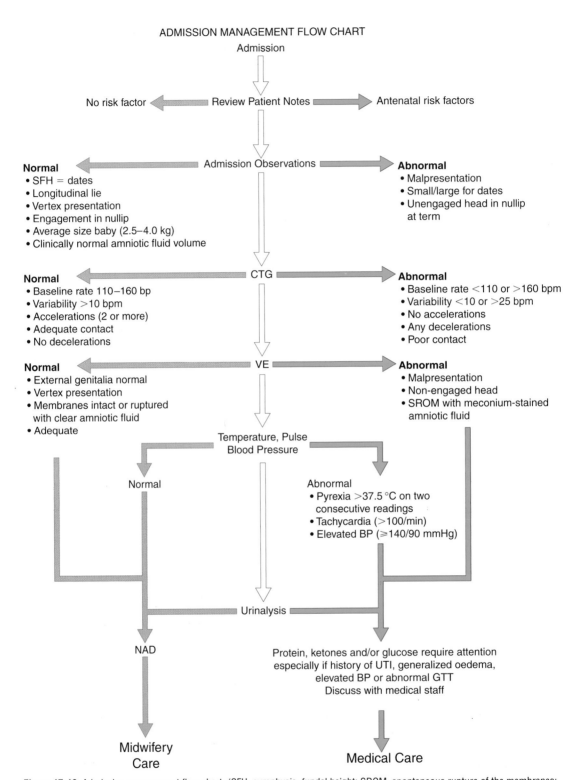

Figure 17.18 Admission management flow chart. (SFH, symphysis–fundal height; SROM, spontaneous rupture of the membranes; BP, blood pressure; UTI, urinary tract infection; GTT, glucose tolerance test; NAD, no abnormality detected; CTG, cardiotocograph; VE, vaginal examination.)

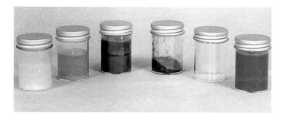

Figure 17.19 Samples of amniotic fluid. From left to right: clear/whitish amniotic fluid; slight meconium staining (grade 1); moderate meconium staining (grade 2); thick meconium (grade 3); no fluid obtained; bloodstained amniotic fluid.

EFM. This can be achieved by using an abdominal transducer or a fetal scalp electrode, which is inserted through the cervix and fixed to the fetal head.

The interpretation of the fetal heart rate pattern on a CTG is discussed in Chapter 8. In brief, features of a normal fetal heart rate pattern include: baseline rate 110–160 bpm, baseline variability 10–25 bpm, two accelerations in 20 minutes, and no decelerations.

A healthy term fetus is usually able to withstand the rigors of a normal labour. However, with each contraction, placental blood flow and oxygen transfer are temporarily interrupted, and a fetus that is already compromised before labour will become increasingly so. Insufficient oxygen delivery to the fetus causes a switch to fetal anaerobic metabolism and the generation of lactic acid and hydrogen ions. In excess, these saturate the buffering systems of the fetus and cause a metabolic acidosis which, in the extreme, can cause neuronal damage and permanent neurological injury. Hypoxia and acidosis cause a characteristic change in the fetal heart rate pattern, which can be detected by the CTG. Unfortunately, these CTG changes can be difficult to interpret and carry a significant false-positive rate, i.e. they often suggest fetal compromise when in fact the fetus is still in good condition. In order that the use of CTG does not lead to unnecessary intervention, an FBS may be performed during labour to measure fetal pH and base excess directly (see p. 244). Often, these results are normal even when the CTG is abnormal.

The use of electronic fetal monitors, only introduced in the 1970s, has been controversial and their value in 'low-risk' labours is doubtful. Education and training are crucial in the proper use of all equipment. Unfortunately, these devices were introduced before their understanding was fully developed. There is little doubt that babies' lives have been saved by the use of electronic fetal monitors, but they have contributed to the rise in the Caesarean section and instrumental delivery rates and they lead to reduced mobility in labour and increased parental anxiety. This remains a challenge.

The partogram

The introduction of a graphic record of labour in the form of a partogram has been an important development. This record allows an instant visual assessment of the rate of cervical dilatation and comparison with an expected norm, according to the parity of the woman, so that slow progress can be recognized early and appropriate actions taken to correct it where possible. Other key observations are entered onto the chart, including the frequency and strength of contractions, the descent of the head in fifths palpable, the amount and colour of the amniotic fluid draining, and basic observations of maternal well-being such as blood pressure, pulse rate and temperature (Fig. 17.20).

A line can be drawn on the partogram at the end of the latent phase demonstrating progress of 1 cm dilatation per hour (the alert line). This line predicts 'ideal' progress during the active phase (1 cm dilatation per hour). If the plot of progress falls beyond an 'action' line drawn 2–4 hours to the right of this line, progress is described as slow and the cause of this should be sought. What constitutes normal progress in the active phase is much debated. Many women, especially multiparous women, will make faster progress than 1 cm of dilatation per hour.

The first stage

Key management principles of first stage of labour

The first stage of labour is timed from the diagnosis of onset of labour to full dilatation of the cervix.
- Provision of continuity of care and emotional support to the mother.
- Observation of the progress of labour with timely intervention if it becomes abnormal.
- Monitoring of fetal well-being.
- Adequate and appropriate pain relief consistent with the woman's wishes.
- Adequate hydration to prevent ketosis.

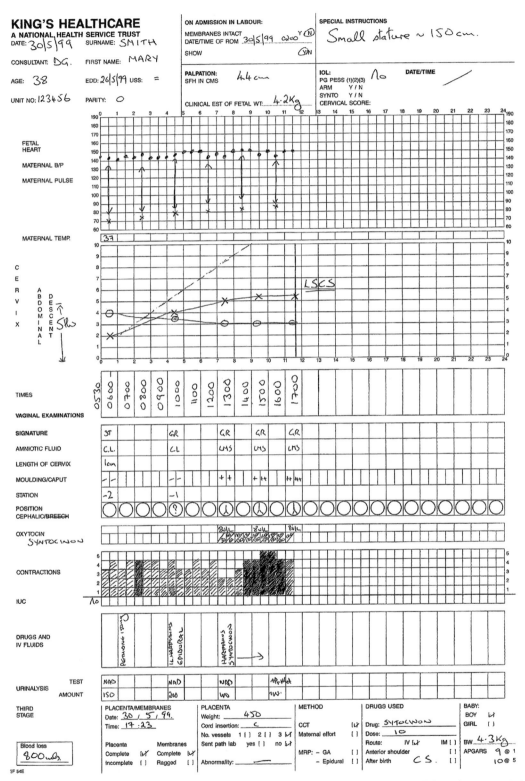

Figure 17.20 A typical partogram. This is a partogram of a nulliparous woman of short stature with a big baby and an augmented labour. The labour culminates in an emergency Caesarean section for cephalopelvic disproportion.

Women who are in the latent phase of labour should be encouraged to mobilize and should be managed away from the labour suite where possible. Indeed, they may well go home, to return later when the contractions are stronger or more frequent. Encouragement and reassurance are extremely important. Intervention during this phase is best avoided unless there are identified risk factors. Simple analgesics are preferred over nitrous oxide and epidurals. There is no reason to restrict eating and drinking, although lighter foods and clear fluids may be better tolerated. Vaginal examinations are usually performed every 4 hours to determine when the active phase has been reached (approximately 3 cm dilatation and full effacement). Thereafter, the timing of examinations should be decided by the midwife. Four-hourly is standard practice; however, this frequency may be increased if the midwife thinks that progress is unusually slow or fast. Remember that progress of 1 cm dilatation per hour (or more) is considered 'normal'. Descent of the presenting part through the pelvis is another crucial component of progress and should be recorded at each vaginal examination. Full dilatation may be reached, but if descent is inadequate, vaginal delivery will not occur.

During the first stage, the membranes may be intact, may have ruptured spontaneously or may have been ruptured artificially. Generally speaking, if the membranes are intact, it is not necessary to rupture them if the progress of labour is satisfactory.

A woman in the first stage of labour should undergo intermittent monitoring of both her condition (blood pressure, pulse rate, temperature) and that of her fetus by intermittent auscultation of the fetal heart rate. This is sufficient provided she is progressing normally. If labour is abnormal (see later), continuous CTG monitoring, antacid administration to the mother, epidural and urinary catheter insertion may be required.

Mobility is encouraged throughout. The posture adopted by the woman is a matter of choice, although it is likely that standing upright encourages progress. Unfortunately, many women adopt a supine position, especially if there is a need for continuous EFM (i.e. the CTG).

Second stage

If the labour has been normal, the first sign of the second phase of the second stage is an urge to push experienced by the mother. Full dilatation of the cervix should be confirmed by a vaginal examination if the head is not visible. The woman will get an expulsive reflex with each contraction, and will generally take a deep breath, hold it, and strain down (the Valsalva manoeuvre). The pushing needs to be organized so that it is effective, and the midwife has an important role to play here. Early in the second stage it does not matter what position the woman adopts, but if she is well propped up with her head upright and her hands behind her knees, she will be in a comfortable position to push effectively with some assistance from gravity. Alternatively, pushing can be quite effective in the left lateral position, which has the advantage of removing the weight of the uterus from the inferior vena cava and aorta (so maximizing cardiac output and uterine artery blood flow). There may be requests by women to deliver in different positions, or in water. There are differences of opinion regarding this. In general, as long as mother and baby are well, and there is good progress in labour, then the outcome will be good. Possible risks or disadvantages should be explained to the mother.

Descent and delivery of the head

The progress of the descent of the head can be judged by watching the perineum. At first there is a slight general bulge as the woman strains. When the head stretches the perineum, the anus will begin to open, and soon after this the baby's head will be seen at the vulva at the height of each contraction. Between contractions, the elastic tone of the perineal muscles will push the head back into the pelvic cavity. The perineal body and vulval outlet will become more and more stretched, until eventually the head is low enough to pass forwards under the subpubic arch. When the head no longer recedes between contractions (crowning), this indicates that it has passed through the pelvic floor, and delivery is imminent. If delivery of the baby is left entirely to nature, laceration of the perineum often occurs during the birth. Therefore, at this stage the midwife must control the head to prevent it being delivered suddenly. Once the head has crowned the woman should be discouraged from bearing down by telling her to take rapid, shallow breaths. The head may now be delivered carefully by pressure through the perineum onto the forehead by means of a finger and thumb placed one each side of the anus, pushing the head forward slowly before it is allowed to extend and complete its delivery, and controlling the rate of escape with the other hand.

If extension of the head begins before the biparietal diameter has passed through the vulval orifice, a larger diameter than the suboccipital–frontal diameter will distend the vulva and a tear may result, unless an episiotomy is performed. Even if the head has crowned gradually, perineal rupture may occur if the head is allowed to expel suddenly and rapidly.

Delivery of the shoulders and rest of the body

Once the fetal head is born, a check is made to see whether the cord is wound tightly around the neck, thereby making delivery of the body difficult. If this is the case, the cord may need to be clamped and divided before delivery of the rest of the body. If there is any meconium staining of the amniotic fluid, nasopharyngeal suction should be performed to prevent meconium aspiration. With the next contraction, there is external rotation of the head and the shoulders can be delivered. To aid delivery of the shoulders, the head should be pulled gently downwards and forwards until the anterior shoulder appears beneath the pubis. The head is then lifted gradually until the posterior shoulder appears over the perineum and the baby is then swept upwards to deliver the body and legs. If the infant is large and traction is necessary to deliver the body, it should be applied to the shoulders only, and not to the head. Shoulder dystocia (difficulty in delivering the shoulders) is discussed in Chapter 19.

Immediate care of the neonate

After the infant is born, it lies between the mother's legs and usually takes its first breath within seconds. There is no need for immediate clamping of the cord, and indeed about 80 mL of blood will be transferred from the placenta to the baby before cord pulsations cease, reducing the chances of neonatal anaemia and iron deficiency. The baby's head should be kept dependent to allow mucus in the respiratory tract to drain, and oropharyngeal suction should be applied if necessary. After clamping the cord, the baby should have a 1-minute Apgar score (see Chapter 22) assessed and then be placed on the mother's abdomen for cuddling and suckling. This will help bonding, and the release of oxytocin will encourage uterine contractions. Before being taken from the delivery room, the first dose of vitamin K should be given and the infant should have a general examination for abnormalities and a wrist label attached for identification.

Third stage

This is timed from the delivery of the baby to the expulsion of the placenta and membranes. This normally takes between 5 and 10 minutes. If longer than 30 minutes, it should be regarded as prolonged.

Separation of the placenta occurs because of the reduction of volume of the uterus due to uterine contraction and the retraction (shortening) of the lattice-like arrangement of the myometrial muscle fibres. A cleavage plane develops within the decidua basalis and the separated placenta lies free in the lower segment of the uterine cavity. Signs of separation are:

- lengthening of the cord protruding from the vulva,
- a small gush of blood from the placental bed, which normally stops quickly due to a retraction of the myometrial fibres,
- rising of the uterine fundus to above the umbilicus (Fig. 17.21),

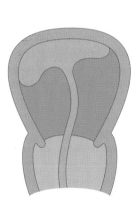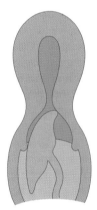

Figure 17.21 Signs of separation and descent of the placenta. After separation, the uterine upper segment rises up and feels more rounded.

- the fundus becomes hard and globular compared to the broad, softer fundus prior to separation.

The normal spontaneous expulsion of the placenta can take as long as 20 minutes and is associated with a 5 per cent risk of postpartum haemorrhage.

The modern management of the third stage is active and involves a procedure called controlled cord traction (Fig. 17.22). This technique is as follows.

- Synthetic oxytocin 10 iu (Syntocinon) or Syntometrine (5 iu oxytocin, 0.5 mg ergometrine) is given by intramuscular injection following delivery of the anterior shoulder. Syntometrine gives a more sustained contraction due to the

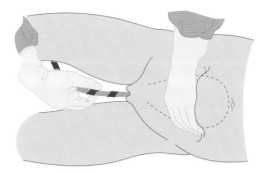

Figure 17.22 Delivering the placenta by controlled cord traction.

ergometrine, but should not be given if the woman is hypertensive. This injection will cause the uterus to contract soon after delivery of the baby.

- After delivery of the baby, the attendant should place the left hand on the uterus to identify when a contraction has occurred. During this time, the vulva should be observed for any haemorrhage. The cord should be double clamped approximately 1–2 minutes after delivery of the baby. It is wise to place a clamp close to the vulva so that lengthening of the cord can be better identified.
- When a contraction is felt, the left hand should be moved suprapubically and the fundus elevated with the palm facing towards the mother. At the same time, the right hand should grasp the cord and exert steady traction so that the placenta separates and is delivered gently, care being taken to peel off all the membranes, usually with a twisting motion.

In approximately 2 per cent of cases, the placenta will not be expelled by this method. If no bleeding occurs, a further attempt at controlled cord traction should be made after 10 minutes. If this fails, the placenta is 'retained' and will require manual removal under general or regional anaesthesia in the operating theatre.

Controlled cord traction is the favoured way of managing the third stage in most hospitals as it shortens the third stage and is associated with a significant reduction in postpartum haemorrhage. It is of crucial importance that controlled cord traction is not performed in the absence of a uterine contraction, otherwise uterine inversion may occur (see Chapter 19).

After completion of the third stage, the placenta should be inspected for missing cotyledons or a succenturiate lobe. If these are suspected, manual removal of the placenta (possibly under ultrasound guidance) should be arranged, for in this situation the risk of postpartum haemorrhage is high.

Finally, the vulva of the mother should be inspected for any tears or lacerations. Minor tears do not require suturing, but tears extending into the perineal muscles (or, indeed, an episiotomy) will require careful repair (see Chapter 18).

Key Points

Normal labour

The key features of normal labour are:

- spontaneous onset,
- single cephalic presentation,
- 37–42 weeks' gestation,
- no artificial interventions,
- unassisted spontaneous vaginal delivery,
- duration of <12 hours in nulliparous women, and <8 hours in multiparous women,
- a retrospective diagnosis.

A labour which deviates from these key features can be described as 'abnormal'.

CASE HISTORY

Mrs W is a 32-year-old para 1 (previous normal vaginal delivery at term), with no medical or obstetric history of note, who realized she was pregnant at approximately 6 weeks' gestation. An appointment was arranged with her GP, who confirmed the pregnancy and referred her to one of the local community midwives. Due to the absence of risk factors, she was booked under midwifery care. A dating scan organized by the midwife agreed with the menstrual estimated delivery date (EDD), and screening tests in the second trimester were all reassuring. Regular visits through the second and third trimesters did not reveal any new problems.

At 39 weeks' gestation, after a week of increasingly uncomfortable but irregular uterine tightenings, Mrs W experienced a 'show'. Her contractions remained irregular for a further 24 hours. Finally, they began to come frequently and, when they reached every 5 minutes, she phoned her midwife, who recommended assessment at the local maternity unit. Mrs W called her own parents, who came to look after her first child, and she and her husband drove to the hospital.

On admission, the midwife took a history and performed an abdominal examination. The head was well engaged and the contractions were coming every 3 minutes. A CTG on admission was normal, as were the maternal observations. A vaginal examination showed the membranes to be intact and the cervix to be fully effaced and 4 cm dilated. The vertex was found to be 1 cm above the spines. Mrs W therefore remained 'low risk' and under the care of the midwives. She was not reviewed by the doctors on their labour suite round.

She remained mobile and continued to drink whilst in labour, but did not want anything to eat. She spent some time in the bath, as this helped her cope with the pain of the contractions. The midwife listened regularly to the fetal heart with a Pinard stethoscope, during and after contractions, and this remained steady and of a normal rate. Maternal observations also remained normal. Three hours later, her membranes ruptured. Permission was given for an internal examination and Mrs W was found to be 9 cm dilated. She was finding the contractions much more painful, but, with support and reassurance from her partner and the midwife,

did not require anything more than nitrous oxide for analgesia.

One hour later, she was aware of a strong urge to 'bear down' and began involuntarily pushing. The midwife confirmed second stage with another vaginal examination and the pushing continued. Mrs W elected to lie in a supine position on the bed from this point onwards. The fetal heart was listened to during and after each and every contraction during the second stage. Twenty minutes later, the maternal anus began to dilate slightly and the vertex became visible soon after at the vaginal introitus. Three further contractions and the head had delivered and, with the fourth, the rest of the body. The midwife delivered the baby onto the maternal chest and clamped and cut the cord a few minutes later. An intramuscular injection of Syntometrine was given by a second midwife as the baby was born, and the placenta delivered 5 minutes later. Vitamin K was given to the baby and the first breastfeed established. A check by the paediatrician suggested all was well and Mrs W left hospital 7 hours later with her husband and new baby.

Abnormal labour

Labour becomes abnormal when there is poor progress (as evidenced by a delay in cervical dilatation or descent of the presenting part) and/or the fetus shows signs of compromise. Similarly, by definition, if there is a malpresentation, a uterine scar or if labour has been induced, labour cannot be considered normal.

Poor progress in labour

Poor progress in the first stage of labour
Progress in labour is dependent on three variables:
1. the powers, i.e. the efficiency of uterine contractions,
2. the passenger, i.e. the fetus (with particular respect to its size, presentation and position),
3. the passages, i.e. the uterus, cervix and bony pelvis.

Abnormalities in one or more of these factors can slow the normal progress of labour. Plotting the findings of serial vaginal examinations on the partogram will help to highlight poor progress in the first stage.

Inefficient uterine action
This is the most common cause of poor progress in labour. It is more common in primigravidae and

perhaps in older women and is characterized by weak and infrequent contractions. The assessment of uterine contractions is most commonly carried out by clinical examination and by using external uterine tocography. However, this can only provide information about the frequency and duration of contractions. Intrauterine pressure catheters are available and these do give an accurate measurement of the pressure being generated by the contractions, but they are rarely necessary. A frequency of four to five contractions per 10 minutes is usually considered ideal. Fewer contractions than this does not necessarily mean progress will be slow, but more frequent examinations may be indicated to detect poor progress earlier. Treatment is by maternal rehydration, ARM and intravenous oxytocin (Syntocinon). Uterine contractions may also be extremely irregular and may occur close together in twos and threes, followed by longer periods of inertia. Syntocinon is also effective in correcting this 'inco-ordinate' uterine activity and usually succeeds in spacing the contractions out more evenly.

Cephalo-pelvic disproportion
This implies anatomical disproportion between the fetal head and maternal pelvis. It can be due to a large head, small pelvis or a combination of the two. Women

of small stature (<1.60 m) with a large baby in their first pregnancy are likely candidates to develop this problem. The pelvis may be unusually small because of previous fracture or metabolic bone disease. Relative CPD can also occur with malposition of the fetal head together with deflexion such as occurs in the OP position (Fig. 17.23).

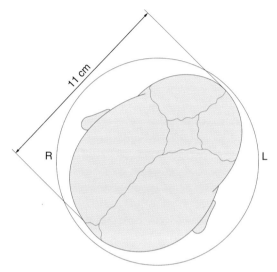

11 cm

R   L

Figure 17.23 Vaginal palpation of the head in the right occipito-posterior position. The circle represents the pelvic cavity, with a diameter of 12 cm. The head is poorly flexed so that the anterior fontanelle is easily felt.

Cephalo-pelvic disproportion is suspected in labour if:

- progress is slow or arrested despite efficient uterine contractions,
- the fetal head is not engaged,
- vaginal examination shows severe moulding and caput formation,
- the head is poorly applied to the cervix.

Oxytocin can be given carefully to a primigravida with mild to moderate CPD as long as the CTG is reactive. Relative disproportion may be overcome if the malposition is corrected (i.e. conversion to a flexed OA position). Using oxytocin in a multiparous woman with slow or obstructed labour carries the risk of causing uterine rupture (see below).

Malpresentations

Vital to good progress in labour is the tight application of the fetal presenting part onto the cervix. Breech and face presentations (see later) may fail to do this and the resulting progress in labour may be poor. Brow presentations are associated with the mento-vertical diameter, which is simply too large to fit through the bony pelvis unless flexion occurs or hyperextension to a face presentation. Brow presentation therefore often manifests as poor progress in first stage, often in a multiparous woman. Shoulder presentations cannot deliver vaginally and once again poor progress will occur. Malpresentations are more common in women of high parity and they carry a risk of uterine rupture if the labour is allowed to become obstructed.

Abnormalities of the passages

The bony pelvis may cause delay in the progress of labour as discussed above (CPD). Abnormalities of the uterus and cervix can also delay labour. Unsuspected fibroids in the lower uterine segment can prevent descent of the fetal head. Delay can also be caused by cervical dystocia, a term used to describe a non-compliant cervix which effaces but fails to dilate because of severe scarring, usually as a result of a previous cone biopsy. Caesarean section may be necessary.

Poor progress in the second stage of labour

The second stage of labour is the time of descent of the presenting part and lasts from full dilatation to delivery of the baby. It is important to be certain that the woman is fully dilated before delay in the second stage is diagnosed. In the first phase of the second stage, the woman has no urge to push, so vaginal examination is the only means of determining that she is fully dilated. Even when she has the urge to push, it is not certain that full dilatation has occurred. A persistent OP position, for example, often gives an urge to bear down before full dilatation.

The causes of second stage delay can again be classified as abnormalities of the powers, the passenger and the passages. Secondary uterine inertia is a common cause of second stage delay, and may be exacerbated by epidural analgesia. Having achieved full dilatation, the uterine contractions become weak and ineffectual and this is sometimes associated with maternal dehydration and ketosis. If no mechanical problem is anticipated, the treatment is with rehydration and intravenous oxytocin. Delay can also occur because of a persistent OP position of the fetal head. In this situation, the head will either have to undergo a long rotation to OA or be delivered in the OP position, i.e. face to pubes. Either way, the second stage is usually prolonged and if the contractions are not strong, oxytocin infusion may help to speed up the process.

Delay in the second stage can also occur because of a narrow mid-pelvis (android pelvis), which prevents internal rotation of the fetal head. This results in the fetal head being arrested at the level of the ischial spines in the transverse position, a condition called deep transverse arrest (Fig. 17.24). Under these

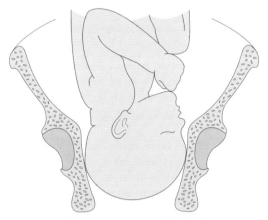

Figure 17.24 Deep transverse arrest of the head.

circumstances, delivery may be achieved by means of rotational forceps (Kielland's) or ventouse extraction, but frequently Caesarean section is required. When there is doubt as to whether vaginal delivery is achievable, the obstetrician may decide to perform a trial of forceps in the operating theatre. If any difficulty is encountered, Caesarean section is performed.

In the past, obstetricians regarded delivery of a baby in an obstructed second stage as a test of their prowess in the art of instrumental delivery. Nowadays, it is regarded as prudent not to attempt to deliver the baby if there is any chance of a difficult delivery that may cause trauma to the baby's skull and brain, for example intracranial haemorrhage, torn falx cerebri or skull fractures.

Risk factors for poor progress in labour

- Small woman
- Big baby
- Malpresentation
- Malposition
- Early membrane rupture
- Soft-tissue/pelvic malformation

Patterns of abnormal progress in labour

The use of a partogram to plot the progress of labour improves the detection of poor progress. Indeed, three patterns of abnormal labour are commonly described on the partogram (Fig. 17.25).

Prolonged latent phase occurs when the latent phase is longer than the arbitrary time limits discussed previously. It is more common in primiparous women and probably results from a delay in the chemical processes that occur within the cervix which

Figure 17.25 Abnormalities of the partogram.

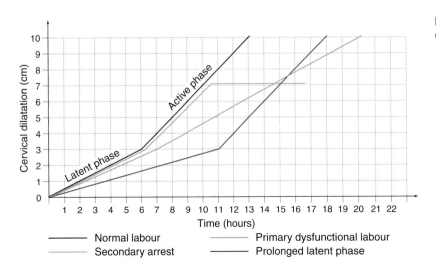

soften it and allow effacement. Prolonged latent phase can be extremely frustrating and tiring for the woman. However, intervention in the form of ARM or oxytocin infusion will increase the likelihood of poor progress later in the labour and the need for Caesarean birth. It is best managed away from the labour suite with simple analgesics, mobilization and reassurance.

Primary dysfunctional labour is the term used to describe poor progress in the active phase of labour (<1 cm/h cervical dilatation) and is also more common in primiparous women. It is most commonly caused by inefficient uterine contractions, but can also result from CPD and malposition of the fetus. **Secondary arrest** occurs when progress in the active phase is initially good but then slows, or stops altogether, typically after 7 cm dilatation. Although inefficient uterine contractions may be the cause, fetal malpositions, malpresentations and CPD are more common.

When poor progress is detected in first or second stage, it is vital to make a diagnosis (i.e. consider the cause). ARM followed by an oxytocin infusion is the treatment of choice for primary dysfunctional labour in a primiparous labour caused by poor contractions or malposition. Great care must be exercised in the use of oxytocin if CPD, malposition or malpresentation is suspected in a multiparous labour, as it may cause uterine rupture in these situations. Multiparous women with poor progress are probably best treated by ARM and further time to see if the malposition, or even malpresentation, corrects itself. Uterine rupture is an extremely rare event in primiparous women.

Augmentation of contractions with oxytocin (Syntocinon) should only ever be commenced if the CTG (or FBS) is normal. If progress fails to occur over the next 4–6 hours of augmentation with Syntocinon, a Caesarean section will be necessary.

The 'active management of labour' is a philosophy of labour management originating from Ireland, the main tenet of which is the early diagnosis of poor progress in labour corrected by early ARM and use of Syntocinon. In fact, the most important factor in the apparent success of active management in limiting Caesarean sections is the provision of one-to-one care by an experienced birth attendant.

Management of failure to progress in women with a breech presentation or previous Caesarean section is discussed later.

Key Points

The use of oxytocin
- The use of oxytocin is relatively safe in nulliparous women. It is less safe in multiparous women because of the risk of uterine hyperstimulation, fetal compromise and uterine rupture in the face of obstruction.
- Women with breech presentation or previous Caesarean section require careful consideration. Oxytocin treatment can be appropriate but should be used with great caution.

Presumed fetal compromise in labour

Concern for the well-being of the fetus is one of the most common reasons for medical intervention during labour. The fetus may already be compromised before labour, and the reduction in placental blood flow associated with contractions may uncover this and ultimately lead to fetal hypoxia and eventually acidosis. Fetal compromise may present as fresh meconium staining to the amniotic fluid, or an abnormal CTG. However, neither of these factors confirms fetal hypoxia/acidosis. Meconium can be passed for benign reasons, such as fetal maturity, and it is well recognized that the abnormal CTG carries a very high false-positive rate for the diagnosis of fetal compromise. The use of the term 'fetal distress' as a reason for intervention is therefore often inaccurate. In fact, intervention often occurs only because of *presumed* fetal compromise. After delivery, the condition of the baby is often found to be good. Only an FBS can definitely diagnose fetal hypoxia and acidosis in labour.

Risk factors for fetal compromise in labour

- Placental insufficiency – intrauterine growth restriction (IUGR) and pre-eclampsia
- Prematurity
- Postmaturity
- Multiple pregnancy
- Prolonged labour
- Uterine hyperstimulation
- Precipitate labour
- Intrapartum abruption
- Cord prolapse
- Uterine rupture/dehiscence
- Maternal diabetes

- Cholestasis of pregnancy
- Maternal pyrexia
- Chorioamnionitis
- Oligohydramnios

Management of possible fetal compromise

If there is concern regarding the well-being of the fetus in labour, a number of resuscitative manoeuvres should be considered.

- Maternal dehydration and ketosis can be corrected with intravenous fluids.
- Maternal hypotension secondary to an epidural can be reversed by a fluid bolus, although a vasoconstrictor such as ephedrine is occasionally necessary.
- Uterine hyperstimulation from excess Syntocinon can be reduced by turning off the infusion temporarily and using tocolytic drugs such as salbutamol and ritodrine.
- Venocaval compression and reduced uterine blood flow can be eased by turning the woman into a left lateral position.
- Oxygen is often given to the mother by a facemask; however, there is conflicting evidence as to whether this improves fetal oxygenation.

If meconium staining of the liquor is noted a CTG must be commenced. Fresh, thick meconium in the presence of a reassuring CTG is still cause for concern, and although the labour should be allowed to continue, the threshold for intervention will be lowered and a paediatrician should be present at delivery to aspirate the meconium from the airways immediately after birth.

If a CTG becomes suspicious or abnormal, it is important to carry out an immediate vaginal examination to exclude malpresentation and cord prolapse and to assess progress of the labour. If the cervix is fully dilated, it may be possible to deliver the baby vaginally using the forceps or ventouse. Alternatively, if the cervix is not fully dilated, an FBS can be considered (usually only possible at 2–3 cm dilatation or more). A normal result will permit labour to continue, although it may need to be repeated every 45–60 minutes if the CTG abnormalities persist or worsen. If there is another indication for Caesarean section, such as failure to progress, a normal result will allow the delivery to be performed with slightly less urgency, allowing a spinal anaesthetic, for example, instead of a general. An abnormal result mandates immediate delivery, by Caesarean section if the woman is not fully dilated.

Women with a uterine scar

Some women will have a pre-existing uterine scar, mostly because of a previous Caesarean section. The uterus is usually incised through the lower segment

CTG signs suggestive of fetal compromise
(see Figs 17.26–17.30)

- Fetal tachycardia (>160 bpm, or a steady rise over the course of the labour)
- Loss of baseline variability (<5 bpm)
- Loss of accelerations
- Recurrent late decelerations
- Persistent variable decelerations
- Fetal bradycardia (<100 bpm for more than 3 minutes)

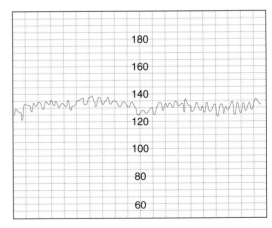

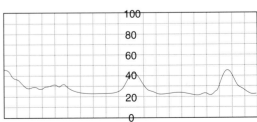

Figure 17.26 Normal trace. The upper record is of the fetal heart rate; the lower record shows uterine activity.

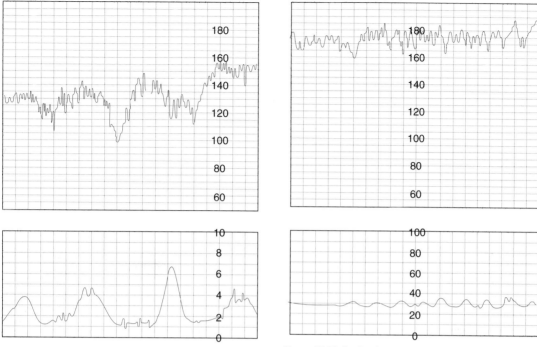

Figure 17.27 Fetal heart rate: late decelerations.

Figure 17.29 Fetal tachycardia.

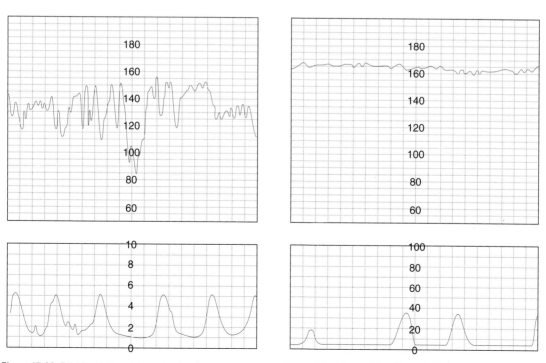

Figure 17.28 Fetal heart rate: variable decelerations.

Figure 17.30 Loss of baseline variability in fetal heart rate.

- An amnioscope is inserted into the vagina and its distal end is placed at right-angles on to the fetal head. The scalp is cleaned and a small cut is made using a blade with a guard. The resulting blood is collected into a microtube. The amount of blood required is approximately 25 μL.
- The normal pH would be above 7.25. A pH below 7.20 is confirmation of fetal compromise.
- The base deficit can also be useful in interpretation of the fetal scalp pH. A base excess or more than -10

demonstrates a significant metabolic acidosis, with increasing risk of fetal neurological injury beyond this level.
- One fetal scalp pH in labour is not as useful as several. A downward trend in the fetal scalp pH values is significant and should be assessed together with how the labour is progressing.
- If an abnormal CTG persists in labour, then, despite normal values, fetal scalp sampling should be repeated every 30–60 minutes.

CASE HISTORY

Mrs S is a 30-year-old gravida 2 para 1. She is 153 cm tall. Her previous baby weighed 3.2 kg at term and was delivered by forceps after a prolonged second stage. The father of this second baby is a new partner.

She has been admitted in spontaneous labour 10 days past her due date. Her hand-held records show concern from her midwife that this is a significantly larger baby than last time. Indeed, a scan at 36 weeks' gestation placed the abdominal and head circumference measurements on the 97th centiles. A subsequent glucose tolerance test was normal.

Despite good progress in the earlier part of the labour, dilatation has arrested at 7 cm. On examination, the head is found to be 3/5 palpable per abdomen; the position is left occipito-transverse and the contractions are poor. There is meconium-stained amniotic fluid.

What risks do Mrs S and her baby face?

The large fetal size and the short maternal stature raise the possibility of CPD. The previous need for a forceps delivery of only an average-size baby may indicate small pelvic diameters. There is a risk of obstructed labour, poor progress and the need for a Caesarean section. The meconium may simply be a sign of fetal maturity, but it may also indicate a degree of fetal compromise. At the very least, it poses the risk of meconium aspiration at delivery.

What care should Mrs S receive?

She should be informed of the concerns and provided with adequate pain relief. Fetal monitoring with a continuous CTG should begin (fortunately, this proves to be reactive and therefore reassuring). There is no need for an FBS at this point.

She should then be assessed by an experienced obstetric registrar, who must make a diagnosis as to the cause of this secondary arrest in first stage. Has the delay in labour occurred simply because of poor uterine contractions? Is there CPD, exacerbated by a fetal malposition?

If there is no caput or moulding, and the contractions do indeed prove to be poor and infrequent, a cautious trial of oxytocin can be considered. However, this woman has significant risk factors for CPD, and augmenting the labour with Syntocinon risks uterine rupture if the labour becomes truly obstructed.

What subsequent assessment should be undertaken?

A repeat examination should be performed by the same registrar 2 hours later. If the augmentation has been unsuccessful and the cervix is no further dilated, a Caesarean section is indicated. Even if full dilatation is reached, a vaginal delivery cannot be guaranteed. The obstetric registrar must be confident that the head has descended appropriately, without the development of excessive moulding or caput.

during Caesarean section because blood loss is reduced, healing is better and the risk of subsequent rupture is less than that following an upper segment or 'classical' Caesarean section. There are still a few indications for upper segment Caesarean section and it is important that these women are counselled appropriately. It is estimated that uterine rupture or

dehiscence (partial rupture) occurs in approximately 1 in 200 women who labour spontaneously with a pre-existing lower segment uterine scar. The risk is two to three times higher than this in women with a previous upper segment incision. As about 20 per cent of all deliveries in developed countries are by Caesarean section (>99 per cent lower segment

Caesarean sections), the care of such women in a subsequent pregnancy has become a significant problem.

Rupture of the uterus is particularly likely to occur:
- late in the first stage of labour,
- with induced or accelerated labour,
- in association with a large baby.

Signs of uterine rupture include severe lower abdominal pain, vaginal bleeding, haematuria, cessation of contractions, maternal tachycardia and fetal compromise (often a bradycardia). Uterine rupture carries serious maternal risks (shock, need for blood transfusion and operative repair, possibly a hysterectomy) and also serious fetal risks (including hypoxia and permanent neurological injury and intrapartum death).

Labour after a previous Caesarean section is known as 'vaginal birth after Caesarean' (VBAC), 'trial of vaginal delivery' or 'trial of scar'.

Relative contraindications to VBAC include:
- two or more previous Caesarean section scars,
- a high head at term,
- induction of labour (IOL).

There remains a debate over these issues. However, all obstetricians agree that a previous upper segment Caesarean section is an absolute contraindication to a trial of vaginal birth.

If a woman with a previous history of a Caesarean section delivery is admitted in labour, intense surveillance is required to identify early signs of uterine rupture. Continuous CTG monitoring is vital in labour and there should be a low threshold for urgent delivery by repeat Caesarean section.

Some women will have scars on the uterus as a result of a previous myomectomy. In general, there is minimal danger of rupture of a myomectomy scar unless the uterine cavity has been extensively opened during the procedure.

Malpresentations

Breech presentation

The antenatal management of breech presentation is discussed in Chapter 11 and the mechanics of the delivery are discussed in Chapter 18. For this discussion, it is sufficient to list some of the complications of a breech labour, which include the following.
- Increased risk of prolapsed cord: this is especially so with footling breech presentations, and to a lesser extent with the flexed breech. This can cause rapid and severe hypoxia in the fetus (see Chapter 19).

- Increased risk of CTG abnormalities: cord compression is common during a breech vaginal delivery.
- Mechanical difficulties in the delivery of the shoulders and/or head: damage to the visceral organs or the brachial plexus can occur if traction is exerted on the breech. Delay in the delivery of the head may occur with the larger fetus, leading to prolonged compression of the umbilical cord and asphyxia. An uncontrolled rapid delivery of the head may occur with a smaller fetus and this predisposes to tentorial tears and intracranial bleeding.

The majority of breech presentations recognized antenatally are delivered by Caesarean section, to avoid these risks. Although this is evidence based, and it is probably safer for breech babies to be delivered this way, the most frequent cause of harm in breech labours is the failure to recognize and respond to CTG abnormalities, rather than mechanical problems at the very end of the labour. There is still a place for the vaginal delivery of a breech presentation. Maternal choice and the failure to detect breech presentation until very late in labour will mean that there will continue to be a need for obstetricians to be expert in the skills of breech vaginal delivery.

Poor progress in a breech labour is taken by most to be an indication for Caesarean section. However, a few would support the use of augmentation with oxytocin if contractions are infrequent.

Face presentation

This malpresentation occurs in about 1:500 labours and is due to complete extension of the fetal head (Fig. 17.31). In the majority of cases, the cause for the extension is unknown, although it is frequently attributed to excessive tone of the extensor muscles of the fetal neck. Certainly, during the antenatal period, full extension of the fetal neck can frequently be identified by ultrasound, which may last for a few hours. Rarely, extension may be due to a fetal anomaly such as a thyroid tumour. The presenting diameter is the submento-bregmatic, which measures 9.5 cm, i.e. approximately the same as the suboccipito-bregmatic (vertex) presentation. Despite this, engagement of the fetal head is late and progress in labour is frequently slow, possibly because the facial bones do not mould. It is diagnosed in labour by palpating the nose, mouth and eyes on vaginal examination. If progress in labour is excellent, and the chin remains mento-anterior, vaginal delivery

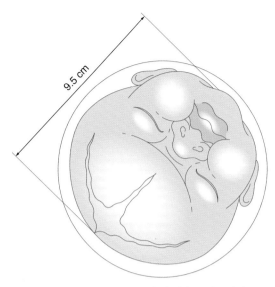

Figure 17.31 Vaginal examination in the left mento-anterior position. The circle represents the pelvic cavity, with a diameter of 12 cm.

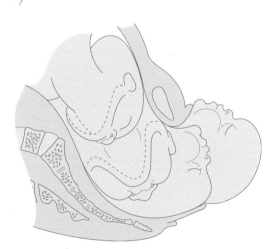

Figure 17.32 The mechanism of labour with a face presentation. The head descends with increasing extension. The chin reaches the pelvic floor and undergoes forward rotation. The head is born by flexion.

is possible, the head being delivered by flexion (Fig. 17.32). If the chin is posterior (mento-posterior position), delivery is impossible, as extension over the perineum cannot occur. In this circumstance, Caesarean section is performed. Oxytocin should not be used, and if there is any concern about fetal condition, Caesarean section should be carried out.

Brow presentation

This arises when there is less extreme extension of the fetal neck than that with a face presentation. It can be considered a midway position between vertex and face. It is the least common malpresentation, occurring in 1:2000 labours. The causes of this are similar to those of face presentation, although some brow presentations arise as a result of exaggerated extension associated with OP position. The presenting diameter is mento-vertical (measuring 13.5 cm) (Fig. 17.33). This is

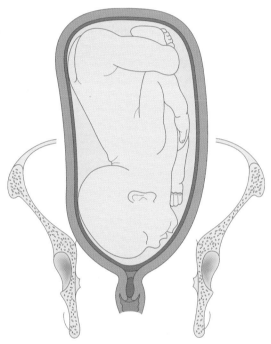

Figure 17.33 Brow presentation. The head is above the brim and not engaged. The mento-vertical diameter of the head is trying to engage in the transverse diameter at the brim.

incompatible with a vaginal delivery. It is diagnosed in labour by palpating the anterior fontanelle, supra-orbital ridges and nose on vaginal examination (Fig. 17.34). If this presentation persists, delivery will only be achieved by Caesarean section.

Shoulder presentation

This is frequently reported as occurring in 1:300 deliveries, but few of these women will go into labour. Shoulder presentation occurs as the result of a transverse or oblique lie of the fetus and the causes of this abnormality include placenta praevia, pelvic tumour and uterine anomaly. Occasionally, a woman, usually

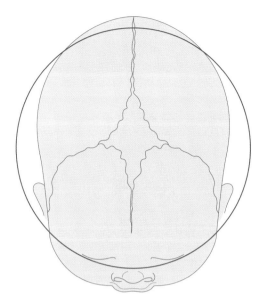

Figure 17.34 Vaginal examination with brow presentation. The circle represents the pelvic cavity, with a diameter of 12 cm. The mento-vertical diameter of 13 cm is too large to permit engagement of the head.

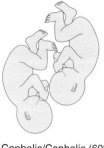
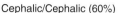

Cephalic/Cephalic (60%)   Cephalic/Breech (20%)

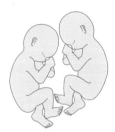
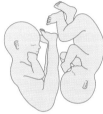
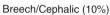

Breech/Cephalic (10%)   Breech/Breech (10%)

Figure 17.35 The four major presentations of twin pregnancy.

of high parity, will present in labour with a shoulder presentation as a result of an uncorrected unstable lie due to uterine laxity. Normally, the antenatal problem of unstable lie will have been recognized and the woman admitted for observation. Delivery should be by Caesarean section. Delay in making the diagnosis risks cord prolapse or uterine rupture.

Multiple gestations

About 1:80 pregnancies at term are multi-fetal. High-order multiples such as triplets and quadruplets are now invariably delivered by Caesarean section, because of the risks to the last fetus if vaginal delivery is attempted. Elective (i.e. planned) Caesarean section is frequently performed in twin pregnancies also, mostly for fetal reasons.

Indications for elective Caesarean section in twin pregnancy

- Malpresentation of the first twin
- Second twin larger than the first
- Evidence of IUGR in one or both twins
- Monoamniotic twins

There are four principal combinations of presentation (Fig. 17.35):
- cephalic/cephalic – 60 per cent,
- cephalic/breech – 20 per cent,
- breech/cephalic – 10 per cent,
- breech/breech – 10 per cent.

Essentially, the lie and the presentation of the second twin are not crucially important. However, planned Caesarean section will usually be performed if the first twin presents by the breech, and certainly if it is transverse.

The ideal criteria for a twin labour are:
- spontaneous onset,
- cephalic presentation of twin 1,
- twin 1 larger than twin 2,
- dichorionic pregnancy.

The mechanics of the delivery of twins is discussed in greater detail in Chapter 18. Suffice to say that CTG abnormalities, fetal compromise, malpresentations, cord prolapse, need for emergency Caesarean section and postpartum haemorrhage all occur more commonly than in singleton labours.

⚓ Key Points

Labour
- Most labours are uncomplicated and the outcomes are good.
- Labour can be a hazardous journey for the baby.

- Abnormalities of the uterine contractions (the 'powers'), the fetus (the 'passenger') and the pelvis and lower genital tract (the 'passages') can cause abnormal labour.
- The term 'fetal distress' is unhelpful and often misleading. If there are concerns for fetal well-being in labour, 'presumed fetal compromise' should be used instead.
- Augmentation of labour with oxytocin will often correct poor uterine contractions and fetal malposition.
- Augmentation of labour with oxytocin can be dangerous in multiparous women, in those with a uterine scar and in cases of malpresentation.

Induction of labour

Induction of labour is the planned initiation of labour prior to its spontaneous onset. Between 15 and 25 per cent of all pregnancies in the UK end as an IOL. The reasons for IOL are listed below. Broadly speaking, an IOL is performed when the risks to the fetus and/or the mother of the pregnancy continuing outweigh those of bringing the pregnancy to an end. It should only be performed if there is a reasonable chance of success and if the risks of the process to the mother and/or fetus are acceptable. If either of these is not the case, a planned Caesarean section should be performed instead.

Common indications for induction of labour

- 'Post dates' (i.e. 12 days or more beyond EDD)
- Fetal growth restriction
- Other evidence of placental insufficiency, e.g. oligohydramnios
- Pre-eclampsia
- Other maternal hypertensive disorders
- Deteriorating maternal illnesses
- Prolonged prelabour rupture of membranes
- Unexplained antepartum haemorrhage
- Diabetes mellitus
- Twin pregnancy continuing beyond 38 weeks
- Rhesus iso-immunization
- 'Social' reasons (see text)

The most common reason for IOL is 'post-dates' or 'post-maturity'. There is evidence that prolonged pregnancies extending beyond 42 weeks' gestation are associated with a higher risk of stillbirth, fetal compromise in labour, meconium aspiration and mechanical problems at delivery. Because of this, women are usually recommended IOL at 10–12 days past their expected due date. Another common indication for IOL is prolonged prelabour rupture of membranes (PPROM). It is not uncommon for the membranes to rupture and the subsequent onset of labour to be significantly delayed. The longer this situation is left to continue, the greater the risk of ascending infection (chorioamnionitis). Women whose membranes rupture at term before going into labour are usually advised to undergo IOL if their labour has not commenced within the next 24–72 hours (opinions vary as to how long women can be safely left). At preterm gestations this period of time is much longer, but intense fetal and maternal surveillance for signs of infection is necessary. Pre-eclampsia is another common indication for IOL. However, if the pre-eclampsia is severe and/or of early onset, it may be considered safer for mother and baby for the delivery to occur by Caesarean section.

'Social' induction of labour is controversial and is performed to satisfy the domestic and organizational needs of the woman and her family. It is mostly discouraged, and there must be careful counselling as to the potential risks involved. These are determined essentially by the parity and the cervical condition. If the situation is favourable for vaginal birth, with higher parity and a favourable cervix (see below), 'soft' indications are more acceptable. In any circumstance, an induced labour cannot be considered 'normal' and should be carefully supervised.

The Bishop score

As the time of spontaneous labour approaches, the cervix becomes softer, shortened, moves forward and starts to dilate. This reflects the natural preparation for labour. If labour is induced before this process is nearly complete, the induction process will tend to be correspondingly longer. Bishop produced a scoring system (Table 17.1) to quantify how far this process had progressed prior to the IOL. High scores (a 'favourable' cervix) are associated with an easier, shorter induction that is less likely to fail. Low scores (an 'unfavourable' cervix) point to a longer IOL that is more likely to fail and result in Caesarean section.

Table 17.1 – Modified Bishop score

Score	0	1	2	3
Dilatation of cervix (cm)	0	1 or 2	3 or 4	5 or more
Consistency of cervix	Firm	Medium	Soft	–
Length of cervical canal (cm)	>2	2–1	1–0.5	<0.5
Position of cervix	Posterior	Central	Anterior	–
Station of presenting part	−3	−2	−1 or 0	Below spines

Methods

Induction of labour was traditionally performed by ARM. In the mid-1950s, synthetic oxytocin became available and was then used as an intravenous adjunct after rupture of the membranes. In favourable cases, this would succeed in inducing labour and often in effecting vaginal delivery. However, in unfavourable cases, it was not so successful and sometimes it was impossible to rupture the membranes. In the late 1960s, prostaglandin became available. Various routes and various preparations have been used, but the most common formulation in current use is inserted vaginally into the posterior fornix as a tablet or gel.

Women with an unfavourable cervix will require between one and three doses of vaginal prostaglandin. It is usually possible after this to perform an ARM and then to commence Syntocinon if the contractions are still poor (as is usually the case in primiparous women). Women with a more favourable cervix may not require pre-treatment with prostaglandin, and an ARM with or without Syntocinon may be sufficient to establish labour.

Complications of induction of labour

A CTG should be performed at the start of every induction and is normally continued throughout the process. Many indications for IOL will be associated with a higher risk of fetal compromise in labour, as is the use of prostaglandins and oxytocin.

Induction of labour may fail and result in Caesarean section. An induction is said to have failed if an ARM is still impossible after the maximum number of doses of prostaglandin have been given, or if the cervix remains uneffaced and <3 cm dilated after an ARM has been performed and Syntocinon has been running for 6–8 hours. Hyperstimulation of the uterus (from prostaglandin administration or use of Syntocinon) may result in fetal asphyxia and the need for Caesarean section. IOL in the presence of a uterine scar may lead to uterine rupture. ARM performed when the presenting part is still high risks cord prolapse. IOL is associated with a longer duration of labour, greater use of epidurals and more assisted vaginal deliveries. Long labours augmented with Syntocinon predispose to postpartum haemorrhage due to uterine atony after delivery of the placenta.

CASE HISTORY

Mrs B is a 33-year-old woman in her first pregnancy. She is 42 weeks' gestation and a report of reduced fetal movements has prompted an ultrasound scan. Although the growth parameters of the fetus are on the 50th centile there is oligohydramnios (reduced amniotic fluid). A CTG is reactive.

An IOL has been discussed and a vaginal examination performed. The Bishop score is 2.

What risks do Mrs B and her baby face?

There are three reasons to think that there is placental insufficiency of recent onset. First, prolonged pregnancy is associated with histological placental changes ('ageing') that reduce placental nutrient and gas exchange. Second, the liquor volume is reduced; and third, the fetus is less active than previously. Continuation of the pregnancy will increase the risks of intrauterine hypoxia, acidosis or even death. Labour will carry a higher risk of compromising the fetus and there is a greater risk of meconium passage and aspiration by the newborn. The reactive normal CTG gives no guarantee of future fetal well-being or its ability to tolerate contractions.

The unfavourable cervix increases the chances of long induction, which may ultimately be unsuccessful. Whether the labour is induced or spontaneous, this scenario carries a greater risk of assisted delivery, either instrumental or Caesarean section.

What care should Mrs B receive?

She should be given full psychological support from the midwifery and medical team. She should be counselled against delaying the delivery of the fetus any further. Despite the concerns regarding the possible outcomes, IOL would be recommended. Mrs B should receive prostaglandin gel administered per vaginam at 6-hourly intervals. Recent guidelines recommend using only two doses of prostaglandin. Electronic fetal heart rate monitoring should

be instituted when significant contractions begin. ARM should be performed and an oxytocin infusion used if labour fails to establish or progress following the ARM. Pain relief should be offered as usual, although epidural anaesthesia might be encouraged in these circumstances, as the labour process may be long.

What ongoing care should she receive?

Attention should be paid to the need for continuity of care despite staff shift changes. A senior doctor should be involved and should review the situation at intervals to determine if it is safe to continue or whether emergency Caesarean section should be performed. If labour is prolonged and difficult, an H2-blocker and an anti-emetic should be given orally to suppress gastric acid secretion and reduce the risks in the event of a general anaesthetic becoming necessary. Caesarean section should be performed if induction fails, the labour establishes but fails to progress, or fetal monitoring (the CTG or FBS) suggests compromise.

Women and their partners should be advised of these risks before embarking on the procedure.

Pain relief in labour

The provision of analgesia in childbirth varies between cultures. Some women and their carers believe that there is an advantage in avoiding analgesia, whereas other women will use all methods on offer to limit their pain. Professionals who are knowledgeable about labour and are sympathetic to the labouring woman should give advice regarding pain relief in labour. The method of pain relief is to some extent dependent on the previous obstetric record of the woman, the course of labour and also the estimated length of labour. Just as one woman's labour can be made into an unhappy experience by unsolicited and unnecessary analgesia, pain relief that is inadequate, or offered too late, can ruin another's. It should be remembered that the final decision rests with the woman, although there are certain circumstances in which particular forms of analgesia are contraindicated and should not be offered.

Non-pharmacological methods

Relaxation and breathing exercises may help the woman to manage her pain. Prolonged hyperventilation can make the woman dizzy and can cause alkalosis. Homeopathy, acupuncture and hypnosis are sometimes employed, but their use has not been associated with a significant reduction in pain scores or with a reduced need for conventional methods of analgesia, and they are probably not widely applicable.

Transcutaneous electrical nerve stimulation (TENS) is frequently used. It works on the principle of blocking pain fibres in the posterior ganglia of the spinal cord by stimulation of small afferent fibres (the 'gate' theory). It also has not been shown to reduce pain scores or the need for other forms of analgesia. It does not have any adverse effects, but is often disappointing. It can be of use early in labour.

Relaxation in warm water during the first stage of labour often leads to a sense of well-being and allows women to cope much better with the pain. Clearly, a woman in labour cannot use an opiate or have an epidural sited whilst in water.

Pharmacological methods

Opiates such as pethidine are still used in most obstetric units and indeed can be administered by midwives without the involvement of the medical staff. This may be one of the reasons for their popularity. However, on the whole, women do not regard them as any better than TENS. They cause a degree of sedation and this may be interpreted by onlookers as a successful reduction in pain, which is not actually experienced by the woman. In conventional doses, opiates also cause nausea and vomiting and an anti-emetic is often given in tandem. They have a prolonged effect on the newborn and can cause respiratory depression, which may affect bonding and breastfeeding. Giving naloxone to the newborn can counteract these effects. Possibly the most serious adverse effect of pethidine and all the opiate analgesics is delayed maternal gastric emptying. This represents a danger to mothers if they require general anaesthesia. In the presence of a full stomach, under general anaesthesia, regurgitation and pulmonary aspiration can occur unless skilled cricoid pressure is applied. Therefore ranitidine should be given to women in labour who opt for pethidine, and to all other women who are at risk of needing a Caesarean section.

Diamorphine is a better analgesic than pethidine, but has potentially a greater respiratory depressant effect on the newborn. Opiates tend to be given as intramuscular injections; however, a more effective way is to give a subcutaneous or intravenous infusion by patient-controlled analgesia (PCA). This allows the woman, by pressing a dispenser button, to determine the level of analgesia that she requires. If a very short-acting opiate is used, e.g. remifentanil, the opiate doses can be timed with the contractions.

Inhalational analgesia

Nitrous oxide (NO) in the form of Entonox (an equal mixture of NO and oxygen) is used on most labour wards. It has a quick onset, a short duration of effect, and is more effective than TENS or pethidine. Its adverse effects are light-headedness and nausea. It is not suitable for prolonged use from early labour because hyperventilation may result in hypocapnoea, dizziness and ultimately tetany and fetal hypoxia. Its most suitable use is late in labour or while awaiting epidural analgesia.

Epidural analgesia

Epidural (extradural) analgesia is the most reliable means of providing effective analgesia in labour. Failure to provide an epidural is one of the most frequent causes of anxiety and disappointment among labouring women. The epidural service must be well organized to be effective, and fortunately resources are now in place so that a significant delay in the siting of an epidural is unusual.

Indications
The decision to have an epidural sited should be a combined one between the woman, her midwife, the obstetric team and the anaesthetist. The final decision in most cases rests with the woman unless there is a definite contraindication. The main contraindications are:
- coagulation disorders,
- local or systemic sepsis,
- hypovolaemia,
- a lack of trained staff (both anaesthetic and midwifery).

The main indication is for effective pain relief. There are other maternal and fetal conditions in which epidural analgesia would be advantageous in labour. These are:
- prolonged labour,
- maternal hypertensive disorders,
- multiple gestation,
- certain maternal medical conditions,
- where there is a high risk of operative intervention.

Advanced cervical dilatation on its own is not a contraindication to an epidural. It is more important to assess the rate of progress, the anticipated length of time to delivery and the type of delivery expected. Careful counselling is required before the epidural is sited, and the potential complications should be explained to the mother. It is important to warn the woman that she may temporarily lose sensation and movement in her legs.

Technique
An intravenous infusion of crystalloid (e.g. Hartmann's solution or normal saline) needs to be set up prior to insertion of the epidural. This is to give intravenous access in case of a problem, and may also be used to give a preload of 500–1000 mL crystalloid in order to prevent hypotension.

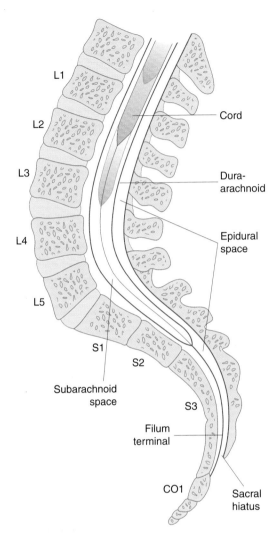

Figure 17.36 Sagittal section of the lumbo-sacral spinal cord.

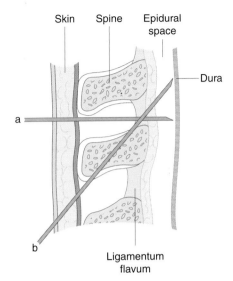

Figure 17.37 Needle positioning for an epidural anaesthetic. Midline (a) and paramedian (b) approaches.

The epidural catheter is normally inserted at the L2–L3, L3–L4 or L4–L5 interspace and should come to lie in the epidural space, which contains blood vessels, nerve roots and fat (Fig. 17.36). The catheter is aspirated to check for position and, if no blood or cerebrospinal fluid is obtained, a test dose is given to confirm the catheter position (Fig. 17.37). This test dose is a small volume of dilute local anaesthetic (e.g. 2 mL 0.5 per cent bupivacaine). If it has no obvious effect on sensation in the lower limbs, the catheter is correctly sited. If there is a sensory block, leg weakness and peripheral vasodilatation, the catheter has been inserted too far and into the subarachnoid (spinal) space. Inserting the normal dose of local anaesthetic into the spinal space by accident would risk complete motor and respiratory paralysis. If none of these signs is observed 5 minutes after injection of the test dose, a loading dose can be administered.

After the loading dose is given, the mother should be kept in the right or left lateral position, and her blood pressure should be measured every 5 minutes for 30 minutes. A fall in blood pressure may result from the vasodilatation caused by blocking of the sympathetic tone to peripheral blood vessels. This hypotension is usually short lived, but may cause a fetal bradycardia due to redirection of maternal blood away from the uterus. It should be treated with intravenous fluids and, if necessary, vasoconstrictors such as ephedrine. The mother should never lie supine, as aorto-caval compression can reduce maternal cardiac output and so compromise placental perfusion. Opioids such as fentanyl may be used to supplement the epidural block and allow a reduction in the amount of local anaesthetic required. This has the added advantage of impairing motor function in the lower legs to a lesser degree.

Regional analgesia can be maintained throughout labour with either intermittent boluses or continuous infusions, or, occasionally, a combination of both.

Spinal analgesia

A fine-gauge atraumatic spinal needle is passed through the epidural space, through the dura and into the subarachnoid space, which contains the cerebrospinal fluid. A small volume of local anaesthetic is injected, after which the spinal needle is withdrawn. This may be used as the anaesthetic for Caesarean sections, trial of instrumental deliveries (in theatre), manual removal of retained placentae and the repair of difficult perineal and vaginal tears. Spinals are not used for routine analgesia in labour.

Combined spinal–epidural analgesia

Combined spinal–epidural (CSE) analgesia has gained in popularity. This technique has the advantage of producing a rapid onset of pain relief and the provision of prolonged analgesia.

Complications of regional analgesia

- Hypotension is the most common complication and can usually be rectified easily (see above).
- Accidental dural puncture during the search for the epidural space should occur in <1 per cent of cases. Because the needle used for an epidural is wider bore than that used for a spinal, if the subarachnoid space is accidentally reached with an epidural needle there is a risk that the hole left afterwards in the dura will be large enough to allow the leakage of cerebrospinal fluid. This results in a 'spinal headache', which is characterized by relief when lying flat but exacerbation by sitting upright. If the headache is severe or persistent, a blood patch may be necessary. This involves injecting a small volume of the woman's blood into the epidural space at the level of the accidental dural puncture. The resulting blood clot is thought to block off the leak of cerebrospinal fluid.
- Accidental total spinal anaesthesia (injection of epidural doses of local anaesthetic into the subarachnoid space) causes severe hypotension, respiratory failure, unconsciousness and death if not recognized and treated immediately. The mother requires intubation, ventilation and circulatory support. Hypotension must be treated with intravenous fluids, vasopressors and left uterine displacement, though urgent delivery of the baby may be required to overcome aortocaval compression and so permit resuscitation.

- Neurological complications are rare, and are usually associated with other factors.
- Drug toxicity can occur with accidental placement of a catheter within a blood vessel. This is normally revealed by aspiration prior to injection.
- Bladder dysfunction can occur if the bladder is allowed to overfill because the woman is unaware of the need to micturate whilst the spinal or epidural is wearing off. Over-distension of the detrusor muscle of the bladder can permanently damage it and leave long-term voiding problems. To avoid this, catheterization of the bladder should be carried out early or prophylactically if the woman has difficulty in passing urine.
- Backache during and after pregnancy is not uncommon. There is now good evidence that epidural analgesia does not cause backache.
- The effect of epidural analgesia on labour and the operative delivery rate has been the most controversial issue of all. The evidence is now clear that epidural analgesia does not increase Caesarean section rates, but instrumental delivery rates (ventouse and forceps) do increase unless the second stage is actively managed with a more aggressive use of Syntocinon in primiparous women. In certain clinical situations, an epidural in the second stage of labour may assist a vaginal delivery by relaxing the woman and allowing time for the head to descend and rotate.

Clinical risk management

Risk management is an approach to healthcare provision that aims to limit harm occurring to patients. Clinical risk management (CRM) can be applied to all areas of medicine, but the labour ward provides one of the best illustrations of its importance to modern health care.

Labour and delivery carry a serious risk of harm. Maternal trauma (both physical and psychological) and infant neurological injuries are examples of poor outcomes from labour suite that can potentially be avoided in many cases. Legal action is frequently taken after outcomes such as these, and this is expensive for the National Health Service in litigation payments and distressing for the staff involved. The aim of CRM is to improve standards of care and subsequently reduce the harm occurring to women and their babies. This in turn should reduce the number of complaints made against hospital trusts and the financial costs of litigation.

Shoulder dystocia, for example, can result in Erb's palsy, intrapartum asphyxial damage and serious maternal perineal trauma. In the majority of cases, these poor outcomes of shoulder dystocia can be avoided by appropriate management. Regular staff education and the performance of shoulder dystocia 'drills' should limit these outcomes. In these drills, the manoeuvres used to safely overcome shoulder dystocia are rehearsed to aid with recollection in the event of a real emergency. The use of guidelines and protocols drawn from evidence-based medicine is another tool of CRM. These help to reduce errors and to prevent bizarre or unusual decision making.

Once a 'near-miss' or a poor outcome has occurred, careful documentation is vital if claims of negligence are to be defended. Good communication between the patient and the staff involved may help to clear up misunderstandings and minimize the chances of a formal complaint or legal action.

Audit of labour ward outcomes is an important tool in risk management. If guidelines are not being followed, and certain standards are not being met, this will be detected by audit and steps taken to address the problem. A repeat audit should show improvements have occurred as a result of the actions taken.

Key Points

Induction of labour and clinical risk management

- Every induction of labour should have a valid indication.
- The most common indication for induction of labour is 'postmaturity'.
- A high Bishop score predicts an easier induction of labour.
- The alternatives for intrapartum analgesia each have advantages and disadvantages and should be discussed with the woman and her birthing partner.
- Clinical risk management aims to improve standards of intrapartum care and to reduce the harm of poor obstetric outcomes for women, babies, hospital trusts and medical staff.

Operative intervention in obstetrics

OVERVIEW

The best outcome of pregnancy is a healthy mother and baby, ideally following a normal vaginal delivery with an intact perineum. Sadly, for many women and babies, the hazards of childbirth are a serious risk. Indeed, operative obstetric intervention to manage these hazards has come to be regarded as a mainstay of safe motherhood.

Millions of women have died and more women continue to die in childbirth. Although now not a problem seen frequently in Western labour wards, in the nineteenth century maternal mortality in England was called a 'dark continuous stream'. The risk of dying then was nearly a hundred times greater than it is today. In the absence of skilled attendants and facilities for intervention, this figure remains accurate today for 'death in childbirth' in many parts of the world.

Introduction

Sepsis, haemorrhage and eclampsia were, and remain, the leading causes of death. There can be no doubt that operative vaginal and abdominal delivery and surgical management of placental and uterine complications have all contributed to the dramatic improvements seen in maternal risk and outcome in the West.

Ironically, at the close of the twentieth century, the issues of 'over-intervention' were more topical in the West. Indeed, as operative interventions carry their own risks of mortality and morbidity, this chapter maintains the principle of 'avoiding unnecessary operative intervention wherever possible' (primum non nocere).

The material included in this chapter is based on a systematic review of the literature. It is intended to give the reader an introduction to operative procedures in as relevant and practical a way as possible. For that reason, a large component of each section is 'how to do it'.

The general principles that should be adhered to in all situations in which interventions are contemplated are as follows.

- A diagnosis should be recorded and examination or operative findings clearly documented.
- The most appropriate intervention should be chosen.
- At all stages, details of planned procedures should be discussed with the mother, who should remain free to make informed choices.
- Documentation should be legible, timed, dated and signed.

- Full details of operative procedures and complications should be recorded.
- A rectal examination should be performed before and after perineal repair to exclude injury.
- Swabs should always be counted and both swabs and needles recorded.

Perineal care

Episiotomy

Definition
Episiotomy is a surgical incision of the perineum made to increase the diameter of the vulval outlet during childbirth.

History and epidemiology
Although introduced as an obstetric procedure more than 200 years earlier, in general, obstetricians only came to favour episiotomy at the beginning of the twentieth century. It was then thought that all primigravidae should receive an episiotomy to protect the fetal head and the pelvic floor. By the 1970s, episiotomy rates were as high as 90 per cent. Further research carried out over the last 20 years has shown the problems associated with the procedure, which include unsatisfactory anatomical results, increased blood loss, perineal pain and dyspareunia. These studies have concluded that the routine use of episiotomy should be abandoned. The World Health Organization (WHO) recommends an episiotomy rate of 10 per cent for normal deliveries.

How to avoid an episiotomy/perineal trauma
Alternative positions of the woman during labour may prevent perineal damage, e.g. kneeling, a supported squat or all fours. Physiological pushing and an upright position may allow the presenting part to descend and stretch the perineum gently. Fetal distress can sometimes be rectified by a change in the maternal position and this may also prevent a ventouse or forceps delivery. The presence of a caring companion through labour reduces the incidence of episiotomy and perineal trauma. Alternatives to epidurals for pain relief should be considered. When instrumental delivery is required, the use of the vacuum extractor rather than forceps is associated with a decrease in perineal trauma.

Technique
There are two different techniques that are widely used (Fig. 18.1):
1. midline (common in USA): this is cut vertically from the fourchette down towards the anus,
2. mediolateral (standard in the UK): this starts in the midline position at the fourchette but is then directed diagonally outwards to avoid the anal sphincter.

The advantages of the midline episiotomy are:
- less blood loss,
- it is easier to repair,
- the wound heals quicker,
- there is less pain in the postpartum period,
- the incidence of dyspareunia is reduced.

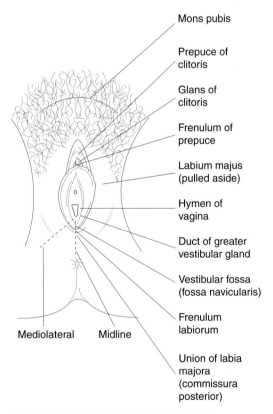

Figure 18.1 Mediolateral and midline episiotomies.

However, the major disadvantage that it carries a more than six-fold risk of it extending to involve the anal sphincter (third/fourth-degree tear).

Anaesthesia
Prior to an episiotomy being performed, adequate anaesthesia must be administered. If the woman has

an epidural, it must be topped-up accordingly or the perineum must be infiltrated with local anaesthetic.

Possible indications for an episiotomy

- Fetal distress
- Short or inelastic perineum
- Shoulder dystocia
- Fetal malposition, e.g. occipito-posterior
- An instrumental or breech delivery
- Previous pelvic floor surgery

Performing the episiotomy

Large, sharp, straight scissors are the instrument of choice. If the episiotomy is performed too far laterally, it will not increase the diameter of the vulval outlet, but may cause damage to the right Bartholin's gland. This could predispose to a decrease in vaginal lubrication or cyst formation. If it is made too small, it will not increase the diameter of the vulval outlet sufficiently to facilitate delivery and it may form a weak point in the perineal tissues from which a tear could extend.

The episiotomy must be made in one single cut. If it is enlarged by several small cuts, a zigzag incision line will be produced which will be difficult to repair. The episiotomy should begin in the midline at the fourchette.

Complications

Cuts that begin more laterally are likely to be more painful and more complicated to suture. Any episiotomy may extend and cause a third-degree tear to the anal sphincter. An episiotomy can bleed heavily. Haemostasis should be achieved, with pressure or arterial clamps if necessary. Infection is more likely when the episiotomy is contaminated. Prophylactic antibiotics may be indicated.

Key Points

Episiotomy
- The episiotomy rate should be kept under 20 per cent.
- Use a mediolateral cut – but this must begin in the midline.
- Refer for experienced opinion if episiotomy extends.

Perineal repair

Definition of perineal injury (Fig. 18.2)
- First degree: involves skin only.
- Second degree: involves perineal muscle and therefore includes episiotomy.
- Third degree: second-degree tear with disruption of the anal sphincter, further subdivided into:
  - 3a: less than 50 per cent of external sphincter thickness torn,
  - 3b: more than 50 per cent of external sphincter thickness torn,
  - 3c: internal anal sphincter also torn.
- Fourth degree: third-degree tear with torn anal epithelium.

On rare occasions, the rectal mucosa can tear through the vagina with an intact anal sphincter, but this is not included in the above classification.

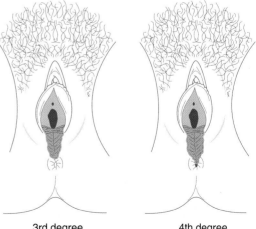

| 1st degree | 2nd degree | 3rd degree | 4th degree |

Figure 18.2 Perineal anatomy with schematic graded injuries.

History and epidemiology

Perineal injuries have occurred since childbirth began, and surgical attempts at repair have been documented across a wide range of cultures, starting with crude juxtaposition described in ancient Egypt.

In the UK today, approximately 750 000 women give birth each year and of these, 525 000 (70 per cent) will sustain perineal trauma and will require stitches. The majority of these women will experience perineal pain in the immediate period following delivery and more than 100 000 will have long-term problems such as superficial dyspareunia. If the repair is performed perfunctorily or inadequately, it may leave women suffering from perineal pain, which they describe as being far worse than the pain of childbirth.

Long-term perineal morbidity, associated with failure to recognize or to repair adequately trauma to the external anal sphincter, can lead to major physical, psychological and social problems.

Technique

The skill of the operator, repair technique and suture material are contributing factors to perineal pain during the healing process.

Some first-degree tears will not require suturing and others will simply require one or two interrupted sutures. A loose, continuous, non-locking suture technique to appose each layer (vaginal epithelium, perineal muscle and skin) is associated with less short-term pain and need for suture removal compared to the traditional interrupted method.

Complications

Missing the apex of the tear or episiotomy may allow continued bleeding or the development of a paragenital haematoma. Deep sutures including the rectal mucosa could lead to fistula formation. Over-enthusiastic tight suturing can lead to significant later discomfort. Closure of the skin over the fourchette sometimes leads to formation of a bridge of tissue that can make intercourse very uncomfortable. Mal-aligned repairs lead to distortions in healing and increased scarring.

Over-zealous repairs can, paradoxically, lead to more complications.

Third/fourth-degree tear repair

History and epidemiology

Traditionally, this has been thought to be a complication affecting relatively small numbers of women (0.5–2 per cent). More recent work has shown that unrecognized complete disruption of the anal sphincter is much more common than this. Overall, long-term incontinence affects 5 per cent of women.

Technique

As the anal sphincter (like the levator ani muscle) is normally in a state of tonic contraction, even at rest, disruption will result in retraction of the muscle ends. In order to bring the muscle ends together, adequate muscle relaxation with regional or general anaesthesia is essential. Some surgeons juxtapose the ends of the sphincter (end-to-end), whereas others overlap them. Current evidence suggests that the short-term outcome is similar with both techniques. Antibiotics and laxative agents are prescribed to prevent secondary infection and constipation.

Complications

Up to half the women who sustain a third/fourth-degree tear develop bowel symptoms (including incontinence) despite a postpartum primary anal sphincter repair. The most probable explanation for the poor outcome is either the operator's lack of expertise or inappropriate repair technique. It is for this reason that the most experienced person available should be involved.

Assisted delivery

Instrumental vaginal delivery

Definition

Delivery of a baby vaginally using an instrument for assistance.

History and epidemiology

Instrumental vaginal delivery is the hallmark of the specialty of obstetrics and the 'man-midwife'. Prior to the sixteenth century, childbirth was predominantly

---

Key Points

Perineal repair

- An absorbable synthetic suture is preferable.
- If possible, do a subcutaneous stitch.
- If there is extensive tear, regional/general anaesthetic may be needed.

the domain of traditional (female) birth attendants. Barber-surgeons and others with appropriate skills were involved in the management of obstructed labour (usually by destructing the fetus). A variety of single-bladed instruments was also used as levers to deliver the fetal head. With the discovery of forceps (first used, and kept secret, by the Chamberlen family in London), a means to end the suffering of obstructed labour and a tool for delivering babies alive became available. Used exclusively by men, this allowed them to achieve, and maintain, a position of authority until the twentieth century.

Hundreds of different sorts of forceps have been invented and continue to be used around the world. Some forceps in current use were designed in Victorian times and others in the nineteenth century, e.g. 'Simpson' (Fig. 18.3) and 'Neville–Barnes'. Although they have undoubtedly been used to save many lives, they are also associated with many maternal deaths. Particularly dangerous were 'high-forceps' deliveries; sometimes these were attempted by GP obstetricians at home. Where the delivery failed, the woman would be referred to the hospital as an 'FFO' ('failed forceps outside'). To ensure that GPs did not try high deliveries, Wrigley, before the Second World War, introduced a new design with short shanks/arms. Kjelland's forceps (see Fig. 18.3) are another important development from the turn of the twentieth century. These forceps did not have a 'pelvic curve' and could be turned around in the vagina to rotate an occipito-posterior position.

In the 1950s, the vacuum extractor (or ventouse) was invented in Sweden and is now more widely used worldwide than forceps. Current evidence suggests that when assisted vaginal delivery is required, the ventouse should be chosen first, principally because it is significantly less likely to injure the mother.

Worldwide, assisted vaginal delivery remains an integral part of the obstetrician's duties. Although it may occur as infrequently as in 1.5 per cent of deliveries (Czech Republic), in other countries it occurs as often as in 15 per cent (Australia and Canada). Discrepant rates may be related to differing management of labour.

Reduction of instrumental vaginal delivery rates

Various techniques may help in achieving low instrumental delivery rates, e.g. companionship in labour, active management of the second stage with Syntocinon, upright posture in the second stage, and undertaking fetal scalp sampling (rather than a delivery) when fetal heart rate decelerations occur. Letting the epidural wear off or having a more liberal attitude to the length of the second stage when an epidural is being used will also reduce the likelihood of needing an assisted delivery.

Ventouse delivery

Types of ventouse cup

The metal cups most widely used are the 'Bird-modification' ones. These have a central traction chain and a separate vacuum pipe. The anterior cups come in 4, 5 and 6 cm sizes. The posterior cup is designed to be inserted higher up in the vagina than the anterior cups. This is to allow correct placement over the occiput when the head is deflexed. More recently, a number of soft cups have been developed, one example of which is the silicone-rubber cup (Fig. 18.4). The soft cups are smoothly applied to the contour of the baby's head and do not develop a 'chignon'.

It has been shown that successful delivery is most likely with the ventouse when the cup is applied in the midline over the occiput. A well-placed cup will result in a well-flexed head, whilst failure to put the cup far enough back will result in deflexion.

Technique

To minimize the chances of any fetal damage, the prerequisites and basic rules for delivery with the ventouse should be followed.

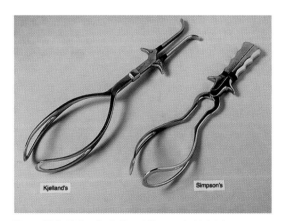

Figure 18.3 Kjelland's (left) and Simpson's (right) forceps.

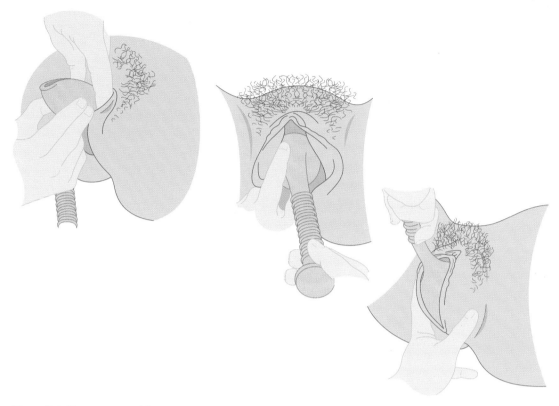

Figure 18.4 Sil-cup ventouse delivery.

Indications and contraindications for delivery with the ventouse

Indications and contraindications for delivery with the ventouse

Indications
- Delay in the second stage
- Fetal distress in the second stage
- Maternal conditions requiring a short second stage

Contraindications
- Face presentation
- Gestation less than 34 weeks
- Marked active bleeding from a fetal blood sampling site

Prerequisites for delivery with the ventouse
- Dilatation of the cervix and full engagement of the head.
- Co-operation of the patient.
- Good contractions should be present.

Basic rules for delivery with the ventouse
- The delivery should be completed within 15 minutes of application.
- The head, not just the scalp, should descend with each pull.
- The cup should be reapplied no more than twice.
- If failure with the correctly placed ventouse occurs despite good traction, the forceps should not be tried as well.

Examination

First, the patient should be carefully examined. The size of the baby should be estimated per abdomen and the head should be fully engaged (none of the head should be palpable above the pubic symphysis). The position of the vertex and the amount of caput should be determined by vaginal examination, and no attempt should be made to deliver the baby vaginally if the presenting part is above the ischial spines. In a 'flexed' attitude, only the posterior fontanelle can be felt, whilst any situation in which the anterior fontanelle can be felt or the posterior fontanelle cannot be found is 'deflexed'.

Preparation

There is no need to catheterize the patient (unless there is another indication, e.g. epidural). No additional anaesthetic is required (perineal infiltration will suffice if an episiotomy is planned). Lithotomy is the commonest position used, but delivery may be possible in dorsal, lateral or squatting positions. The appropriate cup should be chosen. It should be connected to the pump and a check should be made for leakages prior to commencing the delivery.

Delivery with the ventouse

The vacuum extractor cup is gently inserted into the vagina with one hand whilst the other hand parts the labia. The pressure is taken to $0.8\,kg/cm^2$, beginning traction with the next contraction after this pressure has been achieved.

Traction should be along the pelvic axis (downwards at 45°) for the duration of the contraction (Fig. 18.5). One hand should rest on the bell of the cup whilst the other applies traction. Malmstrom, who invented the ventouse, said, 'Vacuum extraction is a matter of co-operation between the traction hand and the backward-pressing hand'. The hand on the cup detects any early detachment and also indicates whether the head moves downwards with each pull. The fingers on the head can promote flexion and can help to guide the head under the arch of the pubis by using the space in front of the sacrum. As the head crowns, the angle of traction changes upward through an arc of over 90°. At this point, either an episiotomy is cut or, if the

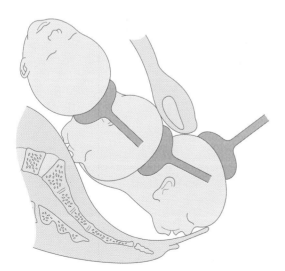

Figure 18.5 Traction down the pelvic axis.

perineum is stretching as normal, it is simply supported with the hand that was on the bell.

The difficult ventouse

Each of the following factors contributes to failures.

- Failure to use the correct cup type. Failures with the silicone-rubber cup group will be common if it is used inappropriately when there is deflexion of the head, excess caput, a big baby or a prolonged second stage of labour.
- Inadequate initial assessment of the case.
  - The head being too high: a classic mistake is to assume that because caput can be felt below the ischial spines, the head must be engaged.
  - Misdiagnosis of the position and attitude of the head: attention to simple detail will minimize the occurrence of this problem.
- Either too anterior or lateral placements will increase the failure rate. If the cup placement is found to be incorrect, it may be appropriate to begin again with correct midline placement over the occiput.
- Failures due to traction in the wrong direction. These may be amenable simply to a change in angle of traction.
- Excessive caput. Rarely, even with the metal cups, adequate traction is not possible because of excessive caput. Careful consideration in these cases must be given to delivery by Caesarean section unless the head is well down, in which case forceps can be used.
- Poor maternal effort. There is no doubt that maternal effort can contribute substantially to the success of the delivery. Adequate encouragement and instruction should be given to the mother.
- The incidence of (true) failure is low and usually secondary to outlet contraction.

Complications

With good technique and adherence to guidelines, the risk of complications to mother or baby is small. Trauma to the genital tract is the commonest maternal complication. Unrecognized injury of the cervix leading to serious haemorrhage has been reported. Most babies will have a chignon (oedematous skin bump) at the site of the cup application. Some will also have a cephalhaematoma (subperiosteal bleed). Rare serious intracranial injuries will be more likely to occur if multiple attempts at delivery are made (especially if a variety of instruments is used).

Ventouse delivery

- Ensure the head is engaged abdominally and the presenting part is not above the ischial spines vaginally.
- Use the correct size and type of ventouse cup.
- If forceps are indicated, ensure the use of a matching pair.
- Unless the head is on the perineum, **do not** use an alternative instrument after failure with ventouse or forceps.
- **Document** carefully; count and document swabs.

Forceps delivery

Technique

- It is essential the head is fully engaged on abdominal palpation. This is particularly true with face presentation (which will appear to be engaged on vaginal examination some time before the head is actually engaged).
- It is generally advised that catheterization and an episiotomy are required for forceps delivery.
- It is essential that the position of the head is carefully noted. If occipito-transverse or occipito-posterior, complications are more likely.
- The operator must check the forceps are a matching pair.
- The left-handed blade is applied first.
- It is held in the operator's left hand (like a pen).

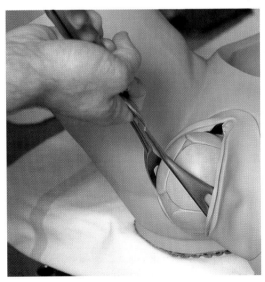

Figure 18.6 Application of forceps (using model).

- Insertion (downwards, then inwards) is guided by the right hand.
- Exactly the same procedure is followed for the other blade.
- The blades must lock easily; they should not be forced to close.
- The first pull is downward and then upward (Fig. 18.6). If the head does not descend, the station may be higher than first thought or the position may be occipito-posterior.

Complications

Traumatic vaginal and uterine injuries can occur with forceps delivery. These can often be the result of undue traction or rotatory forces. As in ventouse delivery, serious injuries to the baby can occur when excessive force is used or when multiple attempts are made.

Indications and contraindications for forceps instead of ventouse

Indications
- Face presentation
- Bleeding from fetal blood sampling site
- After-coming head of the breech
- Delivery before 34 weeks' gestation

Contraindications to a vaginal assisted delivery
- Head not fully engaged
- Cervix not fully dilated

Breech delivery

Definition

When the fetal buttocks occupy the lower part of the uterus it is referred to as breech presentation. The three different types of breech presentation (extended, flexed and footling) are illustrated in Figure 18.7.

History and epidemiology

Three per cent of all term pregnancies present as breech. This may be due to fetal (congenital abnormality), placental (cornual or praevia), amniotic fluid (increased) or uterine (bicornuate or septate) factors.

Breech delivery has an important part in the history of childbirth. Before the discovery of forceps, it was sometimes possible to deliver a baby in obstructed labour by internal podalic version and

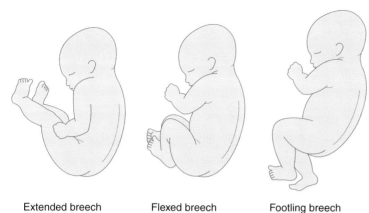

Figure 18.7 Different breech types.

Extended breech   Flexed breech   Footling breech

breech extraction. This technique was also used, prior to the use of Caesarean section, to try to stem the bleeding from a placenta praevia. Internal version and breech extraction are no longer practised except in very specialized situations. Indeed, clinicians skilled in the art of breech delivery are becoming rarer as more women with a term breech pregnancy have an elective Caesarean section. Provided that there are no contraindications, external cephalic version should be offered to all antenatal women who have a breech presentation at term (see Chapter 11).

Caesarean section or vaginal breech?

A large, prospective, multi-centre trial comparing Caesarean section and vaginal delivery for the term breech presentation has revealed that planned Caesarean section is better than planned vaginal birth, with no difference in maternal complications between the groups. However, when a woman presents in advanced labour and delivery is imminent, there would be no choice but to perform a vaginal delivery. There is inadequate evidence to determine the appropriate mode of delivery in the preterm breech.

Prerequisites for vaginal breech delivery

Feto-maternal
- The presentation should be either extended (hips flexed, knees extended) or flexed (hips flexed, knees flexed but feet not below the fetal buttocks).
- There should be no evidence of feto-pelvic disproportion with a pelvis clinically thought to be adequate and an estimated fetal weight of ≤3500 g (ultrasound or clinical measurement).

- There should be no evidence of hyperextension of the fetal head, and fetal abnormalities should have been searched for.

Management of labour
- Fetal well-being and progress of labour should be carefully monitored.
- An epidural analgesia is not essential and may be associated with prolongation of the second stage; it can prevent pushing before full dilatation.
- In selected cases, induction or augmentation may be justified.
- Fetal blood sampling from the buttocks provides an accurate assessment of the acid–base status (when the fetal heart rate trace is suspect).
- There should be an operator experienced in delivering breech babies available in the hospital.
- A symphysiotomy (division of the symphysis pubis) may be necessary should the head be entrapped.

  Although much emphasis is placed on adequate case selection prior to labour, a survey of outcome of the undiagnosed breech in labour managed by experienced medical staff showed that safe vaginal delivery can be achieved.

Technique

Breech delivery epitomizes the position of 'masterly inactivity' (hands-off). Problems are more likely to arise when the obstetrician tries to speed up the process (by pulling on the baby).

Delivery of the buttocks
In most circumstances, full dilatation and descent of the breech will have occurred naturally. When the

buttocks become visible and begin to distend the perineum, preparations for the delivery are made. The buttocks will lie in the anterior–posterior diameter. Once the anterior buttock is delivered and the anus is seen over the fourchette (and no sooner than this), an episiotomy can be cut.

Delivery of the legs and lower body

If the legs are flexed, they will deliver spontaneously. If extended, they may need to be delivered using Pinard's manoeuvre. This entails using a finger to flex the leg at the knee and then extend at the hip, first anteriorly then posteriorly. With contractions and maternal effort, the lower body will be delivered. Usually a loop of cord is drawn down to ensure that it is not too short.

Delivery of the shoulders

The baby will be lying with the shoulders in the transverse diameter of the pelvic mid-cavity. As the anterior shoulder rotates into the anterior–posterior diameter, the spine or the scapula will become visible. At this point, a finger gently placed above the shoulder will help to deliver the arm. As the posterior arm/shoulder reaches the pelvic floor, it too will rotate anteriorly (in the opposite direction). Once the spine becomes visible, delivery of the second arm will follow. This can be imagined as a 'rocking boat' with one side moving upwards and then the other. Loveset's manoeuvre essentially copies these natural movements (Fig. 18.8). However, it is unnecessary and meddlesome to do routinely (one risks pulling the shoulders down but leaving the arms higher up, alongside the head).

Figure 18.8 Loveset's manoeuvre.

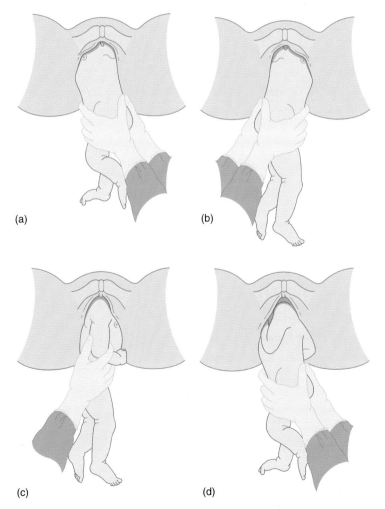

(a)   (b)

(c)   (d)

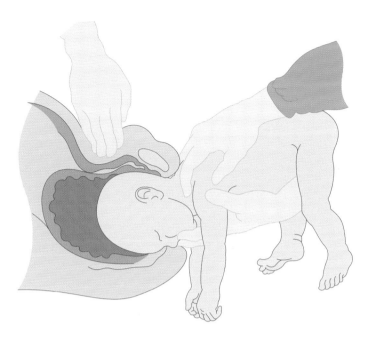

Figure 18.9 Mauriceau–Smellie–Veit manoeuvre for delivery of the head.

Delivery of the head

The head is delivered using the Mauriceau–Smellie–Veit manoeuvre: the baby lies on the obstetrician's arm with downward traction being levelled on the head via a finger in the mouth and one on each maxilla (Fig. 18.9). Delivery occurs with first downward and then upward movement (as with instrumental deliveries). If this manoeuvre proves difficult, forceps need to be applied. An assistant holds the baby's body aloft whilst the forceps are applied in the usual manner (Fig. 18.10).

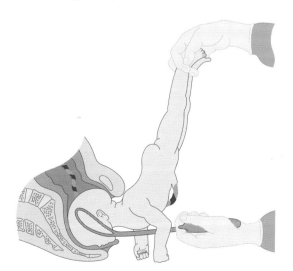

Figure 18.10 Delivery of the aftercoming head with forceps.

Complications

The greatest fear with a vaginal breech is that the baby will get 'stuck'. Interference in the natural process by the inappropriate use of oxytocic agents or by trying to pull the baby out (breech extraction) will (paradoxically) increase the risk of obstruction occurring. When delay occurs, particularly with delivery of the shoulders or head, the presence of an experienced obstetrician will reduce the risk of death or serious injury.

Caesarean section

Definition

Caesarean section refers to an operation that is performed to deliver a baby via the transabdominal route.

History and epidemiology

Caesarean section to deliver the baby of a mother who has died has been documented in ancient Egypt, Asia and Europe. The first Caesarean carried out on a live woman is thought to be that of the wife of Jacob Nufer, a sixteenth-century Swiss pig farmer. She was in obstructed labour and her life was saved by the procedure. The history of the operation thereafter is fascinating, with a wide range of isolated cases being documented and various techniques being investigated to try to lower the enormous risks of death due to haemorrhage and sepsis. By the early twentieth century, the 'classical' (midline vertical uterine incision) operation had become quite widespread for obstructed labour and placenta praevia. When Munro-Kerr introduced the concept of a 'lower segment operation' in the 1920s, the profession was derisive. Nevertheless, he persisted with the new procedure, which has now become the standard intervention for complicated labour worldwide.

Preparation for Caesarean section

All patients being transferred to theatre must be in the left lateral position with a wedge under the right buttock (to prevent 'supine hypotension' and fetal distress). Premedication with antacid is standard. In theatre, the operating table must also be kept in the left lateral tilt position until after the delivery. Thromboprophylaxis should be considered for all patients and prophylactic antibiotics should be given.

Operative procedure

Double-gloving reduces the likelihood of needle puncture and use of a clear plastic shield reduces exposure of the face. A transverse suprapubic skin incision should be used. The bladder should be reflected inferiorly before incising the uterus. It is possible to injure the baby as the uterine wall is opened; therefore considerable care needs to be taken. Delivery of the placenta should be by continuous cord traction. The uterus should be left inside the abdomen for repair. Securing both angles of the uterine incision first will reduce the risk of 'missing an angle' and having post-surgical bleeding. Re-peritonealizing may cause more harm than good and is not required.

Post-mortem Caesarean section

If a pregnant woman has a cardiac arrest and the fetus is viable, post-mortem Caesarean section should be carried out without delay. For speed, this would be best done via midline skin and uterine ('classical') incisions. Not only can a baby's life be saved, but also resuscitation of the mother is facilitated (less pressure on the diaphragm and improved venous return).

Complications

Overall, the risks of both early and long-term complications are increased in women delivered by Caesarean section, when compared with the outcomes after normal vaginal delivery. The risks are surgical and anaesthetic. The main problems are thromboembolism, infection and haemorrhage, which can be minimized by appropriate prophylaxis and surgical skill. Women are increasingly demanding Caesarean section to minimize the risk of pelvic floor trauma and its sequelae. Although they have a right to choose their mode of delivery, they need to be counselled regarding the increased mortality and morbidity associated with Caesarean section.

Indications for Caesarean section

- Obstructed labour, malpresentation, malposition, multiple gestation
- Fetal distress/prolapsed cord
- Maternal medical conditions requiring urgent/controlled delivery
- Obstetric complications, e.g. placenta praevia
- Previous Caesarean section

The 'classical' operation is still undertaken occasionally (less than 1 per cent of cases), for specific indications (shown below).

Classical Caesarean section: possible indications

- Preterm delivery with poorly formed lower segment
- Placenta praevia/abruptio with large vessels in lower segment
- Premature rupture of membranes, poor lower segment and transverse lie
- Transverse lie with back inferior
- Large cervical fibroid
- Severe adhesions in lower segment reducing accessibility
- Post-mortem Caesarean section

Twin delivery

Twin pregnancies account for approximately 1.5 per cent of all pregnancies in the UK population but, with increasing numbers of babies resulting from artificial conception, the incidence of twins and greater multiple gestation is increasing (see Chapter 12). Overall, perinatal mortality is increased and the risks are greater for monozygotic than dizygotic twins. Complications in labour are more common with multiple gestations. These include premature birth, abnormal presentations, prolapsed cord, premature separation of the placenta and postpartum haemorrhage. Judiciously managed, labour is generally considered to be safe. It may require considerable expertise and is the only situation in which internal podalic version is still practised in obstetrics.

Analgesia during labour

Epidural analgesia is recommended. Indeed, if the presentation of twins is anything other than vertex–vertex, the use of an epidural can be justified in terms of analgesia for possible intrauterine manipulations required in the second stage for delivery of the second twin. Contrary to recommendations for the management of a singleton labour, the epidural should be kept running throughout the second stage, as it is most likely to be required after the delivery of twin 1. Having an anaesthetist present and ready to administer anaesthesia if complications arise is a satisfactory alternative. However, many obstetric units now opt to deliver twins in the operating theatre.

Fetal well-being in labour

Fetal heart rate monitoring should be continuous throughout labour, ideally using a specialized twin monitor. An abnormal fetal heart rate pattern in twin 1 may be assessed using fetal scalp sampling, as for a singleton pregnancy. However, a non-reassuring pattern in twin 2 will usually necessitate delivery by Caesarean section. The condition of twin 2 must be carefully monitored after the delivery of twin 1, as acute complications such as cord prolapse and placental separation are well recognized.

Vaginal delivery of vertex–vertex

Although this combination is considered low risk and will most frequently be delivered by a midwife, an obstetrician should be present, as complications with delivery of the second twin can occur. Delivery of the first twin is undertaken in the usual manner and thereafter the majority of second twins will be delivered within 15 minutes. However, there is no urgency to deliver the second twin within a set time period, providing both mother and baby remain well.

After the delivery of the first twin, abdominal palpation should be performed to assess the lie of the second twin. It is helpful to use ultrasound for confirmation, which is also useful for checking the fetal heart rate. If the lie is longitudinal with a cephalic presentation, one should wait until the head is descending and then perform amniotomy with a contraction. If contractions do not ensue within 5–10 minutes after delivery of the first twin, an oxytocin infusion should be started. If an assisted delivery becomes necessary, the vacuum extractor has a number of advantages.

Delivery of vertex–non-vertex

If the second twin is non-vertex, which occurs in about 40 per cent of twins, numerous studies have shown that vaginal delivery can be safely considered.

If the second twin is a breech, the membranes can be ruptured once the breech is fixed in the birth canal. A total breech extraction may be performed if fetal distress occurs or if a footling breech is encountered, but this requires considerable expertise. Complications are less likely if the membranes are not ruptured until the feet are held by the operator. Where the fetus is transverse, external cephalic version can be successful in more than 70 per cent of cases. The fetal heart rate should be closely monitored, and ultrasound can be helpful to demonstrate the final position of the baby. If external cephalic version is unsuccessful, given that the operator is experienced, an internal podalic version can be undertaken.

Internal podalic version (Fig. 18.11)
A fetal foot is identified by recognizing a heel through intact membranes. The foot is grasped and pulled gently and continuously into the birth canal. The membranes are ruptured as late as possible. This procedure is easiest when the transverse lie is with the back

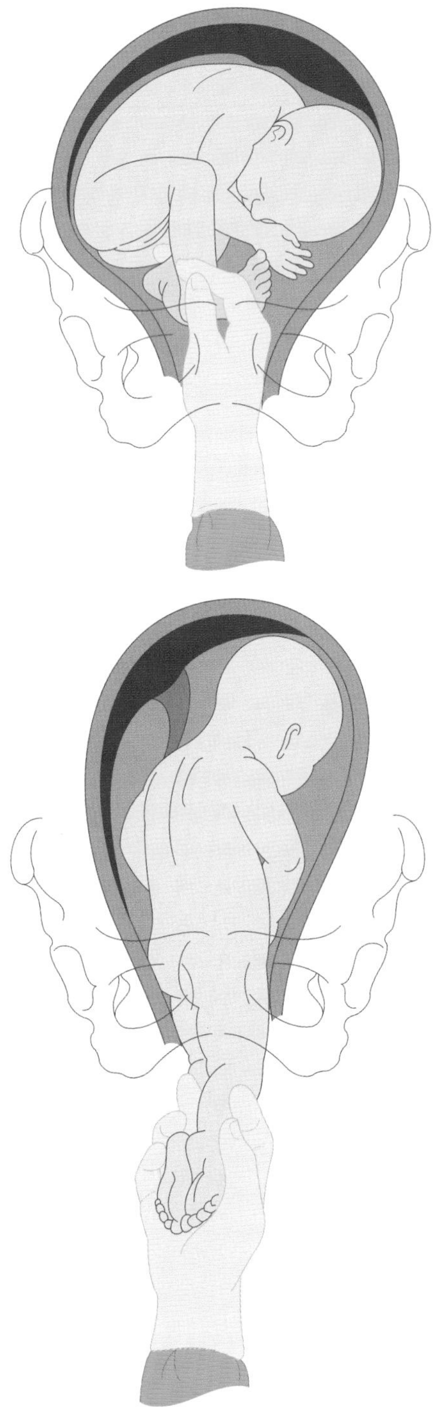

Figure 18.11 Internal podalic version.

superior or posterior. If the back is inferior or if the limbs are not immediately palpable, ultrasound may help to show the operator where they would be found. This will minimize the unwanted experience

of bringing down a fetal hand in the mistaken belief that it is a foot.

Non-vertex first twin

When twin 1 presents as a breech, clinicians usually recommend delivery by elective Caesarean section. This is largely because of the increased risks associated with singleton breech vaginal delivery. Other factors include dwindling experience of breech delivery and the rarely seen phenomenon of 'locked twins'. In this latter case, the chin of the first (breech) baby locks against the chin of the second (cephalic) twin.

Preterm twins

Even in low-birth-weight twin gestations, the method of delivery in relation to fetal presentation will have little or no effect on neonatal mortality and subsequent neonatal developmental outcome. No significant differences in perinatal outcome exist when comparing breech-extracted second twins to those delivered by Caesarean section.

Requirements for twin delivery

- Large delivery room
- Operating theatre and staff ready
- Anaesthetist present
- Senior obstetrician present
- At least two midwives present
- Twin resuscitaires
- Ventouse/forceps to hand
- Blood grouped and saved
- Intravenous access
- Neonatologists present
- Pre-mixed oxytocin infusion ready

Placental complications

Retained placenta

Incidence
Retained placenta is found in 2 per cent of deliveries. The frequency of retained placenta is markedly

increased (twenty-fold) at gestations <26 weeks, and even up to 37 weeks it remains three times more common than at term. At term, 90 per cent of placentas will be delivered within 15 minutes. Once the third stage exceeds 30 minutes, there is a ten-fold increase in the risk of haemorrhage.

Management

When the placenta is delivered, it should be inspected for completeness because if there is a suggestion of retained segments, manual exploration of the uterine cavity is required. This will need to be undertaken under anaesthesia.

If the placenta is retained as a whole, it is often worth checking prior to induction of anaesthesia that it has not detached spontaneously. Not infrequently, a placenta is found in the cervical canal or vagina at this time. If it is still within the uterus, the operator (wearing a 'gauntlet' glove) should use the fingers of one hand, held as a 'spatula', to lift the placenta, whilst the hand on the abdomen balances these movements with downward pressure on the uterus. If there are retained fragments, further manual exploration (with a gauze swab around the exploring fingers) of the uterine cavity will need to be undertaken. If retained fragments cannot be removed in this manner, curettage with a blunt instrument may be required. Small remaining fragments of placenta can be left if there is no haemorrhage, provided there is adequate antibiotic cover and follow-up. Antibiotics should be routinely administered, as there is a significant association between manual removal of the placenta and postpartum endometritis.

Placenta accreta

Definition

Placenta accreta is a retained placenta that is morbidly adherent to the uterine wall.

Epidemiology

Placenta accreta is a serious cause of haemorrhage. It is becoming more common, and over the last 40 years, the incidence has increased ten-fold. This phenomenon is due to the fact that lower segment Caesarean section appears to increase the risk of subsequent placenta praevia, and there is a well-documented association between placenta praevia and previous Caesarean section and placenta accreta. In recent reviews, up to a quarter of women undergoing Caesarean section for placenta praevia, in the presence of one or more scars, subsequently underwent Caesarean hysterectomy for placenta accreta.

Management

If placenta accreta with haemorrhage is encountered, and if the woman has no intention to bear further children, hysterectomy is the procedure of choice. However, if hysterectomy is considered a last resort, then other measures may be successful in up to 50 per cent of women. These procedures range from simple excision of the site of trophoblast invasion with oversewing of the area to uterine or internal iliac artery ligation.

🔑 Key Points

Retained placenta

- Anticipate haemorrhage, insert an intravenous infusion line, take blood for full blood count, group, save and catheterize.
- Check that the placenta is not in the cervical canal or vagina prior to giving anaesthetic.
- Give prophylactic antibiotics.
- Carry out manual removal – call senior help if there is accreta and/or heavy bleeding.

Haematomas

Vulval and paravaginal haematomas

Definition

Haematomas are divided into those that lie above and those that lie below the levator muscle (Fig. 18.12). Infralevator haematomas include those of the vulva and perineum, as well as paravaginal haematomas and those occurring in the ischiorectal fossa. Supralevator haematomas spread upwards and outwards beneath the broad ligament or partly downwards to bulge into the walls of the upper vagina. These haematomas can also track backwards into the retroperitoneal space.

Incidence and associations

Criteria used to define a haematoma vary widely and, because of this, a range of frequencies has been reported. An acceptable definition would be any haematoma >4 cm in diameter. The incidence of these is approximately 1:1000 deliveries.

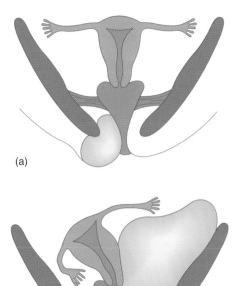

(a)

(b)

Figure 18.12 (a) Vulval and (b) paravaginal haematomas.

The injury is frequently related to episiotomy, but in some series nearly 20 per cent of patients developed a significant haematoma despite delivery with an intact perineum. Overall, half of the women who develop a genital haematoma do so following a spontaneous delivery.

Diagnosis
Although a vulval haematoma is usually obvious, a paravaginal haematoma may be missed, with no symptoms until shock develops. In general, the symptoms depend upon the size and rate of haematoma formation. Some genital haematomas may be up to 15 cm in diameter.

Management
The management of an infralevator haematoma usually necessitates, in addition to resuscitative measures, surgical evacuation of the haematoma. However, this depends on the size. If the haematoma is <5 cm in diameter and not expanding, most obstetricians would simply recommend observation using ice-packs and pressure dressings to limit haematoma expansion. Appropriate analgesia should be given and markings should be made on the skin to establish whether the peripheral margins of the mass are expanding. For haematomas >5 cm in diameter or

those that are rapidly expanding, surgical intervention is recommended.

Technique
Where possible, the incision should be made via the vagina to minimize scar formation. If distinct bleeding sites are seen, these can be clamped, but, more commonly, there is no distinct bleeding. If a figure-of-eight suture does not achieve haemostasis, either a drain or a pack can be used.

🔑 Key Points

Management of haematomas
- A trap for the unwary – beware occult haemorrhage in a 'collapsed' postpartum patient.
- Large vulval haematomas benefit from drainage:
  - leave the wound open,
  - leave a drain.
- Broad ligament haematomas are usually managed conservatively.

Subperitoneal haematomas

Incidence and associations
Subperitoneal haematomas (broad ligament) are much less common than genital haematomas: 1 in 20 000 deliveries. They follow spontaneous vaginal delivery, Caesarean section or forceps operations. Approximately 50 per cent of subperitoneal haematomas are discovered virtually immediately, whereas the other half only present after 24 hours. Patients presenting immediately tend to show signs of lower abdominal pain and haemorrhage.

Management
A conservative approach is recommended, with 'expectant' management. If it is not possible to maintain a stable haemodynamic state, prompt surgical exploration is recommended and a hysterectomy may be indicated.

Injuries to the cervix

After a vaginal delivery, the majority of women will have lacerations and/or bruising of the cervix. Minor cervical lacerations are therefore extremely common. Usually these remain undetected. However, bleeding which does not appear to be arising from the vagina or perineum and which continues despite a well-contracted uterus is an indication for examining the cervix. Deep lacerations, and particularly those that involve the vaginal vault, need to be managed in theatre under anaesthesia. A laceration into the vault could extend forward to the bladder or laterally towards the uterine artery at the base of the broad ligament.

Management

Prompt recognition of the injury and action to control the bleeding are essential.

Repair

For repairing a cervical tear, good visibility using right-angle retractors is essential. Using two pairs of ring forceps applied to the cervix at any one time, it is possible to inspect the whole circumference accurately. Identification of the apex of the tear is essential before commencing repair.

🔑 Key Points

Injuries to the cervix
- The cervix often looks damaged but is very rarely associated with bleeding.
- Ventouse prior to full dilatation has been implicated in injury to the cervix.

Caesarean hysterectomy

Incidence

Emergency indications for Caesarean hysterectomy are less common than in the past, as there are now alternative treatments available (0.01–0.05 per cent).

Indications

The relative risk of emergency hysterectomy is increased with Caesarean delivery, previous Caesarean birth, placenta praevia, placenta accreta and uterine atony.

The majority of hysterectomies are done for haemorrhage when conservative medical and surgical measures have been unsuccessful. Increasingly, placental problems account for a larger proportion of cases.

🔑 Key Points

Emergency hysterectomy
- Anticipate problems that may lead to hysterectomy, e.g. accreta in placenta praevia and previous Caesarean section.
- Try medical (and possibly surgical) alternatives.
- If in doubt, obtain the patient's consent for the possibility of hysterectomy, prior to inducing anaesthesia.

Rarely performed but important operative interventions

Symphysiotomy

Symphysiotomy is considered of some value for the management of cephalo-pelvic disproportion in selected situations in developing countries and it has also been recommended as the treatment of choice for a trapped after-coming head of a breech.

It has a very low maternal mortality, with no procedure-related deaths in a series of nearly 2000 women. In contrast, Caesarean section in rural developing-world hospitals may be associated with a mortality of up to 5 per cent and a reported incidence of uterine scar rupture in subsequent pregnancies of up to 6.8 per cent. However, after a symphysiotomy, subsequent symptoms such as pain in the symphysis pubis and groin are common. A major advantage is that the majority of women (73 per cent) will have an uncomplicated vaginal delivery in a subsequent pregnancy.

Indication
Symphysiotomy can be considered in cases of cephalopelvic disproportion with a vertex presentation and a living fetus. At least one-third of the fetal head should have entered the pelvic brim. It may also be indicated for the trapped after-coming head of a breech and has been described as an intervention in a 'desperate case' scenario of shoulder dystocia.

Destructive operations

Destructive operations may be required where the fetus is dead and where a vaginal delivery is either the only delivery that can be managed in that particular situation or is the only route by which the mother wishes to be delivered. The three commonest destructive procedures are craniotomy, perforation of the after-coming head and decapitation.

Craniotomy

Craniotomy is indicated for the delivery of a dead fetus when labour is neglected and obstructed in a cephalic presentation.

After-coming head of the breech

This can be managed similarly, by craniotomy with perforation of the head through the occiput. Where there is hydrocephalus and accompanying spina bifida, either cerebrospinal fluid can be withdrawn, by exposing the spinal canal and passing a catheter into the canal and up into the cranium, or the hydro-cephalic head can be decompressed transabdominally using a spinal needle.

Decapitation

In cases of neglected obstructed labour with shoulder presentation and a dead fetus, decapitation might be the treatment of choice.

CASE HISTORY

Miss S is 1.80 m tall and weighed 76 kg at booking for her second pregnancy. Her first pregnancy ended in spontaneous labour at 39 weeks' gestation. Abdominal examination indicates an average-sized baby, estimated to weigh around 3.6 kg, and vaginal examination a vertex presentation. Labour is slow, with full dilatation of the cervix being reached after 10 hours. There is a normal reactive CTG baseline of 135/min and clear liquor draining. After 1.5 hours of active pushing, the station of the head is +1 cm below the ischial spines (0/5 palpable on abdominal examination) and there is caput and moulding. The position of the head is occipito-anterior.

Should Miss S have an assisted delivery?

After a long labour and prolonged maternal efforts at pushing in the second stage of labour, an assisted delivery is quite appropriate. It should be possible to deliver the baby vaginally, as there is no evidence of fetal compromise and the vertex is at station +1 below the ischial spines.

What features suggest that an assisted delivery might be difficult?

Caput and moulding suggest that the baby's head is being squeezed tightly through the pelvis; this might mean an assisted delivery would be trickier than first thought, and the operator must be sure of the exact position of the head prior to attempting delivery.

Which instrument should be chosen?

Either ventouse or forceps would be reasonable. Many obstetricians would use ventouse in the first instance to reduce maternal soft-tissue trauma. Equally, it could be argued that the presence of caput would make ventouse more likely to fail, and a non-rotational forceps (such as Neville–Barnes) could be used.

Should the delivery be performed in the obstetric theatre?

If there is any concern that the delivery might not succeed easily, or there is fetal distress, Miss S should be moved to the operating theatre for a 'trial of ventouse/forceps'. Should the delivery not be completed simply and rapidly, a Caesarean section might be required. In this situation, a Caesarean section would be most unlikely unless the fetus were to become compromised and attempted vaginal delivery was more difficult than at first thought. One important question depends on the skill of the obstetrician. Is the true position of the vertex (taking into account the boggy caput) at +1 cm and is the fetal head really occipito-anterior? If this was in fact occipito-posterior, and the baby's head was at the spines (0 cm), many operators might perform a Caesarean section.

What risks are there for Miss S after delivery?

Postpartum haemorrhage is always more common after an assisted delivery due to the risk of uterine atony and vaginal or cervical lacerations. In this situation, these risks are compounded by a long labour. The appropriate steps should be taken to anticipate and deal with this: intravenous access, blood sent for haemoglobin estimation and grouping and saving, oxytocin/ergometrine at delivery and an intravenous oxytocin infusion for 4 hours after delivery.

Additional reading

Myerscough PR. *Munro-Kerr's operative obstetrics*, 10th edn. London: Baillière Tindall, 1982.

Pregnancy and childbirth reviews. In: The Cochrane database of systematic reviews. *The Cochrane library*. Oxford: Update Software (four issues each year).

Obstetric emergencies

OVERVIEW

Obstetric emergencies cause damage and death to mothers and babies. They require quick, decisive and effective action from the staff immediately available. In the UK, the maternal mortality rate is around 11.4 per 100 000 (*Why women die*, 2001 – see Chapter 3), apparently representing relatively few deaths due directly to pregnancy complications, a tribute to the management of obstetric emergencies. However, in many cases, care could and should have been better, resulting in fewer deaths. Worldwide the situation is much worse, with around 600 000 maternal deaths reported each year, mainly due to haemorrhage, sepsis, eclampsia and obstructed labour.

In the UK, the main causes of maternal death directly attributable to pregnancy are embolism (thrombotic and amniotic fluid), hypertensive disorders, haemorrhage and sepsis. As the obstetric population ages, coincidental medical conditions make a progressively larger contribution to mortality and morbidity. All of these conditions may present to obstetric staff as an emergency.

Definition

An emergency is an occurrence of a serious and dangerous nature, developing suddenly and unexpectedly, demanding immediate attention. Although the actual emergency itself will occur unexpectedly, in some cases pre-existing risk factors will be present.

Obstetric emergencies related directly to pregnancy include, for instance, pre-eclampsia and eclampsia, antepartum and postpartum haemorrhage and amniotic fluid embolism. Other emergencies may be coincidental, or associated with or made worse by pregnancy, for instance caused by congenital heart disease or epilepsy.

Emergencies may primarily affect the mother in the first instance, but if they occur antenatally or intrapartum, there will always be two patients (mother and fetus) to consider. Postpartum complications will affect only the mother in the short term, but potentially the baby as well in social and psychological terms. Finally, complications may be primarily fetal, such as severe fetal distress in utero or shoulder dystocia as a complication of delivery.

Management

The ideal management of a potential emergency situation is in its avoidance. Although most cases cannot

Table 19.1 – Principles of managing obstetric emergencies

Avoidance	Assessment	Action
Address and manage risks	Need for ABC	Resuscitate as necessary
Adopt good obstetric practice	Obvious causes	Intravenous access (2×14 gauge)
		Oxygen
		Remove obvious causes
		Seek and manage other causes

be anticipated, adequate thromboprophylaxis in high-risk cases, effective management of worsening hypertensive disorders and proper management of medical disorders in pregnancy will all reduce the occurrence of emergencies. Similarly, so will good obstetric practice, for instance avoiding prolonged labour and having staff of appropriate experience available for known potential problems, such as Caesarean section for placenta praevia.

When an emergency does occur, management must always begin with an assessment of the maternal and then, when appropriate, fetal condition. As ever, airway, breathing and circulation (ABC) must be managed. Prior to introduction of an artificial airway, tilting the head and lifting the jaw will be effective. If the mother is breathing spontaneously, she must be moved to the left lateral position; aspiration of stomach contents is a more common problem in pregnancy. If there is no spontaneous respiration, give two breaths and then check the circulation at the carotid or femoral pulse prior to chest compression if necessary. A rate of 100 compressions per minute with a ratio of 15:2 with artificial respiration is required if managing a case alone. Obtain as much help as is possible immediately. In most delivery suites, an obstetric anaesthetist will be available, and in hospitals summon the cardiac arrest team immediately.

In the majority of obstetric emergencies, respiratory or cardiac arrest has not yet occurred when management begins. Assess the situation quickly, including the need for ABC (Table 19.1). Large-calibre intravenous access is almost always required, as may be oxygen. Take blood for haematological and biochemical analysis and for cross-matching. Is there an obvious cause (for instance revealed blood loss as in postpartum haemorrhage due to an atonic uterus) that can be quickly halted? Then move on to consider the likely cause and remedy.

Obstetric haemorrhage

Definition

Any blood loss from the vagina greater than a show during pregnancy or excessive blood loss after delivery.

Understanding the pathophysiology

The haemochorial nature of the human placenta places the pregnant women at particular risk of haemorrhage (Fig. 19.1). The placenta cotyledons are directly bathed in maternal blood. Any disruption of this interface may lead to blood loss. Initially this is retroplacental or periplacental. It will often be concealed and may extend. Extension to the edge of the placenta leads to revealed blood loss. Resolution of the haemorrhage depends upon haemostasis in the placental bed, achieved by myometrial contraction. Coagulation factors are secondary to this process. Final resolution can only be achieved if the uterus is empty; antepartum, this means delivery of the baby. Effective management of major haemorrhage requires aggressive supportive measures at the same time as measures to resolve the bleeding (Table 19.2).

Obstetric blood loss is almost always maternal. The fetus may be affected by maternal hypoxia or hypotension or by the secondary effects of placental separation reducing the available interface for oxygen delivery. An unusual exception is vasa praevia, where blood vessels on the fetal surface of the placenta are

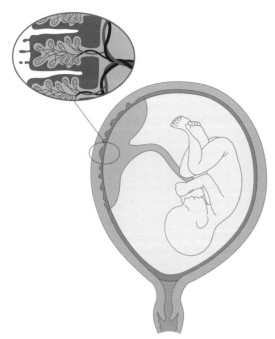

Figure 19.1 Haemochorial placentation.

Table 19.2 – Severe haemorrhage

- Summon help:
  - senior obstetrician
  - anaesthetist
- Notify blood bank and consult haematologist
- Cross-match at least 6 units of blood
- Full blood count and clotting studies
- Test for renal function and liver function tests
- Oxygen by mask initially
- 2 × 14-gauge intravenous lines
- Foley catheter into the bladder and fluid balance chart
- Plasma expander
- Transfuse blood as soon as possible – uncross-matched same group as mother or, in extreme cases, O negative
- Central venous pressure and arterial lines
- May need fresh frozen plasma, platelets and cryoprecipitate (consult haematologist)
- Eliminate the cause – deliver the baby and placenta, manage postpartum haemorrhage

---

ruptured. Losing even small quantities of fetal blood may be catastrophic.

Antepartum haemorrhage

Epidemiology and aetiology

Antepartum haemorrhage (APH) complicates 2–5 per cent of pregnancies. Most cases involve relatively small quantities of blood loss, but may still have sequelae relating to poor placental function, intrauterine growth restriction and premature delivery (see also Chapter 11). Some cases are life threatening: six maternal deaths were recorded in the last UK triennial report and there will have been many more near-misses.

There are two major causes of APH threatening the life of the mother and fetus, placental abruption and placenta praevia. Both involve placental separation. The placenta praevia becomes detached because the cervix is taken up or dilated in late pregnancy. Abruption is separation of a normally sited placenta. In UK practice, in the majority of cases, the placental site will have been established by routine ultrasound scan before major bleeding occurs. If this is not the case, there are clinical differences between placenta praevia and abruption that will aid diagnosis (Table 19.3). Do not perform a digital vaginal examination until the diagnosis is established, either by ultrasound scan or by overwhelming clinical evidence.

Whatever the cause, the standard assessment of need for resuscitation and basic management strategies has to be gone through. Thereafter, management will depend upon the maternal state, the fetal state, the cause of the condition and the gestation of the pregnancy.

Placenta praevia

A placenta that is praevia occupies part of the lower uterine segment. Major degrees of placenta praevia cover, at least in part, the internal os of the cervix. The incidence in the UK is 5:1000 and is increasing. Patients with placenta praevia present with recurrent APH in late pregnancy. It is inevitable that bleeding will occur as the cervix takes up and dilates. In major degrees of placenta praevia, safe vaginal delivery is impossible. The risk to the fetus is mainly prematurity due to early Caesarean section. However, if a case is neglected, there is also a risk of hypoxia due to placental separation as the cervix dilates, but this would usually be accompanied by torrential maternal haemorrhage.

Table 19.3 – Comparison of haemorrhage from placental praevia with that from placental abruption

Placenta praevia	Placental abruption
Painless	Painful
Patient is less distressed	Patient is distressed
Soft abdomen	Tender, tense abdomen
Abnormal lie and presentation	Normal lie and presentation
CTG usually normal	Abnormal CTG likely
No particular association with pre-eclampsia	May be associated with pre-eclampsia
No coagulation defect initially	Coagulation defect may occur early

CTG, cardiotocography.

The risk to the mother is haemorrhage, either as APH or during Caesarean section when the placental bed may not contract or there may be morbid adherence, especially in the case of an anterior placenta praevia over an old Caesarean section scar. This may lead to massive postpartum haemorrhage (PPH).

Delivery is by Caesarean section, performed by a senior, preferably consultant, obstetrician. The risk of excess bleeding is particularly great when the placenta is situated anteriorly. The indications for delivery are reaching 37–38 weeks' gestation, a massive (>1500 mL) bleed, or continuing significant bleeding of lesser severity.

Placental abruption

A placental abruption is separation of a normally situated placenta from the uterine wall. In more than two-thirds of cases, the separation reaches the edge of the placenta, tracks down to the cervix and is revealed as vaginal bleeding. The remaining cases are concealed, and present as uterine pain and potentially maternal shock or fetal distress without obvious bleeding. The fetus is at risk because of hypoxia following placental separation and premature delivery. The mother is at risk of hypovolaemic shock, clotting disorders and consequent more widespread organ damage. The aetiology and pathophysiological consequences of placental abruption are discussed in further detail in Chapter 13.

Management depends upon recognition of the problem, realization that true blood loss may be far greater than the blood loss seen, and rapid institution of major haemorrhage management (see Table 19.2). In very severe cases, the fetus will be dead and vaginal delivery can be accelerated by artificial rupture of the membranes once the mother is reasonably stable. Occasionally, oxytocics will be required as well. If the fetus is alive, delivery without compromising the mother's resuscitation is urgent and this will usually be by Caesarean section.

Vasa praevia

Vasa praevia, rupture of vessels on the fetal side of the placenta, is a much rarer condition than abruption or placenta praevia. It is fetal blood that is lost. Risk factors include placenta praevia and multiple pregnancy. The vessels are usually in a velamentous insertion of the cord, i.e. there is an aberrant feto-placental vessel running in the membrane. In these cases the fetal vessels cross the cervix and they may rupture at spontaneous rupture of membranes or be damaged at artificial rupture of membranes. Relatively slight bleeding is seen, but can cause acute fetal exsanguination and death; major fetal heart rate changes soon become apparent. Fetal tachycardia develops, followed by deep decelerations. Although tests for fetal haemoglobin are possible, the best solution is a high index of suspicion and rapid Caesarean section. The fetus may be dead by the time tests are completed.

Postpartum haemorrhage

Definition

Excess blood loss after delivery is defined as primary PPH in the first 24 hours and secondary PPH up to

6 weeks. Traditionally, excess loss is described as >500 mL, but this is seen after more than 10 per cent of pregnancies and is probably unrealistic as a useful definition. Modern obstetric practice using Syntocinon alone to control uterine contraction, together with the higher numbers of Caesarean sections being performed, mean that many young, fit women may be classified as having PPH without being in danger.

A loss of >1 L occurs in 1 per cent of cases. As well as the volume of blood loss, it is the speed with which it may be lost that is so problematic. Massive PPH may be truly terrifying and its management requires experience and a calm sense of purpose that is best obtained by a thorough knowledge of protocols and participation in obstetric haemorrhage practice drills.

Aetiology and management

The most important cause of massive PPH is uterine atony when the uterus is not contracted. This accounts for 90 per cent of cases. In these cases, the first step to take is to stop the bleeding, by massaging the uterus to cause it to contract, or by bimanual compression. This allows time for other standard measures for dealing with massive haemorrhage to be instituted. Uterine contraction is maintained by ergometrine and high-dose intravenous Syntocinon. The bladder should be emptied. Prostaglandin F2-alpha (Haemabate) may be injected systemically or directly into the myometrium through the anterior abdominal wall.

It may be necessary to maintain bimanual compression until clotting disorders have been corrected, as fibrin degradation products, which are increased in disseminated intravascular coagulation, may themselves act to relax the uterus.

When bleeding persists despite uterine contraction, look for genital tract trauma and repair it. If the patient's haemodynamic status is not improving, or is deteriorating despite apparent control of revealed bleeding, consider hidden bleeding such as broad ligament or paravaginal bleeding or even uterine rupture.

If conservative measures are not succeeding, move to surgical solutions sooner rather than later. Is the uterus empty? Can tamponade be effected by the use of intrauterine balloons such as the Rusch urological catheter? Rarely, bilateral internal iliac artery ligation or hysterectomy may be necessary.

Secondary PPH is a rare cause of massive bleeding. It is usually the result of retained products of conception and/or uterine infection. Although bleeding can be life threatening, it is usually slight or moderate.

Key Points

Massive haemorrhage
- Summon senior multidisciplinary help.
- Resuscitate.
- Replace and maintain fluid volume.
- Investigate status and cause of bleeding.
- Arrest blood loss.

Uterine rupture

Rupture, or tearing, of the uterus occurs most commonly in association with a previous scar on the uterus, typically previous Caesarean section. It may occur in the absence of a scar or in the absence of knowledge of a scar, for instance after unrecognized perforation of the uterus in a previous termination of pregnancy. Almost all cases occur in labour.

The patient complains of continuous abdominal pain and there is usually some vaginal blood loss, which may be slight. Contractions cease. The fetal heart rate pattern becomes abnormal and without immediate laparotomy and delivery, the fetus will usually die.

If rupture occurs in the second stage of labour, it is frequently not recognized. The fetus is usually delivered by ventouse or forceps for 'fetal distress'. The mother will bleed internally and start to show signs of circulatory collapse whilst complaining of abdominal discomfort.

Immediate laparotomy is necessary when uterine rupture is suspected. Sometimes it is possible to repair the uterus, but frequently the only safe way forward is hysterectomy.

Uterine inversion

Uterine inversion (Fig. 19.2) – descent of the uterine fundus into the cavity, through the cervix or even through the vulva – is a very rare event. The inverted uterus may be seen at the vulva, felt in the vagina or, in lesser cases, identified as a dimpling of the uterine fundus on abdominal examination.

The patient may be shocked out of all proportion to visible blood loss. Do not remove the placenta if it is still attached; this will increase the bleeding. Immediately replace the uterus through the cervix by

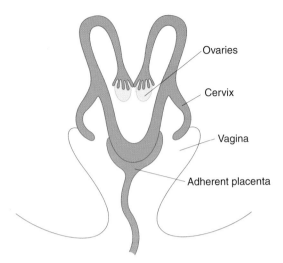

Figure 19.2 Inverted uterus.

manual compression. Do not push with the finger alone, but as much of the hand as possible. If that fails, hydrostatic pressure works well. After replacement, uterine contraction is maintained with an oxytoxic.

Pulmonary embolism

Pulmonary embolism (PE) occurs in association with approximately 3:1000 pregnancies. Two-thirds of cases occur in the puerperium. In the UK, it is the commonest cause of maternal death directly associated with pregnancy. In the 1997–1999 triennial report, 35 deaths were associated with or caused by PE. This is a reduction from previous years, probably related to the publication of thromboprophylaxis guidelines by the Royal College of Obstetricians and Gynaecologists (RCOG).

Diagnosis on clinical grounds alone is not reliable (Table 19.4), but such is the risk of the condition that treatment must be instituted directly; ventilation/ perfusion scans can be performed later.

The diagnosis and management of thromboembolic events is discussed in detail in Chapter 11; rarely, a massive PE may present with sudden cardiorespiratory collapse. Urgent resuscitation (ABC) may be required. Give intravenous crystalloid and administer oxygen. Take blood for clotting studies and to look for thrombophilias and lupus anticoagulant. Give a loading dose of heparin of 5000 iu followed by an infusion of 30 000 iu over 24 hours (postnatal) or low-molecular-weight heparin 2500–5000 iu per day monitored by factor Xa heparin assay (antenatal).

Amniotic fluid embolism

Amniotic fluid embolism is said to occur when amniotic fluid enters the maternal circulation. It causes acute cardiorespiratory compromise and severe disseminated intravascular coagulation (Table 19.5). Rather than being directly caused by amniotic fluid entering the circulation, in some cases there is evidence to suggest an abnormal maternal reaction to amniotic fluid as the primary event.

This is a rare condition, occurring in approximately 1:30 000 pregnancies. In the 1997–1999 *Confidential Enquiries into Maternal Deaths* in the UK, there were eight deaths due to amniotic fluid embolism, more than the number of deaths from haemorrhage.

The prognosis is poor, with around 30 per cent of patients dying in the first hour and only 10 per cent surviving overall.

Table 19.4 – Diagnosis of pulmonary embolism

Symptoms	Signs	Investigations
Acute breathlessness	Tachycardia	Reduced oxygen tension in arterial blood
Pleuritic chest pain	Cyanosis	Electrocardiogram lead 3
Haemoptysis	Hypotension	Large Q waves, inverted T waves
	May be confusion (hypoxia)	Chest X-ray
		Ventilation perfusion scan

Table 19.5 – Clinical presentation of amniotic fluid embolism

Symptoms	Signs	Investigations	Treatment
Sudden severe chest pain Dyspnoea	Hypotension Tachycardia Pulmonary oedema Peripheral shutdown Haemorrhage due to coagulation failure May be seizure secondary to hypoxia or cardiac arrest	Electrocardiogram – right ventricular strain Abnormal coagulation screen Reduced oxygen tension in arterial blood	Urgent resuscitation and circulatory support Intubation and 100% oxygen Treat the coagulopathy aggressively Correct acidosis Dopamine and steroids may be useful Transfer to intensive care unit

Hypertensive disorders: pre-eclampsia and eclampsia

Definition

Pre-eclampsia is a disease of pregnancy characterized by a blood pressure of 140/90 mmHg or more on two separate occasions after the 20th week of pregnancy in a previously normotensive woman. This is accompanied by significant proteinuria (>300 mg in 24 hours). The condition progressively worsens. Eclampsia is the same condition that has proceeded to the presence of convulsions. Imminent eclampsia, or fulminating pre-eclampsia, is the transitional condition characterized by increasing symptoms and signs. Pre-eclampsia is discussed in detail in Chapter 13; the management of severe or fulminating pre-eclampsia and eclampsia is included in this chapter.

Incidence and epidemiology

Eclampsia is relatively rare in the UK, occurring in approximately 1:2000 pregnancies. It may occur antepartum (40 per cent), intrapartum (20 per cent) or postpartum (40 per cent). Severe pre-eclampsia is much more common than eclampsia.

Severe pre-eclampsia is identified by a blood pressure of 160/110 mmHg or more (see boxes below). Proteinuria is identified by routine 'stick' testing.

A 24-hour urine collection for quantification of proteinuria may be started, but in practice there may not be time to wait for its completion before effecting delivery. The patient may feel unwell, restless or nauseated and complaining of right upper quadrant pain.

S Symptoms of severe pre-eclampsia

- Frontal headache
- Visual disturbance
- Epigastric pain
- General malaise and nausea
- Restlessness

Signs of severe pre-eclampsia

- Agitation
- Hyper-reflexia
- Facial and peripheral oedema
- Right upper quadrant tenderness
- Poor urine output

On examination, the blood pressure remains high. Peripheral oedema is too common in pregnancy to be of value as an observation, but facial, usually periorbital, oedema is likely to be of significance. There may be right upper quadrant tenderness, hyperreflexia, clonus and, rarely, papilloedema.

The fetus may appear small, with oligohydramnios and reduced fetal movements.

Eclampsia is obvious as a grand mal convulsion. However, other causes of fits such as epilepsy have to be considered. Preceding pre-eclampsia suggests eclampsia, but in approximately one-third of cases the eclamptic fit precedes other signs. After the convulsion, the blood pressure is frequently normal for a while, but proteinuria will usually still be present. Any convulsion in pregnancy should be considered to be eclamptic until proved otherwise.

Investigations

In the emergency situation:
- test the urine for protein,
- take blood for:
  - full blood count
  - clotting studies
  - liver function tests and urea and electrolytes
  - cross-matching.

Treatment

When a convulsion is occurring or has just occurred:
- turn the woman onto her side with her head down,
- ensure the airway is protected,
- give oxygen,
- give a 5 g bolus of magnesium sulphate intravenously over a few minutes,
- progress to stabilizing the woman's condition (see below).

In severe pre-eclampsia, a convulsion has not yet occurred and it is important to ensure that it does not. The mother's condition needs to be stabilized urgently, before considering delivery in antenatal cases.

Call for help: senior obstetric and anaesthetic staff must be involved. Depending upon the results of clotting studies and the severity of the disease, a consultant haematologist may need to be informed.

Lower the blood pressure to a safe level. Seven of the 15 deaths recorded as due to eclampsia in the last triennial report were due to intracranial haemorrhage, suggesting a failure of antihypertensive therapy. The drug of choice to reduce the blood pressure is either hydralazine, causing direct relaxation of arteriolar smooth muscle, or the alpha- and beta-blocker labetalol. Give a bolus and then a continuous infusion, titrated against the blood pressure. The aim is to return not to normality, but to safety. Even if the blood pressure returns to near normal, this does not mean that the disease process has been stopped, merely that one manifestation of it has been temporarily pharmacologically corrected.

Give anticonvulsants to prevent a fit or further fits. Magnesium sulphate is the drug of choice. This acts as a cerebral vasodilator and membrane stabilizer and has been demonstrated to be very effective. Although it is generally a safe drug, in overdose respiratory depression and even cardiac arrest may occur. Blood levels can be monitored, but adequate observation of the patient's response and testing her reflexes (diminished with magnesium sulphate) are adequate. If necessary, the effects can be reversed with calcium gluconate.

Management of fluid balance can be problematic. In pre-eclampsia, there is intense peripheral vasoconstriction accompanied by a decrease in the plasma volume, together with redistribution of the extracellular fluid. The urine output falls, and over-enthusiastic efforts to provide a fluid challenge may cause pulmonary and cerebral oedema. A strict input/output balance must be maintained, using either blood products or crystalloids, as appropriate. In the absence of bleeding, no more than 100 mL/h of fluids (oral and intravenous) should be given. If oliguria (<20 mL of urine per hour for 4 hours) develops, put a central venous pressure (CVP) line in place to aid management. Renal failure is uncommon. Avoid diuretics.

Timing of delivery depends upon the gestation, the presence of other complicating factors, the severity of the disease and the stability of the patient's condition. In general, if the patient has disease severe enough to warrant antihypertensive and anticonvulsant therapy, delivery should follow stabilization of the maternal condition.

Indications for urgent delivery

- Blood pressure persistently at 160/100 mmHg or more with significant proteinuria
- Elevated liver enzymes
- Low platelet count
- Eclamptic fit
- Anuria
- Significant fetal distress

When it is clear that early delivery is likely, if the gestation is less than 34 weeks, steroids should be given to improve lung maturity and decrease neonatal complications. Steroid administration must not delay delivery that is necessary for the control of severe maternal problems, although recent evidence indicates that steroids also benefit the mother with pre-eclampsia.

Delivery is often by Caesarean section, although if labour is well established, vaginal delivery is possible. If at all possible, clotting disorders must be corrected before delivery (by whatever means) is attempted.

Postpartum, both fulminating pre-eclampsia and eclampsia may occur. Management is as for the antenatal case except that delivery has already taken place.

HELLP syndrome

HELLP syndrome – a combination of **h**aemolysis, **e**levated **l**iver enzymes and **l**ow **p**latelets – is seen in 5–10 per cent of cases of severe pre-eclampsia. It may be associated with disseminated intravascular coagulation, placental abruption and fetal death. This is a serious problem with significant fetal and maternal mortality (5 of 15 eclamptic deaths in the last triennial report).

🔧 Key Points

Hypertensive disorders

- Fulminating pre-eclampsia and eclampsia are dangerous.
- Recognize women at risk.
- Manage minor hypertensive problems to prevent progression.
- In the serious case:
  - prevent or control convulsions,
  - bring down the blood pressure,
  - minimize or avoid organ damage,
  - control coagulopathy,
  - avoid fluid overload,
  - deliver a healthy baby safely.

CASE HISTORY

Mrs B was a 34-year-old Caucasian primigravid teacher. At a gestation of 11 weeks, she was seen in the hospital antenatal clinic for the first time. She was noted to be a non-smoker. There was no relevant past history, but it was known that her mother had been treated for hypertension when in her late forties. Mrs B was 1.56 m tall and weighed 83 kg. Her booking blood pressure was 110/74 mmHg. Nothing abnormal was found on testing her urine. Mrs B was booked for shared care with her GP and for delivery at the hospital under consultant supervision. She was to be seen again in the hospital at 41 weeks if she had not delivered by then.

The antenatal period was uneventful until 37 weeks. Ultrasound examinations were performed at 11 and 19 weeks. The fetal size corresponded to dates and the fetal anatomy was normal. The placenta was in the upper segment of the uterus. At 37 weeks' gestation, a community midwife noted that Mrs B's blood pressure had risen to 150/100 mmHg and that there was + + of protein in the urine. Mrs B was referred to the hospital as an emergency admission.

On arrival at the hospital, Mrs B's blood pressure was 160/110 mmHg and there was + + + of protein in the urine. She was complaining of some epigastric tenderness and there was mild hyper-reflexia. The fetal heart rate was 140 beats per minute (bpm) and was noted to be regular.

What are the risks in this case?

Mrs B was hypertensive and had marked proteinuria, having previously been normotensive. The diagnosis is pre-eclampsia. The level of the blood pressure denotes severe disease. The pregnancy is at term.

Mrs B is at risk of developing a worsening condition. A further rise in her blood pressure will put her at risk of intracranial haemorrhage. She may have an eclamptic fit, develop a coagulopathy and HELLP syndrome, and possibly renal failure. There is a further risk of placental abruption and severe haemorrhage. The fetus is at risk secondary to the mother's condition.

Plan of action

The patient does not require resuscitation. The fetus does not require emergency delivery.

Establish an intravenous line with a wide-bore cannula.

Take blood for clotting studies, full blood count and blood biochemistry and save serum.

- Prevent an eclamptic fit from occurring.
  - Give magnesium sulphate 5 g over 20 minutes via an infusion pump (10 mL of a 50 per cent solution in 200 mL of normal saline).
  - Continue with 2 g/h (20 mL of a 50 per cent solution in 250 mL of normal saline at a rate of 50 mL/h).

- The therapeutic range for magnesium sulphate in serum is 2–3 mmol/L. Check the level at 60 minutes and then 6-hourly. If the blood pressure falls below 110/70 mmHg, the respiratory rate below 16/min, the urine output below 30 mL/h or if the knee-jerk reflexes disappear, the infusion must be stopped and the blood levels checked urgently.
- Lower the blood pressure.
  - The aim is to achieve a diastolic blood pressure of 90–100 mmHg. Check the blood pressure with a Dinamap every 5 minutes.
  - Start by giving hydralazine in intravenous boluses, Slowly inject 2–5 mg up to a total of 10 mg. Repeat after 30 minutes if the blood pressure is not controlled.
  - Continue with an infusion of between 1 and 5 mg/h (20 mg in 40 mL normal saline via a syringe driver).
- Measure input and output of fluids.
  - Put a Foley catheter into the bladder.
  - Restrict input from all sources to <100 mL/h.
  - A CVP line is only necessary if there is profound oliguria.
- If the clotting becomes deranged (platelets <50 000), contact a consultant haematologist for advice regarding further management.

Management of the case

In the case of Mrs B, her blood pressure fell to 145/96 mmHg on treatment with hydralazine. Treatment with magnesium sulphate was started following the stated regimen. The urine output averaged 35 mL/h. Clotting studies and blood biochemistry remained normal. The platelet level was 145 000/mL. The cardiotocograph showed a normal fetal heart pattern.

Once control of the situation had been achieved, delivery was planned. Because the clotting studies were normal, an epidural was put in place. Vaginal examination showed that the cervix was long and closed, with the fetus presenting by the head, which was not engaged.

Clearly, induction of labour was unlikely to lead to early delivery. After discussion with Mrs B and her husband, including an explanation of the risks and benefits of the different modes of delivery, immediate Caesarean section was planned. At operation, a 3.2 kg boy was delivered, with Apgar scores of 6 at 1 minute and 9 at 5 minutes. The estimated blood loss was 600 mL.

After delivery, Mrs B was nursed in the delivery suite for 36 hours. The magnesium sulphate infusion was continued for 24 hours. Atenolol was given by mouth to maintain control of the blood pressure, and the hydralazine infusion was stopped. There was initial concern with regard to the urine output, which remained at 25 mL/h for the first 6 hours after delivery. The position was watched, but no active steps were taken to redress the issue and, between 6 and 12 hours after delivery, the patient began to have a marked diuresis. Seven days after delivery, Mrs B's blood pressure had returned to normal without medication. Mother and baby did well.

Conclusion

This case demonstrates appropriate management of moderate to severe pre-eclampsia at term. Major problems were prevented by swift action. Mrs B is at risk of pre-eclampsia in her next pregnancy, although it is likely to be less severe. She is also at risk of developing hypertension later in life.

The collapsed obstetric patient

Complete or partial loss of consciousness is very uncommon in pregnancy.

Causes of loss of consciousness

- Simple faint
- Epileptic fit
- Hypoglycaemia
- Profound hypoxia
- Intracerebral bleed
- Cerebral infarction
- Cardiac arrhythmia or myocardial infarction
- Pulmonary embolism
- Anaphylaxis
- Septic shock
- Anaesthetic problems
- Major haemorrhage
- Eclampsia
- Amniotic fluid embolus
- Uterine inversion.

Remember the basic life support skills

- Shake and shout
- Airway

- Breathing
- Circulation
- Look for hypovolaemia (tachycardia, pallor)
- Aggressive fluid replacement
- Stop haemorrhage
- Stabilize and seek a cause
- Senior multi-disciplinary assistance throughout.

Fetal emergencies

The fetus may be severely affected by any of the preceding maternal emergencies that occur before delivery. However, there are some emergencies that directly affect the fetus without major immediate physical compromise of the mother.

Major abnormalities of the fetal heart rate, in particular prolonged fetal bradycardia, call for immediate delivery, usually by Caesarean section. Acute fetal distress is discussed in Chapter 17.

It is always said that the decision-to-delivery interval in such cases should not exceed 30 minutes, but in practice many units struggle to meet this deadline, which in some circumstances is unrealistic.

Umbilical cord accidents

Definition and diagnosis
When a loop or loops of umbilical cord are below the presenting part and the membranes are intact, the condition of cord presentation exists. If the membranes rupture, the cord may fall through the cervix and eventually the vulva. Both cord presentation and cord prolapse are associated with prematurity and malpresentations.

The incidence is around 1:500 deliveries. The umbilical vein is compressed between the presenting part and the pelvis, reducing or stopping the flow of oxygenated blood to the fetus. If continuous fetal heart rate monitoring is in progress, deep variable decelerations will be seen, leading to bradycardia if the situation is not relieved.

Management
Vaginal examination will reveal the cord presentation or prolapse. There is little point in feeling for pulsation, which can be difficult to determine; it increases the cord handling, which may cause spasm and is to be avoided.

If the cord is through the vulva, replace it in the vagina to keep it warmer, otherwise avoid handling it.

Urgent Caesarean section is required unless the cervix is fully dilated and an assisted vaginal delivery can be safely performed. There is no place for difficult and consequently prolonged forceps or ventouse delivery. Even if the cervix is fully dilated, if the head is high or there are other factors that suggest that difficulty may be encountered in attempts at vaginal delivery, resort to Caesarean section immediately.

Establish intravenous access with a large-bore cannula, take blood for full blood count and cross-matching and give ranitidine to the mother.

Whilst arranging for Caesarean section to be performed, it is vital to relieve the pressure on the umbilical vein to allow oxygen to reach the fetus. Place the mother in a head-down position. Traditionally, the patient is placed on all fours with the hips elevated. A doctor or midwife keeps a hand in the patient's vagina, pushing the presenting part up and relieving the pressure on the cord. A less intrusive approach that avoids handling the cord is to fill the patient's bladder with 500 mL of saline to displace the fetal presenting part upwards. Empty the bladder before opening the abdomen.

Before commencing Caesarean section, listen to the fetal heart to be sure that the fetus is alive.

Prognosis
Outcome depends upon the gestation, other complicating factors such as intrauterine growth restriction, and for how long the cord has been compressed. With a term baby and when a diagnosis has been made promptly in hospital, the prognosis ought to be excellent. If the cord prolapse is outside of hospital, the fetus is likely to be dead by the time of admission. Total cord compression for longer than 10 minutes will cause cerebral damage and, if continued for around 20 minutes, death. These times will be reduced in an already compromised fetus.

Shoulder dystocia

Definition and aetiology
Difficulty with delivery of the fetal shoulders is termed shoulder dystocia. Quite where minor difficulty becomes true shoulder dystocia is difficult to say. In consequence, the incidence varies from 0.2 to 1.2 per cent depending on the definition.

In passing through the pelvis, the fetal head and shoulders rotate to make use of the widest diameters. After delivery of the head, restitution occurs and the shoulders rotate into the antero-posterior (AP) diameter. This makes use of the widest (AP) diameter of the pelvic outlet. However, if the shoulders have not entered the pelvic inlet, the anterior shoulder may become caught above the maternal symphysis pubis. Occasionally, both shoulders may remain above the pelvic brim.

Management

Shoulder dystocia can only be completely avoided by Caesarean section. Although in some cases the risk of shoulder dystocia may be recognized before delivery, *this is very uncommon*. Even combinations of risk factors have poor predictive value, although if the baby is known to be very large (>4.5 kg) and shoulder dystocia has complicated a previous pregnancy, particularly in a diabetic mother, Caesarean section is prudent (see 'risk factors' box). In the majority of cases, recognition of risk factors should lead to an experienced obstetrician being present at delivery to manage the problem.

Risk factors in shoulder dystocia

- Large baby
- Small mother
- Maternal obesity
- Diabetes mellitus
- Post-maturity
- Previous shoulder dystocia
- Prolongation of late first stage of labour
- Prolonged second stage of labour
- Assisted vaginal delivery

Shoulder dystocia is a very alarming occurrence. Vessels in the fetal neck are occluded after delivery of the head, and cerebral damage will occur if delivery is delayed significantly. The fetus may already be compromised because of the prolongation of labour. After 5 minutes, there is the risk of cerebral damage. However, inappropriate traction, particularly downward traction on the head causing lateral flexion of the head on the neck, will cause stretching of the brachial plexus and nerve damage. Erb's palsy is a likely consequence.

Shoulder dystocia is managed by a sequence of manoeuvres designed to facilitate delivery without fetal damage. This sequence must be part of a prepared plan of action that all obstetric and midwifery staff are familiar with and have practised in labour ward drills (see box below).

- Do not use excess traction on the head to confirm the diagnosis.
- Call for help – the most senior and experienced people available, including obstetrician and paediatrician.
- Remember the time of delivery of the head.
- Get assistance to maximally flex and abduct the patient's hips on her abdomen (McRobert's position).

Shoulder dystocia drill

- Call for help
- Avoid excess traction at all times
- Hyperflex and abduct the hips
- Apply suprapubic pressure
- Rotate the shoulders by internal manipulation
- Deliver the posterior arm
- More dramatic techniques are rarely necessary
- Avoid:
  - fundal pressure
  - turning the patient into the left lateral position
  - inappropriate traction on the head

At this stage, mild to moderate traction on the head will be effective in around 90 per cent of cases.

If this fails, a large episiotomy or extension of the existing episiotomy is usually made. Although the problem is a bony one, this will provide more space at the outlet and is of value.

Apply suprapubic pressure, pushing on the fetal shoulder towards the fetal chest, adducting the shoulders and pushing them into the oblique position and off the symphysis.

The majority of cases will resolve with this management. If not, attempt to rotate the shoulders by putting a hand into the vagina and pushing on the front aspect of the posterior shoulder.

An alternative is to delivery the posterior arm first, pulling on the forearm in such a way as to rotate the fetal body in the pelvis. It may be easier to position the patient on all fours to give greater access, if time permits.

If all of these manoeuvres fail, symphysiotomy, breaking the fetal clavicle or replacing the head in the vagina and giving tocolytics with a view to performing Caesarean section are all theoretically possible. Few doctors in the UK have had experience of these techniques.

Shoulder dystocia is a most alarming emergency for obstetrician and midwife. It is also very frightening for the patient and her partner. Without delaying matters unduly, every opportunity should be taken to explain what is happening and to give a full explanation after delivery.

Finally, a careful record must be made to include the time of the delivery of the head and the body, the manoeuvres used and who was present. The number of attempts of traction on the head and the relationship of these attempts to the other manoeuvres should be recorded. The complication of Erb's palsy commonly leads to subsequent litigation, sometimes 20 or more years later. Accurate and full contemporary records are vital.

Key Points

Obstetric emergencies

An obstetric emergency converts a happy, normal event into a potential catastrophe. The essentials of a successful outcome are as follows.

- Paying attention to risk factors to avoid untoward events.
- A well-organized labour ward with enough experienced staff present.
- Adequate staff training in managing emergencies, with clear protocols and practice drills for all.
- Clear lines of communication and a readiness to involve senior obstetricians, paediatricians, anaesthetists, haematologists and other medical staff as necessary.
- Appropriate hospital facilities, blood bank, intensive care unit.
- Recognition of the frightening nature of obstetric emergencies and a readiness to inform and explain the situation to the patient and her partner.
- Complete and accurate note keeping.

Additional reading

Lewis G (ed.). *Why mothers die 1997–1999*. The Fifth Report of the Confidential Enquiry into Maternal Deaths in the UK. London: RCOG Press, 2001.

The puerperium

OVERVIEW

The puerperium refers to the 6-week period following childbirth, when considerable adjustments occur before return to the pre-pregnant state. During this period of physiological change, the mother is also vulnerable to psychological disturbances, which may be aggravated by adverse social circumstances. Adequate understanding and support from her partner and family are crucial. Difficulty in coping with the newborn infant occurs more frequently with the first baby, and vigilant surveillance is therefore necessary by the community midwife, general practitioner and health visitor. The degree of care provided by the health service varies from country to country. In the UK, a mother may be discharged from hospital within 6 hours of an uncomplicated birth, although she may request to stay longer. Irrespective of duration of hospital stay, however, a midwife must visit her at least once daily for a minimum of 10 days after delivery. Thereafter, the health visitor takes on responsibility for continuing care, particularly of the infant, but the midwife may continue making home visits, if necessary, for up to 4 weeks after delivery. In the Netherlands, a doctor or midwife provides care for the first 5 days, but maternity aides are available to help mothers care for their older children and cope with household duties. In North America, there is more dependence on private health care, and very little organized care after discharge from hospital. There is therefore a lack of consensus as to what constitutes ideal postpartum care, and protocols differ from one centre to the next.

Physiological changes

Uterine involution

Involution is the process by which the postpartum uterus, weighing about 1 kg, returns to its pre-pregnancy state of less than 100 g. Immediately after delivery, the uterine fundus lies about 4 cm below the umbilicus or, more accurately, 12 cm above the symphysis pubis. However, within 2 weeks, the uterus can no longer be palpable above the symphysis. Involution occurs by a process of autolysis, whereby muscle cells diminish in size as a result of enzymatic digestion of cytoplasm. This has virtually no effect on the number of muscle cells, and the excess protein produced from autolysis is absorbed into the bloodstream and excreted in the urine. Involution appears to be accelerated by the release of oxytocin in women who are breastfeeding, as the uterus is smaller than in those who are bottle-feeding. The height of the uterine fundus is measured daily to ascertain the trend in involution.

- Full bladder
- Loaded rectum
- Uterine infection
- Retained products of conception
- Fibroids
- Broad ligament haematoma

A delay in involution in the absence of any other signs or symptoms, e.g. bleeding, is of no clinical significance.

Genital tract changes

Following delivery of the placenta, the lower segment of the uterus and the cervix appear flabby and there may be small cervical lacerations. In the first few days, the cervix can readily admit two fingers, but by the end of the first week it should become increasingly difficult to pass more than one finger, and certainly by the end of the second week the internal os should be closed. However, the external os can remain open permanently, giving a characteristic appearance to the parous cervix. In the first few days, the stretched vagina is smooth and oedematous, but by the third week rugae begin to reappear.

Lochia

Lochia is the bloodstained uterine discharge that is comprised of blood and necrotic decidua. Only the superficial layer of decidua becomes necrotic and is sloughed off. The basal layer adjacent to the myometrium is involved in the regeneration of new endometrium and this regeneration is complete by the third week. During the first few days after delivery, the lochia is red; this gradually changes to pink as the endometrium is formed, and then ultimately becomes serous by the second week. Persistent red lochia suggests delayed involution that is usually associated with infection or a retained piece of placental tissue. Offensive lochia, which may be accompanied by pyrexia and a tender uterus, suggests infection and should be treated with a broad-spectrum antibiotic. Retained placental tissue is associated with increased red blood cell loss and clots, and this may be suspected if the placenta and membranes were incomplete at delivery (see Chapter 19). Management includes the use of antibiotics and evacuation of retained products under regional or general anaesthesia.

Puerperal disorders

Daily maternal observations include temperature, pulse, blood pressure, urinary function, bowel function, breast examination and feeding, assessment of uterine involution, appearance of lochia, perineal inspection, examination of legs and pelvic floor exercises. These observations should be made more frequently in high-risk women or if an abnormality has been detected, e.g. Caesarean section, raised blood pressure, perineal infection, etc. In the UK, it is traditional to check haemoglobin levels on day 3 unless otherwise indicated, and most women who are particularly symptomatic should be transfused if their haemoglobin level at this time is <8 g/dL. However, one study has shown that haemoglobin estimations on day 7 may lead to fewer blood transfusions.

Perineal complications

Perineal discomfort is the single major problem for mothers, and about 80 per cent complain of pain in the first 3 days after delivery, with a quarter continuing to suffer discomfort at day 10. Discomfort is greatest in women who sustain spontaneous tears or have an episiotomy, but especially following instrumental delivery. A number of non-pharmacological and pharmacological therapies have been used empirically with varying degrees of success. However, local cooling (with crushed ice, witch hazel or tap water) and topical anaesthetics such as 5 per cent lignocaine gel provide short-term symptomatic relief. Effective analgesia following perineal trauma can be achieved with paracetamol, but a randomized study has shown that diclofenac suppositories (a non-steroidal anti-inflammatory agent) given at delivery followed by another 12 hours later are significantly more effective than placebo. Codeine derivatives are not preferable, as they have a tendency to cause constipation.

Infections of the perineum are generally uncommon considering the risk of bacterial contamination during delivery; therefore, when signs of infection (redness, pain, swelling and heat) occur, especially when associated with a raised temperature, these must be taken seriously. Swabs for microbiological culture must be taken from the infected perineum, and broad-spectrum antibiotics (see below) should be commenced. If there is a collection of pus, drainage should be encouraged by removal of any skin sutures; otherwise infection would spread, with increasing morbidity and a poor anatomical result.

Spontaneous opening of repaired perineal tears and episiotomies is usually the result of secondary infection. Surgical repair should never be attempted in the presence of infection. The wound should be irrigated twice daily and healing should be allowed to occur by secondary intention. If there is a large, gaping wound, secondary repair should only be performed when the infection has cleared, there is no cellulitis or exudate present and healthy granulation tissue can be seen.

Bladder function

Voiding difficulty and over-distension of the bladder are not uncommon after childbirth, especially if regional anaesthesia (epidural/spinal) has been used. It is now known that after epidural anaesthesia the bladder may take up to 8 hours to regain normal sensation. During this time, about 1 L of urine may be produced and therefore if urinary retention occurs, considerable damage may be inflicted on the detrusor muscle. Over-stretching of the detrusor muscle can dampen bladder sensation and make the bladder hypocontractile, particularly with fibrous replacement of smooth muscle. In this situation overflow incontinence of small amounts of urine may erroneously be assumed to be normal voiding. Fluid overloading prior to epidural analgesia, the antidiuretic effect of high concentrations of oxytocin during labour, increased postpartum diuresis (particularly in the presence of oedema) and increased fluid intake by breastfeeding mothers all contribute to the increased urine production in the puerperium. Therefore an intake/output chart alone may not detect incomplete emptying of the bladder.

Women who have undergone a traumatic delivery such as a difficult instrumental delivery, or who have suffered multiple/extended lacerations or a vulvo-vaginal haematoma, may find it difficult to void because of pain or peri-urethral oedema. Other causes of pain, such as prolapsed haemorrhoids, anal fissures, abdominal wound haematoma or even stool impaction of the rectum, may interfere with voiding. The midwife needs to be particularly vigilant after

an epidural or spinal anaesthetic to avoid bladder distension. The distended bladder should either be palpable as a suprapubic cystic mass or it may displace the uterus laterally or upwards, thereby increasing the height of the uterine fundus.

In order to minimize the risk of over-distension of the bladder in women undergoing a Caesarean section under regional anaesthesia, a urinary catheter may be left in the bladder for the first 12–24 hours. The benefit of leaving a catheter in situ for about 12 hours after epidural insertion should be evaluated against a vigorously enforced postpartum voiding protocol and the small risk of urinary tract infection. However, any woman who has not passed urine within 4 hours of delivery should be encouraged to do so before resorting to catheterization. In general, a clean-catch specimen of urine should be sent for microscopy, culture and sensitivity, and if the residual urine in the bladder is >300 mL, a catheter should be left in to allow free drainage for 48 hours.

Although vaginal delivery is strongly implicated in the development of urinary stress incontinence, it rarely poses a problem in the early puerperium. Therefore any incontinence should be investigated to exclude a vesico-vaginal, urethro-vaginal or, rarely, uretero-vaginal fistula. Obstetric fistulae are rare in the UK, but are a source of considerable morbidity in developing countries. Pressure necrosis of the bladder or urethra may occur following prolonged obstructed labour, and incontinence usually occurs in the second week when the slough separates. Small fistulae may close spontaneously after a few weeks of free bladder drainage; large fistulae will require surgical repair by a specialist.

Bowel function

Constipation is a common problem in the puerperium. This may be due to an interruption in the normal diet and possible dehydration during labour. Advice on adequate fluid intake and increase in fibre intake may be all that is necessary. However, constipation may also be the result of fear of evacuation due to pain from a sutured perineum, prolapsed haemorrhoids or anal fissures. Avoidance of constipation and straining is of utmost importance in women who have sustained a third-degree or fourth-degree tear. A large, hard bolus of stool in this situation would disrupt the repaired anal sphincter and cause anal incontinence. It is

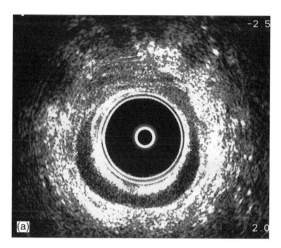
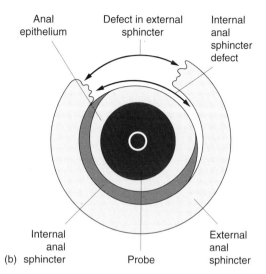

Figure 20.1 (a) Transanal ultrasound showing the anal mucosa and anterior disruption of the internal anal sphincter (dark band) following a third-degree tear at delivery. (b) Diagrammatic representation of part (a).

important to ensure that these women are prescribed lactulose and ispaghula husk (Fybogel, Regulan) or methylcellulose immediately after the repair, for a period of 2 weeks.

The high prevalence of anal incontinence and faecal urgency following childbirth has only recently been recognized. One prospective study using anal endosonography has identified evidence of occult anal sphincter trauma in one-third of primiparous women, although only 13 per cent admitted to defaecatory symptoms by 6 weeks postpartum. Larger, retrospective, short-term studies of parous women indicate a prevalence of between 6 and 10 per cent. Long-term anal incontinence following primary repair of a third-degree or fourth-degree tear occurs in 5 per cent of women, and anovaginal/rectovaginal fistulae occur in 2–4 per cent of these women (Fig. 20.1). It is therefore important to consider a fistula as a cause of anal incontinence in the postpartum period, particularly if the woman complains of passing wind or stool per vaginam. Approximately 50 per cent of small anovaginal fistulae will close spontaneously over a period of 6 months, but larger fistulae will require formal repair, frequently with a covering colostomy.

Secondary postpartum haemorrhage

Secondary postpartum haemorrhage (PPH) is defined as fresh bleeding from the genital tract between 24 hours and 6 weeks after delivery (see Chapter 19 for primary PPH). The most common time for secondary PPH is between days 7 and 14, and the cause is most commonly attributed to retained placental tissue. Associated features include crampy abdominal pain, a uterus larger than appropriate, passage of bits of placental tissue or tissue within the cervix and signs of infection. The management of heavy bleeding includes an intravenous infusion, cross-match of blood, Syntocinon, an examination under anaesthesia and evacuation of the uterus. Antibiotics should be given if placental tissue is found, even without evidence of overt infection. If blood loss is not excessive, the use of pelvic ultrasound to exclude retained products is contentious; distinction between retained products and blood clot can be extremely difficult. Other causes of secondary PPH include endometritis, hormonal contraception, bleeding disorders, e.g. von Willebrand's disease, and choriocarcinoma.

Obstetric palsy

Obstetric palsy, or traumatic neuritis, is a condition in which one or both lower limbs may develop signs of a motor and/or sensory neuropathy following delivery. Presenting features include sciatic pain, footdrop, parasthesia, hypoaesthesia and muscle wasting. The mechanism of injury is unknown and it was previously attributed to compression or stretching of the lumbosacral trunk as it crosses the sacroiliac joint during descent of the fetal head. It is now believed that herniation of lumbosacral discs (usually L4 or L5) can occur, particularly in the exaggerated lithotomy position and during instrumental delivery. An orthopaedic opinion should be sought and management includes bed rest with a firm board beneath the mattress, analgesia and physiotherapy. Peroneal nerve palsy can occur when the nerve is compressed between the head of the fibula and the lithotomy pole, resulting in unilateral foot-drop. Until recently, the development of urinary and faecal incontinence had been attributed largely to pudendal neuropathy following stretching of the pudendal nerve as it leaves Alcock's canal. However, recent evidence indicates that structural damage to the sphincter muscle and supporting fascia is the major aetiological factor.

Symphysis pubis diastasis

Separation of the symphysis pubis can occur spontaneously in at least 1 in 800 vaginal deliveries.

Deliberate surgical separation of the pubis in labour (symphysiotomy) can be performed in cases of borderline cephalopelvic disproportion to increase the pelvic diameter. However, although it may be a safer option in underdeveloped countries (in preference to performing a Caesarean section and risking a ruptured uterus in a subsequent pregnancy because of poor facilities for antenatal care), it is no longer practised in modern obstetrics. Spontaneous separation is usually noticed after delivery and has been associated with forceps delivery, rapid second stage of labour or severe abduction of the thighs during delivery. Common signs and symptoms include symphyseal pain aggravated by weight-bearing and walking, a waddling gait, pubic tenderness and a palpable interpubic gap. Treatment includes bed rest, anti-inflammatory agents, physiotherapy and a pelvic corset to provide support and stability.

Thromboembolism

The risk of thromboembolic disease rises five-fold during pregnancy and the puerperium. The majority of deaths occur in the puerperium and are more common after Caesarean section. If deep vein thrombosis or pulmonary embolism is suspected, full anticoagulant therapy should be commenced and a bilateral venogram and/or lung scan should be carried out within 24–48 hours (see Chapters 11 and 19).

Puerperal pyrexia

Significant puerperal pyrexia is defined as a temperature of 38 °C (100.4 °F) or higher on any two of the first 10 days postpartum, exclusive of the first 24 hours (measured orally by a standard technique). A mildly elevated temperature is not uncommon in the first 24 hours, but any pyrexia associated with tachycardia merits investigation. In about 80 per cent of women who develop a temperature in the first 24 hours following a vaginal delivery, no obvious evidence of infection can be identified. The reverse holds true for women delivering by Caesarean section, when a wound infection should be considered. Common sites associated with puerperal pyrexia include chest, throat, breasts, urinary tract, pelvic organs, Caesarean or perineal wounds and legs (Table 20.1).

Chest complications

Chest complications are most likely to appear in the first 24 hours after delivery, particularly after general anaesthesia. Atalectasis may be associated with fever and can be prevented by early and regular chest physiotherapy. Aspiration pneumonia (Mendleson's syndrome) must be suspected if there is wheezing, dyspnoea, a spiking temperature and evidence of hypoxia.

Genital tract infection

Genital tract infection following delivery is referred to as puerperal sepsis and is synonymous with older descriptions of puerperal fever, milk fever and childbed fever. It was not realized until the mid-nineteenth century that the high maternal mortality and morbidity were due to poor hygiene of the birth attendants; the establishment of lying-in hospitals and overcrowding perpetuated the condition to epidemic proportions. Until 1937, puerperal sepsis was the major cause of maternal mortality. The discovery of sulphonamides in 1935 and the simultaneous reduction in the virulence of the haemolytic *Streptococcus* resulted in a dramatic fall in maternal mortality. Currently, the incidence of puerperal sepsis is approximately 3 per cent (range 1–8 per cent) and, excluding deaths after abortion, it accounts for 7 per cent of all direct maternal deaths (4 per million maternities).

Table 20.1 – Diagnosis and management of puerperal pyrexia

Symptoms	Diagnosis	Special investigations	Management
Cough	Chest infection	Sputum M, C & S	Physiotherapy
Purulent sputum	Pneumonia	Chest X-ray	Antibiotics
Dyspnoea			
Sore throat	Tonsillitis	Throat swab	Antibiotics
Cervical lymphadenopathy			
Headaches	Meningitis	Lumbar puncture	Antibiotics
Neck stiffness (epidural/ spinal anaesthetic)			
Dysuria	Pyelonephritis	Urine M, C & S	Antibiotics
Loin pain and tenderness			
Secondary PPH	Metritis	Pelvic ultrasound	Antibiotics
Tender bulky uterus	Retained placental tissue		Uterine evacuation
Pelvic/calf pain/tenderness	Deep vein thrombosis	Doppler/venogram of legs	Heparin
Chest pain	Pulmonary embolism	Lung perfusion scan angiogram Chest X-ray and blood gases	
Painful engorged breasts	Mastitis Abscess	Milk M, C & S	Express milk Antibiotics Incision and drainage

M, C & S, microscopy, culture and sensitivity; PPH, postpartum haemorrhage.

Aetiology of genital tract infections

A mixed flora normally colonizes the vagina with low virulence. Puerperal infection is usually polymicrobial and involves contaminants from the bowel that colonize the perineum and lower genital tract. In one study of women with endometritis within 48 hours of delivery, two or more organisms were identified in more than 60 per cent of cases. The most frequently identified organisms were facultative Gram-positive cocci, particularly group B *Streptococcus*, frequently co-existing with *Mycoplasma* species. Following delivery, natural barriers to infection are temporarily removed and therefore organisms with a pathogenic potential can ascend from the lower genital tract into the uterine cavity. Placental separation exposes a large raw area equivalent to an open wound, and retained products of conception and blood clots within the uterus can provide an excellent culture medium for infection. Furthermore, vaginal delivery is almost invariably associated with lacerations of the genital tract (uterus, cervix and vagina). Although these lacerations may not need surgical repair, they can become a focus for infection similar to iatrogenic wounds such as Caesarean section and episiotomy.

Organisms commonly associated with puerperal genital infection

Aerobes
- Gram-positive
  - Beta-haemolytic *Streptococcus*, Groups A, B, D
  - *Staphylococcus epidermidis* and *aureus*
  - Enterococci – *Streptococcus faecalis*
- Gram-negative
  - *Escherichia coli*
  - *Haemophilus influenzae*

– *Klebsiella pneumoniae*
– *Pseudomonas aeruginosa*
– *Proteus mirabilis*
- Gram-variable
  – *Gardenella vaginalis*

Anaerobes
  – *Peptococcus* sp.
  – *Peptostreptococcus* sp.
  – *Bacteroides* – *B. fragilis, B. bivius, B. disiens*
  – *Fusobacterium* sp.

Miscellaneous
  – *Chlamydia trachomatis*
  – *Mycoplasma hominis*
  – *Ureaplasma urealyticum*

Haemolytic *Streptococcus* Lancefield Group A and *Staphylococcus aureus* are two exogenous organisms that can cause severe puerperal infection and have been associated with major epidemics and fatalities in the past. The infection usually originates from inpatients or birth attendants who may be asymptomatic carriers or who have an active infection. Transmission can occur by droplet infection, infected dust or direct skin contact. The toxins produced by these organisms can result in a rapid deterioration into septicaemic shock and yet produce minimal local signs. Serious infection has been rare since the advent of penicillin, although penicillin-resistant *Staphylococcus* now poses a new threat.

◉ Signs of puerperal pelvic infection

- Pyrexia and tachycardia
- Uterus – boggy, tender and larger
- Infected wounds – Caesarean/perineal
- Peritonism
- Paralytic ileus
- Indurated adnexae (parametritis)
- Bogginess in pelvis (abscess)

S Symptoms of puerperal pelvic infection

- Malaise, headache, fever, rigors
- Abdominal discomfort, vomiting and diarrhoea
- Offensive lochia
- Secondary PPH

Table 20.2 – Investigations for puerperal genital infections

Investigations	Abnormalities
Full blood count	Anaemia, leukocytosis, thrombocytopenia
Urea and electrolytes	Fluid and electrolyte imbalance
High vaginal swabs and blood culture	Infection screen
Pelvic ultrasound	Retained products, pelvic abscess
Clotting screen (haemorrhage or shock)	Disseminated intravascular coagulation
Arterial blood gas (shock)	Acidosis and hypoxia

Chlamydia trachomatis puerperal parametritis may develop in one-third of women who had a pre-existing infection, but presentation is usually delayed. Investigations for puerperal genital infections are shown in Table 20.2.

There are a number of factors that determine the clinical course and severity of the infection, namely the general health and resistance of the woman, the virulence of the offending organism, the presence of haematoma or retained products of conception and the timing of antibiotic therapy and associated risk factors. The common methods of spread of puerperal infection are outlined below.

- An ascending infection from the lower genital tract or primary infection of the placental site may spread via the Fallopian tubes to the ovaries, giving rise to a salpingo-oophoritis and pelvic peritonitis. This could progress to a generalized peritonitis and the development of pelvic abscesses.
- Infection may also spread by contiguity directly into the myometrium and the parametrium, giving rise to a metritis or parametritis, also referred to as pelvic cellulitis. Pelvic peritonitis and abscesses may also occur.
- Infection may also spread to distant sites via lymphatics and blood vessels. Infection from the uterus can be carried by uterine vessels into the inferior vena cava via the iliac vessels or, directly,

via the ovarian vessels. This could give rise to a septic thrombophlebitis, pulmonary infections or a generalized septicaemia and endotoxic shock.

Common risk factors for puerperal infection

- Antenatal intrauterine infection
- Caesarean section
- Cervical cerclage for cervical incompetence
- Prolonged rupture of membranes
- Prolonged labour
- Multiple vaginal examinations
- Internal fetal monitoring
- Instrumental delivery
- Manual removal of the placenta
- Retained products of conception
- Non-obstetric, e.g. obesity, diabetes, human immunodeficiency virus (HIV)

In contrast to pelvic inflammatory disease unrelated to pregnancy, tubal involvement in puerperal sepsis is in the form of perisalpingitis, which, rarely, causes tubal occlusion and consequent infertility. Tubo-ovarian abscesses are also a rare complication of puerperal sepsis.

Mild to moderate infections can be treated with a broad-spectrum antibiotic, e.g. co-amoxiclav, or a cephalosporin such as cefalexin plus metronidazole. Depending on the severity, the first few doses should be given intravenously.

With severe infections, there is a release of inflammatory and vasoactive mediators in response to the endotoxins produced during bacteriolysis. The resultant local vasodilatation causes circulatory embarrassment and hence poor tissue perfusion. This phenomenon is known as septicaemic/septic/endotoxic shock, and delay in appropriate management could be fatal.

Necrotizing fasciitis is a rare but frequently fatal infection of skin, fascia and muscle. It can originate in perineal tears, episiotomies and Caesarean section wounds. Perineal infections can extend rapidly to involve the buttocks, thighs and lower abdominal wall. A variety of bacteria can be involved, but anaerobes predominate and *Clostridium perfringens* is usually identified. In addition to general signs of infection, there is extensive necrosis, crepitus and inflammation. As well as the measures usually taken to manage septic shock, wide debridement of necrotic tissue under general anaesthesia is absolutely essential to avoid mortality. Split-thickness skin grafts may be necessary at a later date.

Prevention of puerperal sepsis

Increased awareness of the principles of general hygiene, a good surgical approach and the use of aseptic techniques have contributed to the decline in severe puerperal sepsis. However, the risk of sepsis is higher following Caesarean section, particularly when performed after the onset of labour. There is now overwhelming evidence that prophylactic antibiotics during emergency Caesarean section reduce the risk of postoperative infection, namely wound infection, metritis, pelvic abscess, pelvic thrombophlebitis and septic shock. A single intraoperative dose of antibiotics (amoxiclav or cephalosporin plus metronidazole) should be given after clamping of the umbilical cord to avoid unnecessary exposure of the baby to antibiotics. The benefit of prophylaxis for elective Caesarean section is of greater significance in units where the background infectious morbidity is high.

The breasts

Anatomy

The breasts are largely made up of glandular, adipose and connective tissue (Fig. 20.2). They lie superficial to

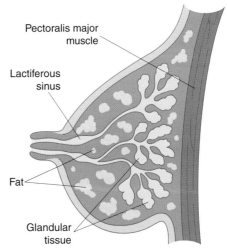

Figure 20.2 The breast during lactation.

the pectoralis major, external oblique and serratus anterior muscles, extending between the second and sixth rib from the sternum to the axilla. A pigmented area called the areola, which contains sebaceous glands, surrounds the nipple. During pregnancy, the areola becomes darker and the sebaceous glands become prominent (Montgomery's tubercles). The breast is comprised of 15–25 functional units arranged radially from the nipple and each unit is made up of a lactiferous duct, a mammary gland lobule and alveoli. The lactiferous ducts dilate to form a lactiferous sinus before converging to open in the nipple. Contractile myoepithelial cells surround the ducts as well as the alveoli.

Physiology

The human species is unique in that most of the breast development occurs at puberty and is therefore primed to produce milk within 2 weeks of hormonal stimulation. It is hypothesized that, unlike animals, female breasts have an erotic role to attract the male to procreate. The control of mammary growth and development is not fully understood and many hormones may contribute to this process. In general, oestrogens stimulate proliferation of the lactiferous ducts (possibly with adrenal steroids and growth hormones), while progesterone is responsible for the development of the mammary lobules. During early pregnancy, lactiferous ducts and alveoli proliferate, while in later pregnancy the alveoli hypertrophy in preparation for secretory activity. The lactogenic hormones prolactin and human placental lactogen probably modulate these changes during pregnancy.

Colostrum

Colostrum is a yellowish fluid secreted by the breast that can be expressed as early as the 16th week of pregnancy but is replaced by milk during the second postpartum day. Colostrum has a high concentration of proteins but contains less sugar and fat than breast milk, although it contains large fat globules. The proteins are mainly in the form of globulins, particularly immunoglobulin (Ig) A, which plays an important role in protection against infection. Colostrum is also believed to have a laxative effect, which may help empty the baby's bowel of meconium.

Table 20.3 – Comparison between human and cow's milk

	Human breast milk	Cow's milk
Energy (kcal/mL)	75	66
Lactose (g/100 mL)	6.8	4.9
Protein (g/100 mL)	1.1	3.5
Fat (g/100 mL)	4.5	3.7
Sodium (mmol/L)	7	22
Water (mL/100 mL)	87.1	87.3

Breast milk

The major constituents of breast milk are lactose, protein, fat and water (Table 20.3). However, the composition of breast milk is not constant; early lactation differs from late lactation, one feed differs from the next, and the composition can even change during a feed. Artificial infant formulas cannot therefore be identical to breast milk. Compared to cow's milk, breast milk provides slightly more energy, has less protein but more fat and lactose. The major protein fractions are lactalbumin, lactoglobulin and caseinogen. Lactalbumin is the major protein in breast milk, whereas caseinogen forms 90 per cent of the protein in cow's milk. The mineral content (particularly sodium) is much higher in cow's milk, which can therefore be dangerous if given to a baby who is dehydrated from gastroenteritis. In addition to IgA, breast milk contains small amounts of IgM and IgG and other factors such as lactoferrin, macrophages, complement and lysozymes. Although breast milk contains a lower concentration of iron, its absorption is better than from cow's milk or iron-supplemented infant formula (>75 per cent, 30 per cent and 10 per cent respectively). The improved bioavailability may be related to lactoferrin, an iron-binding glycoprotein, which also inhibits bacterial growth. With the exception of vitamin K, all other vitamins are found in breast milk and therefore vitamin K is given to the baby to minimize the risk of haemorrhagic disease.

Prolactin

Prolactin is a long-chain polypeptide produced from the anterior pituitary; levels rise up to twenty-fold during pregnancy and lactation. Peak levels of prolactin are reached within 45 minutes of suckling but return to normal immediately after weaning and in non-breastfeeding mothers. The exact mechanism of action is not fully understood, but prolactin appears to have a direct action on the secretory cells to synthesize milk proteins. Prolactin is essential for lactation and it is hypothesized that nipple stimulation prevents the release of prolactin-inhibiting factor from the hypothalamus, thereby initiating the production of prolactin by the anterior pituitary. This theory is supported by the fact that lactation can be arrested with bromocriptine, a dopamine agonist that inhibits prolactin. A similar phenomenon occurs following pituitary necrosis (Sheehan's syndrome) when prolactin production ceases.

Oxytocin

Once milk has been produced under the influence of prolactin, it has to be delivered to the infant. The milk-ejection or let-down reflex is initiated by suckling, which stimulates the pulsatile release of oxytocin from the posterior pituitary. Oxytocin contracts the myoepithelial cells surrounding the alveoli as well as the myoepithelial cells lying longitudinally along the lactiferous ducts, thereby aiding the expulsion of milk. Oxytocin release can also be stimulated by visual, olfactory or auditory stimuli, e.g. hearing the baby cry, but can be inhibited by stress. Oxytocin can also stimulate uterine contractions, giving rise to the 'after-pains' of childbirth.

Breastfeeding

Women who opt to breastfeed tend to decide before or very early in their pregnancy. This decision is usually based on previous experience, influence of family or friends, culture and custom. A new mother who is unprepared for breastfeeding may find it a frustrating task and turn to bottle-feeding. There is now evidence to suggest that antenatal classes and literature on breastfeeding given antenatally may be beneficial.

The most common reasons mothers give for abandoning breastfeeding are inadequate milk production and sore and cracked nipples. Both these problems can be overcome by correct positioning of the baby on the breast (Fig. 20.3). The mouth should be placed over the nipple and areola so that suction created within the baby's mouth draws the breast tissue into a teat which extends as far back as the junction of the soft and hard palate. The tongue applies peristaltic force to the underside of the teat against the support of the hard palate. In this way there should be no to-and-fro movement of the teat in and out of the baby's mouth, thus minimizing friction. The mother should also be taught how to implement the rooting reflex. When the skin around the baby's mouth is touched, the mouth begins to gape. At this point the mother should reposition the baby so that the lower rim of the baby's mouth fits well below the nipple, allowing a liberal mouthful of breast tissue. When the baby is properly attached, breastfeeding should be pain free. The use of creams and ointments for cracked nipples has not been shown to be beneficial and the use of a nipple shield merely reduces milk production.

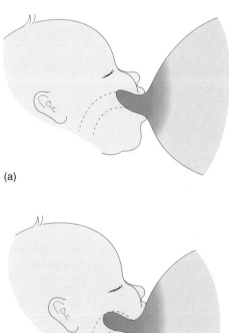

(a)

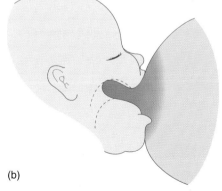

(b)

Figure 20.3 (a) Poor positioning. (b) Good positioning.

Although no study has identified the threshold of the critical time limit for successful breastfeeding, early suckling appears to be beneficial. However, this should not be rushed, and perhaps should be done initially under supervision when the mother is comfortable and in privacy.

There is no scientific evidence to justify a rigid breastfeeding schedule. Babies should be fed on demand and left on the breast until feeding finishes spontaneously. An imposed time limit on feeding can have a deleterious effect on calorie intake.

Supplementary feeds of formula, glucose or water are often given to breastfed infants in the belief that the baby is still hungry or thirsty. However, this is a misconception, as this practice merely increases the risk of total abandonment of breastfeeding.

Test-weighing infants before and after a feed to establish the ideal quantity of milk intake is an archaic practice that should be abandoned, as inappropriate action could prove hazardous.

There is evidence to suggest that dopamine receptor blockers, e.g. metoclopramide, sulpiride and domperidone, may be used to treat women who are temporarily unable to breastfeed. Sublingual or buccal oxytocin may also be used to augment lactation with good effect.

Advantages of breastfeeding
- Readily available at the right temperature and ideal nutritional value.
- Cheaper than formula feed.
- Associated with a reduction in:
  - childhood infective illnesses, especially gastroenteritis,
  - fertility with amenorrhoea,
  - atopic illnesses, e.g. eczema and asthma,
  - necrotizing enterocolitis in preterm babies,
  - juvenile diabetes,
  - childhood cancer, especially lymphoma,
  - pre-menopausal breast cancer.

Non-breastfeeding mothers

There are various reasons why a woman may choose not to breastfeed, ranging from personal choice to stillbirth. The United Nations has issued recommendations intended to discourage women infected with HIV from breastfeeding. In 1997, of the 600 000 HIV-infected children worldwide, up to one-third became infected through breastfeeding. Non-breastfeeding mothers may suffer considerable engorgement and breast pain. Fluid restriction and a tight brassiere have been shown to be equally effective as bromocryptine usage by the second week. Oestrogens are effective,

but not used frequently because of abnormal vaginal bleeding and increased risk of thromboembolism. Dopamine receptor stimulants such as bromocryptine and cabergoline inhibit prolactin and thus suppress lactation. Comparative studies of a single dose of cabergoline versus a twice-daily dose of bromocryptine for 14 days have shown that cabergoline is more effective and associated with fewer side effects and less rebound lactation. It is therefore the drug of choice for the suppression of lactation.

Breast disorders

Bloodstained nipple discharge

Bloodstained nipple discharge of pregnancy is typically bilateral and believed to be due to epithelial proliferation. It usually occurs in the second or third trimester of pregnancy and rarely persists beyond 2 months postpartum. As the condition is self-limiting, no investigation or treatment is necessary, and the woman should be reassured.

Painful nipples

The nipple can become very painful if the covering epithelium is denuded or if a fissure develops giving rise to 'cracked nipples'. The cause is usually attributed to poor positioning of the baby on the breast, although thrush (candidiasis) may also cause soreness. Cracked nipples are also associated with an increased risk of a breast abscess developing. Treatment involves resting the affected nipple and manually expressing milk. Breastfeeding should then be re-introduced gradually.

Galactocele

A galactocele is a retention cyst of the mammary ducts following blockage by inspissated secretions. It is identified as a fluctuant swelling with minimal pain and inflammation. It usually resolves spontaneously but may also be aspirated; with increasing discomfort, surgical excision may become necessary.

Breast engorgement

Engorgement of the breasts usually begins by the second or third postpartum day and if breastfeeding has not been effectively established, the over-distended and engorged breasts can be very uncomfortable. Breast engorgement may give rise to puerperal fever of up to 39 °C in 13 per cent of mothers. Although the fever rarely lasts more than 16 hours, other infective causes must be excluded. A number of remedies for the treatment of breast engorgement, such as manual expression, firm support, applying an ice bag and an electric breast pump, have all been recommended in the past, but allowing the baby easy access to the breast is the most effective method of treatment and prevention.

Mastitis

Inflammation of the breast is not always due to an infective process. Mastitis can occur when a blocked duct obstructs the flow of milk and distends the alveoli. If this pressure persists, the milk extravasates into the perilobular tissue, initiating an inflammatory process. The affected segment of the breast is painful and appears red and oedematous (Fig. 20.4). Flu-like symptoms develop associated with a tachycardia and pyrexia. In the first few postpartum days, about 15 per cent of women will develop a temperature of up to 39 °C, lasting less than 24 hours, due to breast engorgement. By contrast, in infective mastitis, the pyrexia develops later and persists for longer. In general, suppurative mastitis usually presents in the third to fourth postpartum week and is usually unilateral. Symptoms include rigors, fever, pain and reddened, swollen breasts. The most common infecting organism is *Staphylococcus aureus*, which is found in 40 per cent of women with mastitis. Other bacteria include coagulase-negative staphylococci and *Streptococcus viridans*. The most common sources of infection are, first, from the baby's nose or throat and, second, from an infected umbilical cord. Management includes isolation of the mother and baby, ceasing breastfeeding from the affected breast, expression of milk either manually or by electric pump, and microbiological culture and sensitivity of a sample of milk. Flucloxacillin can be commenced while awaiting sensitivity results.

About 10 per cent of women with mastitis develop a breast abscess. Treatment is by a radial surgical incision and drainage under general anaesthesia.

Contraception

The exact mechanism of lactational amenorrhoea is poorly understood, but the most plausible hypothesis is that during lactation there is inhibition of the normal pulsatile release of luteinizing hormone from the anterior pituitary. Breastfeeding therefore provides a contraceptive effect, but it is not totally reliable, as up to 10 per cent of women conceive during this period. However, it has recently been shown that a mother who is still in the phase of postpartum amenorrhoea while fully breastfeeding her baby has a less than 2 per cent chance of conceiving in the first 6 months. Although this is comparable to some of the other methods of contraception (see Chapter 6 in *Gynaecology by Ten Teachers*, 18th edition), most women in developed countries use some form of additional contraception such as barrier methods. If an intrauterine contraceptive device is preferred, it is best to wait at least 4 weeks to allow for involution. Care needs to be exercised in breastfeeding mothers, as there have been reports of increased rates of uterine perforation with the Lippes loop, but not with the T-shaped devices. The combined oral contraceptive pill enhances the risk of thrombosis in the early puerperium and can have an adverse effect on the quality and constituents of breast milk. The progesterone-only pill (the minipill) is therefore preferable and should be commenced about day 21 following delivery, prior to which there may be puerperal breakthrough bleeding. Injectable contraception, such as depot medroxyprogesterone acetate (Depo-Provera) given 3-monthly or Norethisterone enantate (Noristerat) given 2-monthly, is also very effective.

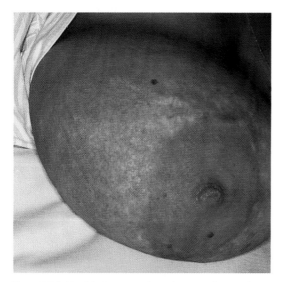

Figure 20.4 Mastitis demonstrating redness, oedema and engorged veins.

However, injectable contraception given within 48 hours of delivery for convenience can cause breakthrough bleeding and therefore should preferably be given 5–6 weeks postpartum.

Sterilization can be offered to mothers who are certain that they have completed their family. Tubal ligation can be performed during Caesarean section or by the open method (mini-laparotomy) in the first few postpartum days. However, it is better delayed until after 6 weeks postpartum, when it can be done by laparoscopy. This allows the mother to spend more time in comfort with her newborn baby and, furthermore, laparoscopic clip sterilization is less traumatic and associated with a lower failure rate.

Women who are not breastfeeding should commence the pill within 4 weeks of delivery, as ovulation can occur by 6 weeks postpartum.

Pelvic floor exercises

It is a widespread belief that pelvic floor exercises tone up the muscles of the pelvic floor and should therefore be advocated in the postpartum period. However, large randomized trials to evaluate their benefit in preventing genital prolapse, urinary incontinence or anal incontinence are lacking. There is also no evidence that antenatal exercises prevent incontinence or prolapse. However, as general exercise is known to strengthen striated muscle and pelvic floor exercises are unlikely to be harmful, women are still taught postnatal exercises. This should also serve to cultivate a feeling of pelvic floor awareness, so that women with pelvic floor dysfunction seek medical help sooner.

Perinatal death

- Stillbirth: a baby born with no sign of life.
- Perinatal death: stillbirth $\geqslant$24 weeks' gestation or death within 7 days of birth.
- Live birth: any baby that shows signs of life irrespective of gestation.

Bereavement counselling following perinatal death requires special expertise and is best left to a senior clinician and a trained bereavement counsellor. Inappropriate management of this traumatic period can have a devastating effect on the woman's emotional and marital life. Effective communication and support are crucial and women should be encouraged to make contact with organizations such as SANDS (Stillbirth and Neonatal Death Society).

The grieving process can be facilitated by practices such as seeing and holding the dead baby, naming the baby, and taking hand/foot prints and photographs. Coming to terms with the perinatal death of a twin is even more difficult because the mother has to mourn one baby and celebrate the arrival of the other.

Table 20.4 – Investigations into perinatal death

Investigations	Reason
Full blood count	Anaemia, leukocytosis
Clotting screen	Disseminated intravascular coagulation
Kleihauer test	Feto-maternal transfusion
Virology, infection screen	Cytomegalovirus, parvovirus
Autoantibody screen (anti-cardiolipin and lupus anticoagulant)	Antiphospholipid syndrome, systemic lupus erythematosus
Blood and placenta culture	Infections such as *Listeria monocytogenes*
Antibodies in rhesus-negative women	Haemolytic disease
Toxoplasma antibodies	Toxoplasmosis
Skin biopsy/cardiac blood/placental biopsy	Chromosome analysis
Full-body X-ray or MRI	To identify congenital defects

MRI, magnetic resonance imaging.

A post mortem is the most important diagnostic test, even though there may be no positive findings. Couples who decline a post mortem may do so because of religious reasons or because they fear mutilation. In this situation, a partial post mortem should be discussed whereby an autopsy of a single organ or a tissue biopsy can be performed. A full-body X-ray or, preferably, magnetic resonance imaging (MRI) may be useful in some cases (Table 20.4).

If the baby was stillborn, a stillbirth certificate should be completed by the attending doctor; otherwise, the paediatrician should complete the certificate. The certificate should be given to the parents to register the death with the Registrar of Births and Deaths. Funeral arrangements can be made privately or by the hospital.

Every mother who has lost a baby should have the 6-week postnatal visit at hospital.

The postnatal examination

This is carried out at about 6 weeks postpartum by the general practitioner or by the obstetrician if delivery had been complicated. The examination includes an assessment of the woman's mental and physical health as well as the progress of the baby. In particular, direct questions must be asked about urinary, bowel and sexual function. Incontinence and dyspareunia are embarrassing issues that women do not volunteer to discuss readily. Weight, urine analysis and blood pressure are checked and a complete general, abdominal and pelvic examination is performed. If a cervical smear is due, it can be taken, although it is preferable to take one after 3 months postpartum. Contraception and pelvic floor exercises are also discussed.

CASE HISTORY

A 42-year-old woman who delivered vaginally 4 days previously presents with heavy, fresh vaginal bleeding and clots. She admits to feeling unwell and experiencing cramp-like abdominal pains.

On examination, she has a temperature of 38.2 °C and there is mild suprapubic tenderness. Vaginal examination revealed blood clots but no products of conception. The cervix admitted only the tip of a finger and the uterus was slightly tender and measured 18 weeks in size. Looking back at her delivery notes, it was noted that the placental membranes were ragged at delivery.

What is the most likely diagnosis?

Secondary PPH due to infected retained products of conception.

How should the patient be managed?

- Blood cultures.
- Intravenous broad-spectrum antibiotics, e.g. cephalosporin and metronidazole.
- Although a pelvic ultrasound may confirm the diagnosis, it has the potential to mislead and is not a prerequisite when the diagnosis is obvious.
- Surgical evacuation of retained products in the uterus.

⚒ Key Points

- The puerperium refers to the 6-week period following childbirth.
- Care during this transition period is crucial before the woman returns to her pre-pregnant state.
- Perineal discomfort is a major complaint following vaginal delivery and therefore adequate analgesia should be prescribed.
- Common disorders include puerperal sepsis, thromboembolism, bowel and bladder dysfunction.

Chapter 21

Psychiatric disorders in pregnancy and the puerperium

OVERVIEW

Pregnancy affects mental illness in a complex way. It is vital for obstetricians, midwives and other healthcare professionals to be alert to the sometimes subtle indicators of impending mental illness and to be aware of the issues surrounding diagnosis and treatment in pregnancy and the puerperium. Remember that pregnancy is one of the greatest risk factors for mental illness in a woman's life.

The importance of psychiatry to obstetrics

Childbirth contributes a substantial risk to the mental health of women. Although the antenatal period is not a particularly high-risk time for the onset of new psychiatric disease, minor disorders do affect a significant minority of pregnant women (see below). More significantly, in the year following childbirth, women who were previously well have a greatly elevated risk of being admitted to a psychiatric hospital, being referred to a psychiatrist, suffering from a psychotic illness or developing severe depression. This risk is higher than their lifetime risk, and is much greater than for other women or men.

Incidence of postpartum mental disorders

- 'Depression'   15–30%
- Major depressive illness   10%
- Moderate/severe depressive illness   3–5%
- Referral to a psychiatrist   1.7%
- Admission to a psychiatric unit   0.4%
- Admission with puerperal psychosis   0.2%

More than 80 per cent of women with postpartum psychiatric disease will be suffering from their first-ever psychiatric illness.

Pregnant women with pre-existing mental illness, or who book with a previous history, also present a challenge to the maternity services. Pregnancy, childbirth and the stresses of life as a new parent may destabilize conditions that had previously been under control. Certain pharmacological treatments may be contraindicated in pregnancy and suitable alternatives have to be found. Optimizing the new relationship between mother and baby may require help from specialist services.

The impact of psychiatric disease in pregnancy has been emphasized by the Confidential Enquiry into Maternal Deaths (*Why mothers die 1997–1999* – see Chapter 3). Twelve per cent of all direct, indirect and late indirect maternal deaths were the fatal consequence of psychiatric illness, with the majority of these accounted for by suicide. Of special note, suicide during pregnancy is unusually violent (shootings, hangings), in contrast with suicide attempts in younger women, which commonly take the form of overdose and are less frequently successful. This highlights the need for specialized healthcare teams who appreciate the unique effect that pregnancy has on mental well-being.

Although not all mental illness associated with pregnancy is predictable, identifiable risk factors do exist, as do screening methods designed to detect early psychiatric disease. Prophylactic treatments can be instituted to prevent the onset of symptoms. It is the responsibility of all healthcare professionals looking after pregnant women to identify these risk factors, institute plans of surveillance and care, and refer to specialist services where necessary.

'Normal' emotional and psychological changes during pregnancy

Diagnosing mental illness in pregnancy is complicated by the wide variety of 'normal' emotional and behavioural changes which can occur. Common patterns include the following.

Antenatal
- Mixed feelings about being pregnant.
- Fears of being unable to cope.
- Increased emotional liability.
- Minor depressive symptoms (most marked in the first trimester).
- Anxiety and fears regarding delivery.
- Obsessional thoughts regarding the safety of the baby (more common in the third trimester, particularly in women who have specific pregnancy complications).

Postnatal
- *The 'pinks'*: for the first 24–48 hours following delivery, it is very common for women to experience an elevation of mood, a feeling of excitement, some over-activity and difficulty sleeping.
- *The 'blues'*: as many as 80 per cent of women may experience the 'postnatal blues' in the first 2 weeks after delivery. Fatigue, short temperedness, difficulty sleeping, depressed mood and tearfulness are common but usually mild and resolve spontaneously in the majority of cases.

The following psychological disruptions should not be considered normal during pregnancy and require further assessment.
- Panic attacks.
- Episodes of low mood of prolonged duration (>2 weeks).
- Low self-esteem.

- Guilt or hopelessness.
- Thoughts of self-harm or suicide.
- Any mood changes that disrupt normal social functioning.
- 'Biological' symptoms (e.g. poor appetite, early wakening).
- Change in 'affect'.

Management of pregnancy in women with pre-existing psychiatric disease

Women with pre-existing mental health issues usually come to the attention of the maternity services at booking. Appropriate screening questions should form part of all routine booking histories. The mental health services should be involved at an early point in the pregnancies of women who have either ongoing disease or a past history of significant mental illness.

Schizophrenia

Although older antipsychotic medications may have impaired fertility, this is not the case with newer drugs. Women with schizophrenia may be at greater risk of unplanned pregnancies as a result of their illness. Fluphenazine and flupenthixol do not have convincing teratogenic effects and the risks to the woman of stopping these drugs suddenly, with the real risk of disease relapse, are considered greater than any theoretical risks of fetal exposure. Under the guidance of a mental health specialist, it may be possible to reduce the dose in the third trimester to minimize levels in the newborn and prevent extrapyramidal and anticholinergic side effects.

Ideally, women with schizophrenia should receive pre-pregnancy counselling from their psychiatrist prior to conception. Issues to discuss are their capacity to be a successful parent in the long term, as well as the effects of pregnancy and the postpartum period on their mental health. Schizophrenia may seriously limit parenting skills and there is a significant risk that an affected mother will not ultimately remain the primary carer of her own child. Extra social support and surveillance will usually be necessary, but this is often tolerated poorly by individuals with schizophrenia. Schizophrenia demonstrates multi-factorial inheritance and the offspring of affected parents are at increased risk of developing the condition.

Postnatally, the woman and her baby may benefit from an inpatient stay in a specialized mother and baby unit under the review and encouragement of a perinatal mental health team. Breastfeeding is to be encouraged to promote bonding with the newborn, and neuroleptic drugs in moderate doses are not a contraindication to this.

Bipolar affective disorder

This condition, also known as 'manic depression', is usually controlled with a combination of mood-stabilizing drugs (lithium, carbamazepine and sodium valproate), antidepressants and neuroleptics. Lithium carries a risk of causing cardiac defects if used in the first trimester and may cause fetal hypothyroidism, polyhydramnios and diabetes insipidus if used in the third trimester. Carbamazepine and valproate are also recognized teratogens. Stopping these medications abruptly before or just after conception carries a risk of causing a relapse, which may be very harmful. If the illness is stable, the mood stabilizers may be reduced and replaced by antidepressants with or without neuroleptics. Ideally, this is done following pre-pregnancy counselling when the decision to stop contraception has been made. Ultimately, the fetal risks of continuing certain preparations may have to be accepted if the maternal risks of stopping treatment are thought to be too great.

Postpartum relapse occurs in approximately 50 per cent of women with bipolar illness and it is important that preventive therapy is commenced immediately after delivery. Lithium is contraindicated in breast-feeding, and the woman may be advised to bottle-feed so that it can be used in the postpartum period. Alternatively, a neuroleptic or antidepressant can be used for prophylaxis.

Depression

At least 1 in 10 women will suffer some form of depression throughout their lifetime. There is no evidence that pregnancy reduces the risk of a relapse or improves the mood of women with active depression. There is ample experience with the use of tricyclic antidepressant drugs during pregnancy and women can be reassured that they carry no teratogenic risk and that they are safe to take whilst breastfeeding.

The situation with selective serotonin reuptake inhibitors (SSRIs) is less clear. Studies have shown a possible increase in the number of minor congenital abnormalities and a link with increased preterm labour risk and low birth weight. However, no causative association with fetal harm has yet been demonstrated and their use in younger women is increasing. Minimization of the dose of all antidepressant drugs in the late third trimester will limit the levels in the newborn infant and help to prevent anticholinergic and extrapyramidal side effects in the neonate.

Women with a history of depression not related to pregnancy carry between a 1 in 3 and 1 in 5 risk of a major postpartum depression. If the previous depressive illness occurred in the postpartum period, the recurrence risk is as high as 50 per cent. At the very least, skilled monitoring should be planned for the postnatal period. Prophylactic medications should be considered.

Anxiety disorders

Pregnancy, the anticipation of labour and the arrival of a new baby may all exacerbate an existing anxiety disorder. Benzodiazepine use during the first trimester may be associated with an increased risk of cleft lip and/or palate, although the evidence is somewhat contradictory. Neonatal withdrawal effects are evident in the babies born to women who have used regular higher doses during pregnancy, and their use should be limited where possible. Breastfeeding may help to reduce the severity of the neonatal withdrawal (neonatal abstinence syndrome), as small amounts do reach breast milk.

New-onset psychiatric disease in pregnancy

Women with no personal history of psychiatric disease are nevertheless at increased risk of mental illness simply because they are pregnant.

Antenatal

Although the antepartum period is not considered a high-risk time for the onset of new psychiatric illness, all conditions may nevertheless present during this time.

The normal emotional changes occurring during pregnancy (see above) may become exaggerated and potentially harmful. Anxiety associated with panic attacks and specific phobias relating to labour (toko-phobia) or needles may require treatment with cognitive or behavioural therapy, benzodiazepines or SSRIs. Depression may have its onset during the pregnancy and is a strong risk factor for postpartum depression. Both pharmacological and non-drug treatment may be necessary.

Postnatal

The greater part of new-onset psychiatric illness presents in the puerperium. Affective (mood) disorders account for the majority and these vary in severity from the mildest (minor postnatal depression) to moderate and severe postnatal depression and, in the extreme, puerperal psychosis (a variant of manic depression or bipolar disorder). As discussed in the overview, the postnatal period represents perhaps the highest risk period in a woman's life for the development of a psychiatric disorder. Although a previous history of moderate to severe depression or bipolar disorder is a significant risk factor, for many women this represents their first episode of mental illness.

Puerperal psychosis
This very severe disorder affects between 1 in 500 and 1 in 1000 women after delivery. It rarely presents before the third postpartum day (most commonly the fifth) but usually does so before 4 weeks. The onset is characteristically abrupt, with a rapidly changing clinical picture.

The aetiology of postpartum psychosis is discussed below but remains unclear.

Risk factors for postpartum psychosis

- Previous history of puerperal psychosis
- Previous history of severe non-postpartum depressive illness
- Family history (first/second-degree relative) of bipolar disorder/affective psychosis

---

S   Symptoms of puerperal psychosis

The characteristic symptoms of puerperal psychosis include:

- restless agitation
- insomnia
- perplexity
- confusion
- fear and suspicion
- delusions (often involving the baby)
- hallucinations
- failure to eat and drink
- thoughts of self-harm
- depressive symptoms (guilt, self-worthlessness, hopelessness)
- loss of insight.

Management
The patient should be referred urgently to a psychiatrist and will usually require admission to a psychiatric unit. If possible, this should be a mother and baby unit under the supervision of a specialist perinatal mental healthcare team. These units prevent separation of the baby from its mother and this may help with bonding and the future relationship.

Treatments include:
- acute treatment with neuroleptics, such as chlorpromazine or haloperidol,
- acute treatment of mania with lithium carbonate,
- electroconvulsive therapy (ECT) – particularly for severe depressive psychoses,
- antidepressants (which will take 10–14 days to be effective) as a second-line treatment.

Recovery usually occurs over 4–6 weeks, although treatment with antidepressants will be needed for at least 6 months. These women remain at high risk of pregnancy-related and non-pregnancy related recurrences. The risk of recurrence in a future pregnancy is approximately 1 in 2, particularly if the next pregnancy occurs within 2 years of the one complicated by puerperal psychosis. Women with a previous history of puerperal psychosis should be considered for prophylactic lithium, started on the first postpartum day.

CASE HISTORY

Mrs A is a 32-year-old teacher with a stable marriage and comfortable social circumstances. Her father had severe depressive illness, aged 50 years, and was treated with ECT.

In her first pregnancy she developed an acute-onset psychosis on the seventh postpartum day following the delivery at 37 weeks' gestation of twins. Her pregnancy had been uncomplicated. She was admitted to a mother and baby unit and for the next 3 days had severe behavioural disturbance and hallucinations, delusions and an elevated mood. This state responded to haloperidol. However, by the 11th postpartum day, her mood and cognitions had become clearly depressed and she would not eat or drink. She was treated with ECT and recovered well. She remained well and was a devoted and competent mother.

Four years later, she was re-admitted to the mother and baby unit on the eighth day postpartum following a full-term normal delivery of a singleton. Her mental state was identical to the previous episode. She and her husband asked for ECT. She recovered fully by the second postpartum week.

Ten years later she has had no further pregnancies and no further psychiatric episodes.

Postpartum (non-psychotic) depression

Depression can be classified as 'minor' or 'major'. Major depression can be divided into 'mild', 'moderate' and 'severe' categories. It is important to distinguish postpartum depression of any degree from the postpartum 'blues'.

Between 10 and 15 per cent of women will suffer with some form of depression in the first year after the delivery of their baby. At least 7 per cent will satisfy the criteria for mild major depressive illness (see symptom box) and many more could be described as having minor depression; 3–5 per cent will suffer severe major postnatal depression. Without treatment, most women will recover spontaneously within 3–6 months; however, 1 in 10 will remain depressed at 1 year.

Risk factors for postnatal depression

- Past history of psychiatric illness
- Depression during pregnancy
- Obstetric factors (e.g. Caesarean section/fetal or neonatal loss)
- Social isolation and deprivation
- Poor relationships
- Recent adverse life events (bereavement/illness)
- Severe postnatal 'blues'

The importance of psychosocial factors in the aetiology of non-psychotic postpartum depression is in contrast to the biological factors predisposing to puerperal psychosis.

Adverse sequelae of postnatal depression

Immediate
- Physical morbidity
- Suicide/infanticide
- Prolonged psychiatric morbidity
- Damaged social attachments to infant
- Disrupted emotional development of infant

Later
- Social/cognitive effects on the child
- Psychiatric morbidity in the child
- Marital breakdown
- Future mental health problems

P Understanding the pathophysiology

Although psychosocial factors are clearly of importance in the aetiology of milder forms of postnatal depression, this is not so clearly the case for severe postnatal depression or puerperal psychosis, in which biological risk factors such as family history predominate. The constancy of incidence across cultures and the temporal relationship with childbirth would tend to suggest a neuroendocrine basis for the more severe conditions. Changes in cortisol, oxytocin, endorphins, thyroxine, progesterone and oestrogen have all been implicated in the causation. Comparable dramatic changes in steroidal hormones outside of the postpartum period have a well-known

(continued)

association with affective psychoses and mood disorders. A plausible recent theory is that the sudden fall in oestrogen postpartum triggers a hypersensitivity of certain dopamine receptors in a predisposed group of women and may be responsible for the severe mood disturbance which follows. The occurrence and the severity of the 'postnatal blues' are thought to be related to both the absolute level of progesterone and the relative drop from a prepartum level. However, there is no clear association between the 'postpartum blues' and affective psychoses, and no evidence as yet to implicate progesterone in the aetiology of puerperal psychosis or severe postnatal depression.

S Symptoms of severe postnatal depression

- Early-morning wakening
- Poor appetite
- Diurnal mood variation (worse in the mornings)
- Low energy and libido
- Loss of enjoyment
- Lack of interest
- Impaired concentration
- Tearfulness
- Feelings of guilt and failure
- Anxiety
- Thoughts of self-harm/suicide
- Thoughts of harm to the baby

Clinical features

In contrast to puerperal psychosis, non-psychotic postpartum depression usually presents later in the postnatal period, most commonly around 6 weeks, with a more gradual onset. The 6-week postnatal check is an ideal opportunity to detect early postnatal depression, but the signs are often missed. The Edinburgh Postnatal Depression Scale is a screening questionnaire which all women should be asked to complete at their postnatal check. Particular attention should be paid to the assessment of women with risk factors for postnatal depression.

Severe postnatal depression may present earlier than milder forms and in this group, biological risk factors may be more important than psychosocial factors.

Treatment options for postnatal depression include:

- remedy of social factors,
- non-directive counselling,
- cognitive–behavioural therapy,
- drug therapy.

The earlier the onset of the depression and the more severe it becomes, the more likely is it that formal psychiatric intervention will be needed. However, randomized trials have demonstrated the benefits of non-directive counselling from specially trained midwives and health visitors. Even simple encouragement to join a local postnatal group may prevent social isolation and limit depression.

If pharmacotherapy is deemed necessary, tricyclic antidepressants or SSRIs are appropriate. There is good evidence to support the safety of the former in breastfeeding, less so for the latter. However, SSRIs in usual doses are probably safe.

There has been a vogue in the past for treating postnatal depression with progestogens in the erroneous belief that the fall in progesterone levels postpartum is the cause of postnatal depression. There is no good evidence to support this, and it may even be harmful if the use of other effective treatments is delayed because of it. This practice should therefore be avoided. High-dose oestrogen regimens have been tried in research trials, but these are not used routinely.

Women with a past history of severe postnatal depression may be candidates for some form of prophylactic treatment, and the help of a specialist in perinatal mental health care should be sought before delivery.

CASE HISTORY

Mrs B is a 42-year-old professional woman who has been married for 16 years and in comfortable circumstances. She has no previous personal or family history of psychiatric disorder. However, she is always anxious, with marked obsessional (perfectionist) personality traits and in the past had not coped well with changes. She had a long history of infertility investigations and had conceived her two children with in-vitro fertilization.

Following the birth of her first child, she found it difficult to adjust to her new lifestyle and suffered from self-doubt and mild anxiety and depression, which spontaneously resolved following her return to work at 6 months postpartum.

Four years later, following the birth of her second child, she became severely depressed. By 6 weeks postpartum she had marked psychomotor slowing and impaired concentration and efficiency. She had early-morning wakening and her mood and coping abilities were worst in the morning (diurnal variation of mood). She was very anxious and had panic attacks triggered by intrusive morbid thoughts of some terrible harm coming to her infant. She had overvalued ideas of guilt and incompetence and actively concealed her state from her health visitor and GP. A good friend insisted that she seek help.

Within 2 weeks of starting a tricyclic antidepressant, Dothiepin, she began to recover and was quite well by 3 months postpartum. She reduced her antidepressants gradually and stopped taking them 6 months later and remained well.

Key Points

- All women should be asked at booking about personal or family history of psychiatric illness.
- Close collaboration is recommended between obstetrician and psychiatrist for women with mental illness, a previous history of severe mental ill-health, or a strong family history of bipolar affective disorder.
- Women with previous serious mental illness should be appropriately counselled regarding the recurrence risks associated with pregnancy.
- Specialist perinatal psychiatric services should be available to all women.
- The prescribing of psychoactive drugs in pregnancy and breastfeeding should be done with care under the guidance of a psychiatrist with particular interest in pregnancy-related mental illness.
- Breastfeeding rarely needs to be avoided in women using psychotropic medications.
- There is an adequate range of drugs available to safely treat the pregnant or lactating woman who is mentally ill.

Neonatology

OVERVIEW

More than half a million babies are born every year in the UK, 4 million in the USA, 25 million in India and over 200 million worldwide. In the industrialized countries of the world, less than 1 per cent of these babies will die, and at least half the deaths are amongst premature babies with a birth weight <1.5 kg. The picture is very different in the least developed countries, where the death rate is between 2 and 8 per cent. The countries of sub-Saharan Africa suffer the highest perinatal mortality rates in the world, around 80 per 1000 live births. Throughout the world, babies are still dying from prematurity, infections, congenital malformations, and hypoxia or trauma acquired intrapartum.

The challenge of neonatology

Neonatology is a relatively new sub-specialty which has achieved some spectacular successes, most notably that of halving the mortality for very premature babies. Complex surgery can be performed safely, artificial nutrition maintained for weeks, and even the tiniest babies can be intubated and ventilated. Challenges remain; for example there has been very little advance in the treatment of hypoxic–ischaemic encephalopathy, and infection is still a problem. Advances in fetal medicine now allow antenatal diagnosis of a whole range of disorders, including cystic adenomatoid malformation of the lung, arachnoid cysts of the brain, and dilatation of the renal pelvis. For many of these conditions there is very little information about the natural history of the disorder if left untreated, and this makes counselling and management difficult. Early discharge ('drive-through' delivery) and choice about the place of delivery have fragmented the provision of 'well baby' care. This means that all those who come into contact with newborns need to be informed about issues such as prophylaxis against vitamin K deficiency bleeding, the promotion of breastfeeding, the management of jaundice, the prevention of hypoglycaemia and the implementation of child health screening policies. The occasional baby with a rare medical condition such as life-threatening congenital heart disease or a small skin lesion overlying a spinal cord defect needs a fast track to highly specialized and appropriate services, and the challenge here lies in early recognition that there is a significant problem.

Organization and provision of neonatal care

About 10 per cent of all babies are admitted to UK neonatal units, with figures for different hospitals ranging from 4 to 35 per cent. Most of these admissions are for 'special care', for example jaundice requiring phototherapy or blood glucose monitoring. About 2 per cent of babies need full intensive care, mainly because they are born very prematurely and need artificial ventilation for respiratory distress syndrome (RDS). Table 22.1 gives examples taken from the current UK definitions of special care, high dependency care and intensive care. The pattern of neonatal intensive care in the UK is fragmented: there are more than 300 maternity units, a quarter of which deliver fewer than 1000 babies each year and hence have a

---

Table 22.1 – Categories of babies requiring neonatal care

Level 1 intensive care (maximal intensive care)

Care given in an intensive care nursery that provides continuous supervision by a suitably trained nurse, ideally 1:1, with immediate medical aid available.
  Examples of babies who need intensive care are those:
1. receiving any respiratory support via a tracheal tube,
2. who are <29 weeks' gestation and <48 hours old.

Level 2 intensive care (high-dependency intensive care)

Care given in an intensive care nursery that provides care by specially trained nursing staff, who may care for two babies at a time.
  Examples of babies who need level 2 intensive care are those:
1. requiring parenteral nutrition,
2. having convulsions,
3. having frequent apnoeic attacks,
4. requiring oxygen treatment and weighing <1500 g.

Special care

Care given in a special care nursery that provides care and treatment exceeding normal routine care. Nurses may care for four babies at a time. Some aspects of special care may be undertaken by a mother supervised by qualified nursing staff.
  Examples of babies who need special care are those:
1. being tube fed,
2. undergoing phototherapy,
3. receiving special monitoring (for example frequent glucose or bilirubin estimations).

Normal care

Provided for babies who themselves have no medical reason to be in hospital.
  Examples include:
1. maternal psychiatric illness requiring close observation of mother and baby,
2. social problems such as homelessness.

Source: British Association of Perinatal Medicine.

very small requirement for intensive care facilities. The UK Department of Health reviewed the service in 2003, and has recommended the development of managed care networks. The aims are to link units in a hub-and-spoke fashion, to develop common guidelines and policies, and to have enough capacity to deliver all levels of neonatal care to the population living within a defined geographical area which a single 'network' will serve, thus reducing long-distance travel. The impact that this considerable restructuring will have on maternity services has not yet been assessed, and there is no doubt that increased cot capacity will be essential if this ideal is to be achieved.

Delivery room care

The transition from intrauterine to extrauterine life

The vast majority of babies achieve a remarkably smooth transition from intrauterine to extrauterine life, making their first respiratory efforts within 10 seconds of birth. Fetal lungs are filled with 'lung liquid', a fluid that is important for normal lung development and growth. During labour, the production of lung liquid ceases and reabsorption begins. Lung liquid is squeezed out of the thorax during vaginal delivery. Finally, the baby takes his first gasp, establishing an air–liquid interface which moves rapidly down through the lungs. The last vestiges of lung liquid are then absorbed by the lymphatics and the pulmonary capillaries. At the same time as the lungs are filled with air, the blood supply to them increases dramatically. Pulmonary blood flow is low in fetal life because a high resistance is actively maintained in the pulmonary capillaries. Immediately after birth, the pulmonary vascular resistance starts to fall. The fall is driven by the release of vasoactive substances, including prostaglandins and nitric oxide, and by the presence of oxygenated blood in the pulmonary capillaries themselves.

Infants who fail to breathe after birth may do so as a result of a deprivation of oxygen and blood supply to the brain before birth (hypoxia–ischaemia, or asphyxia), or because they have a central nervous system or muscle disease, or because they are systemically ill with infection. The possible placental and other mechanisms of hypoxia–ischaemia are discussed on page 323. Our understanding of the newborn's response to asphyxia is based on the classic primate

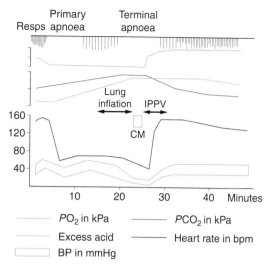

Figure 22.1 The response to asphyxia. (IPPV, intermittent positive-pressure ventilation; CM, cardiac massage.) (Reproduced with permission from the Northern Region handbook.)

experiments of Dawes. The changes in respiration and heart rate following asphyxia are illustrated in Figure 22.1. At birth, the asphyxiated infant may have taken his last gasp (terminal apnoea) or be in the phase of primary apnoea. A baby in terminal apnoea is unlikely to recover without intubation and positive-pressure ventilation, whereas a baby in primary apnoea can auto-resuscitate by gasping, and responds quickly to simple resuscitation.

All professionals who attend deliveries must be able to recognize when a baby is not establishing normal respiration and circulation, and be trained to initiate resuscitation. Certain situations are clearly high risk, and a person with intubation skills should be present at the delivery. Examples of such situations are given in Table 22.2, but about 20–30 per cent of babies who require resuscitation do not fall into high-risk categories. Our inability to predict which babies will fail to make a successful transition to extrauterine life is the reason why all those who attend deliveries have a responsibility to maintain their neonatal resuscitation skills. In the UK, the Resuscitation Council has developed a Newborn Life Support Course, and there are similar such courses in the USA and Europe.

The Apgar score
The Apgar score is a tool which assists in the recognition of an infant who is failing to make a successful transition to extrauterine life. This is exactly what the

Table 22.2 – Deliveries at which a trained neonatal resuscitator should be present

Preterm deliveries
Vaginal breech deliveries
Thick meconium staining of the amniotic fluid
Significant fetal distress
Significant antepartum haemorrhage
Serious fetal abnormality (e.g. hydrops, diaphragmatic hernia)
Rotational forceps or vacuum deliveries
Caesarean section – unless elective and under regional anaesthesia
Multiple deliveries

score was designed to do, and in this respect it performs admirably. The reason for a low Apgar score may not be asphyxia, but the baby certainly has a problem, and the sooner it is recognized and treated the better. The original Apgar score (Table 22.3) includes an item (grimace) that reports the infant's response to a suction catheter. Frequent deep suction of the oropharynx can cause bradycardia, and although regular recording of the Apgar score is to be encouraged, this item carries less weight than the heart rate, colour or breathing pattern. The Apgar score is usually recorded at 1 and 5 minutes. If the Apgar score is still low at 5 minutes, further observations should be made at intervals. The Apgar score cannot replace a detailed narrative describing the baby's condition, the

resuscitative efforts and the response to resuscitation. Recording the Apgar score is helpful because it has become an internationally recognized shorthand way of summarizing the condition of babies at birth and their response to resuscitation.

Resuscitation

Babies fall into one of three categories within a minute of birth.

1. Pink, breathing, with good tone and activity with a heart rate of >100 beats per minute (bpm). Leave this baby alone, preferably with his mother. If the baby has been given to you at the resuscitaire, dry him, wrap him in a warm towel and give him back to his mother. Do not suck him out; this risks producing a vagal bradycardia and cools him.
2. Not breathing regularly, but with a heart rate of >100 bpm and centrally cyanosed. Dry the baby and place him under a radiant heat source wrapped in a warm, dry towel. Drying often provides enough stimulation to induce breathing, but gentle rubbing can also be used. If there is no response, begin active resuscitation using five 'inflation breaths' via a bag and mask (see below), continue with regular breaths, and call for help.
3. Not breathing *or* has a heart rate of <100 bpm *or* is pale. These babies are usually completely floppy. This baby is in need of prompt resuscitation and will not recover without it. Dry him quickly, place him on the resuscitation surface in a warm, dry towel and call for help. Initiate basic resuscitation with mask ventilation. If the heart rate remains

Table 22.3 – The Apgar score

	Score	0	1	2
A	Appearance: central trunk colour	White or blue all over	Pink with blue extremities	Pink all over
P	Pulse rate[a]	Absent	<100 bpm	>100 bpm
G	Grimace (response to stimulation)	Nil	Grimace	Cry or cough
A	Activity (muscle tone)	Limp	Some flexion	Well flexed, active movement
R	Respiratory effort	Absent	Gasping or irregular	Regular or strong cry

[a] Best to record the actual rate.

<60 bpm, commence chest compressions. If there is not a rapid response, proceed to intubation as soon as a person with the necessary skill arrives. Stay to help; a full-blown resuscitation is a job for at least two people.

Remember that, whilst time is of the essence in neonatal resuscitation, this is no excuse for rough handling or sloppy thermal care. Remember, too, that the parents will be extremely anxious; watch what you say to other team members in their hearing and always spare some time to talk to them as soon as possible. Throwing the laryngoscope down, tipping the flat batteries on the floor and stamping on them may seem appropriate at the time, but will create an image that will never fade from the parents' minds. Even if you intubate the baby within seconds with the reserve laryngoscope, if he does badly, the episode will be replayed time and time again, and if you are unlucky, you may be faced with an unpleasant hour or two facing a cross-examination on your actions.

Lung inflation through a facemask

Position the baby face upwards on a resuscitation surface; a head-down slope is not necessary. The head should be supported in a neutral position to keep the tongue from obstructing the back of the pharynx: use a small folded towel under the shoulders if it helps. Gently suction the mouth and nostrils to remove debris. Choose a facemask that covers the baby's mouth and nose but does not press on the eyes or overhang the chin (Fig. 22.2a). Hold the mask over the baby's face with one hand, using some of the fingers of the same hand to lift the chin and support the jaw (jaw thrust; Fig. 22.2b). Begin to ventilate the lungs with air or oxygen using the source provided, but **never, ever** connect a baby directly to the hospital oxygen or air supply without a suitable pressure-limiting device in the circuit. Medical gases are supplied at far too high a pressure for babies, who only need a pressure of about 30 cmH$_2$O to expand their lungs. Make sure the chest is moving with the ventilator breaths and start with about five 'inflation breaths' of 30–35 cmH$_2$O lasting for 1–2 seconds. Then reduce the pressure to that which is just sufficient to move the chest, usually about 20 cmH$_2$O, and continue to give about 30 breaths per minute.

Chest compression

Babies whose heart rate fails to rise above 60 bpm after a minute or two of effective ventilation should

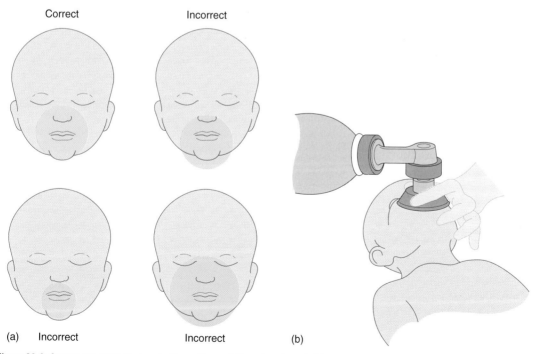

Correct   Incorrect

(a)   Incorrect   Incorrect   (b)

Figure 22.2 Correct use of the facemask. (From *Resuscitation of newborn babies*, 1998. RCPCH and RCOG, BMJ Publications, with permission.)

be given chest compression. Seize the baby's thorax with both hands, and place both thumbs over the lower sternum, just below an imaginary line joining the baby's nipples. Encircle the baby's chest with the rest of both your hands, supporting the spine with your fingers. Press down on the lower sternum sufficiently hard to depress it about one-third of the depth of the baby's chest. Co-ordinate chest compression with ventilatory breaths and give about 90 compressions to 30 breaths per minute (a ratio of 3:1).

Use of drugs during resuscitation

Drugs are very rarely required during neonatal resuscitation and deciding to use them is a job for an experienced operator. Very occasionally, a baby has depressed respiration because the mother was given pethidine between 1 and 6 hours prior to delivery, and these babies can remain sleepy and reluctant to feed for 24–48 hours. Naloxone (Narcan) is a specific opiate antagonist which can reverse the effects of pethidine and should be given in a dose of 100 μg/kg, which is 0.25 mL/kg of the standard-strength solution. 'Neonatal' Narcan has a concentration of 20 μg/mL and should no longer be used. Naloxone is specifically contraindicated in babies born to drug-abusing mothers.

Failure to respond to resuscitation

Most babies who are depressed at birth respond readily to resuscitative efforts. Before considering whether to abandon resuscitation, check the equipment: check the position and size of the endotracheal tube; give intravenous adrenaline twice and consider giving bicarbonate and glucose. Exclude a pneumothorax, if necessary by needling the chest. Consider giving uncross-matched O-negative blood if the baby looks pale, because massive feto-maternal haemorrhage, blood loss at delivery or a failure of an adequate placental transfusion due to extreme cord compression can be a reason for birth depression. If there is no cardiac output after about 20 minutes of adequate cardiopulmonary resuscitation, the prognosis for intact survival is grim, and the most senior person present should consider discontinuing resuscitation. If the baby has a heart rate but is not breathing, intensive care should be offered until more information is available.

Ethical issues surrounding resuscitation

This is an area which generates a great deal of anxiety. A junior doctor suddenly faced with a very preterm or abnormal baby is not in the right place at the right time, nor is he or she sufficiently experienced to make a value judgement about the resuscitation of a very preterm or malformed baby. Ideally, this situation should be avoided by prior warning, so that a discussion can be held between the most senior paediatrician available, a senior obstetrician and the parents and, if possible, the staff who will be present at the delivery. If the parents, after being informed of the chance of intact survival, do not wish active resuscitation of their baby who will be born at 23 or 24 weeks' gestation, or of a severely malformed baby, most neonatologists would support their decision and offer 'comfort care' only. Experience teaches that it is wise to warn the parents beforehand that sometimes there is a surprise and the baby is bigger and more mature than expected, in which case it may be appropriate to offer intensive care on a 'wait and see' basis. If there is not time to consult with the parents beforehand, or there is any conflict or doubt, full resuscitation should be offered. Most tiny babies who die do so very quickly, within 24 hours, and a period of intensive care allows time for the parents to take in the situation and to grieve afterwards because they are certain that 'everything has been done'. This course of action avoids the possibility of anger developing because of doubt about viability remaining in the parents' minds.

Care after resuscitation

Effective resuscitation does not stop once the baby is pink and crying lustily. No matter how well you think the resuscitation has gone, the parents will fear the worst and a full explanation is crucial. Consider whether the baby needs admission to the neonatal unit for observation, or further investigation and treatment for possible sepsis. Use all available information such as the cardiotocogram (CTG), the cord pH, the maternal history and a history of the labour to make a decision about further management. The first seizure in hypoxic–ischaemic encephalopathy often occurs after 12 hours, which makes early discharge risky after resuscitation has been required.

Care of the normal term newborn baby

Examination

A thorough physical examination of every neonate is accepted as good practice and forms a core item of the child health surveillance programme in the UK. The aims of the neonatal examination are:

- diagnosis of congenital malformations (present in about 10–15 per 1000 babies; see Table 22.4),
- diagnosis of common minor problems, with advice about management or appropriate reassurance if no intervention is indicated (e.g. Mongolian blue spots, jaundice, naevi),
- continuing screening, begun antenatally, to identify those babies who should be offered specific intervention, e.g. hepatitis vaccination,
- health education advice, e.g. regarding breastfeeding, cot death prevention, immunization, safe transport in cars,
- general parental reassurance.

Table 22.4 – Prevalence of serious congenital malformations per 1000 live births in England and Wales

Malformation	Prevalence
Congenital heart disease	6–8
Developmental dysplasia of the hip	1.5
Talipes	1.5
Down's syndrome	1.5
Cleft lip and/or palate	1.2
Urogenital (hypospadias, undescended testes)	1.2
Spina bifida/anencephaly	0.5

Source: Office for National Statistics.

For some babies, early diagnosis may make an enormous difference to their subsequent health, for example in congenital cataract and urethral valves. For others, parental reassurance that their infant is normal and general advice are all that is required. Every newborn infant deserves at least one full examination. At present, this is usually carried out by a doctor, although in some areas midwives are being trained to perform this task. For recording purposes, it is useful to have a checklist printed or stamped in the baby's notes to serve as an aide memoire. Items are merely ticked if normal, but any abnormalities are marked distinctively and a full description written

out. The examination should be dated and signed. A suggested order for the examination is as follows.

- Introduce yourself to the mother, ask her about any antenatally diagnosed problems that may need follow-up, and any family problems (deafness, dislocation of hips). Check for risk factors that predispose to neonatal sepsis, such as pyrexia in labour.
- Remove the baby's clothes except the nappy; look at the skin.
- Feel the anterior fontanelle for tension (leave until later if the baby is crying!); palpate the sutures (craniosynostosis is a disorder with premature fusion of the sutures); check the scalp for swellings (a cephalhaematoma is the most common).
- Measure the head circumference.
- Look at the face for colour (cyanosis/pallor/jaundice) or any peculiarities.
- Listen to the heart and estimate the heart rate – normally 110–150 bpm, but can drop to 80 bpm in sleep.
- Count the respiratory rate – normally <60 breaths per minute. The lungs can also be auscultated, but this is seldom informative.
- Palpate the abdomen, feeling for masses, including large bladder or kidneys.
- Examine the eyes, checking that it is possible to obtain a red reflex using an ophthalmoscope to exclude cataract. Fundal examination is not routine.
- Examine the ears, nose and mouth (cleft palate).
- Examine the neck, including the clavicles.
- Examine the arms, hands, legs and feet.
- Remove the nappy.
- Feel for the femoral pulses.
- Examine the genitalia and anus.
- Turn the baby to the prone position and examine his back and spine; assess tone.
- Return the infant to the supine position and evaluate the central nervous system.
- Examine the hips.
- Make sure you have not omitted anything.

Diagnosis of common minor problems

Erythema toxicum (Fig. 22.3)
This is a common rash which usually appears on the second or third day, and takes the form of a white pinpoint 'head' on an oval erythematous base. If the

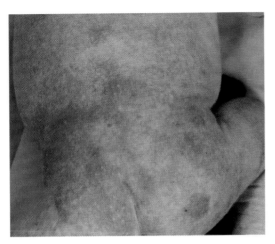

Figure 22.3 Erythema toxicum.

spots are biopsied, massive numbers of eosinophils are found. The rash rarely lasts for more than a few days and is harmless.

Transient neonatal pustular melanosis

This disorder is common in Afro-Caribbean babies. The eruption starts with small, pustule-like spots present soon after birth, which rapidly progress to a hyperpigmented macule resembling a freckle, which fades in a few weeks.

Milia (Fig. 22.4)

These are tiny, yellowish-white spots, especially common on the nose and elsewhere on the face, which disappear spontaneously over a month or two. They represent retention cysts of the pilosebaceous follicles.

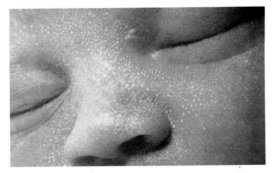

Figure 22.4 Milia. (From *A colour atlas of the newborn*, Milner RDS & Herber SM, 1994. Wolfe Medical Publications, with permission.)

Mongolian blue spots (Fig. 22.5)

Blue spots are blue-black macular lesions, usually situated over the base of the spine and commoner in

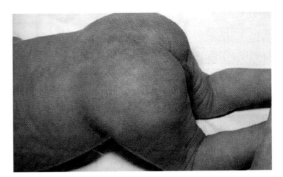

Figure 22.5 Mongolian blue spot. (From *A colour atlas of the newborn*, Milner RDS & Herber SM, 1994, Wolfe Medical Publications, with permission.)

Afro-Carribean or Asian infants. They fade slowly over the first few years.

Port wine stains

These are due to a malformation of the capillaries within the dermis. Port wine stains in the region of the trigeminal nerve are sometimes associated with intracranial vascular abnormalities (Sturge–Weber syndrome). Laser therapy can now produce an excellent cosmetic improvement for large facial lesions.

Skin tags/extra digits

These should be surgically removed; the old practice of tying a silk thread around them produces a cosmetically inferior result. As these are often familial, examination of the parents may provide proof of this.

Spinal birthmarks and sacral pits

Simple midline dimples are common and are not associated with spinal abnormalities. About 5 per cent of babies have some sort of dorsal cutaneous stigmata. Dimples that are large (>5 mm diameter) or high on the back (more than 2.5 cm from the anus) or that occur in combination with other lesions such as haemangiomas, skin tags, hairy patches or subcutaneous masses should arouse suspicion and are an indication for further investigation with ultrasound and/or magnetic resonance imaging (MRI) of the spinal cord. The consequences of missing a lesion that will cause cord tethering or infection can be disastrous.

Genitalia

The foreskin of a male baby cannot be retracted, and it is normal for it to remain non-retractile for up to 4 years. Both testes are usually in the scrotum at term, but it is common for them to be retractile. Scrotal swelling can be due to a hydrocele, inguinal hernia, trauma following breech delivery, or torsion of the testis. Neonatal torsion is usually a prenatal event, and emergency surgery cannot save testicular function. However, many paediatric surgeons believe that it is important to fix the contralateral testis in this situation. If no gonads can be felt in the inguinal region, and the phallus is small (the usual neonatal penis is 3 cm stretched length), the baby may be a female baby with congenital adrenal hyperplasia and urgent investigation is vital to avoid a collapse due to salt loss. If there are palpable gonads and there is a small phallus, the baby is likely to be an under-virilized male wherever the urethral opening is, but it is best not to make any assumptions prior to full investigation.

In female babies, hymenal tags and small amounts of vaginal bleeding are common.

Danger signs in the well-baby nursery

The vast majority of normal babies remain perfectly well and establish feeds, whilst their mothers quickly take on full responsibility for their care. The challenge for healthcare professionals is to spot the baby who is developing a serious illness in order to try to avert a collapse. This can be difficult: the baby who is passed as fit for discharge in the morning can deteriorate so rapidly that he requires ventilation and inotropic support by tea-time. Conditions that can cause such a dramatic deterioration include congenital heart disease (coarctation or hypoplastic left heart syndrome), sepsis, inborn error of metabolism, necrotizing enterocolitis or a gut volvulus, and intracranial haemorrhage.

Danger signs include:

- temperature instability,
- a change in activity, including refusal of feed or having to be wakened for feeds,
- unusual skin colour, mottling,
- an abnormal heart rate or respiratory rate, including grunting or fast breathing,
- apnoea,
- excessive jitteriness or abnormal stereotyped, repetitive movement patterns,
- delayed stooling (beyond 48 hours) or completely dry nappies,
- abdominal distension, green vomit (bilious until proved otherwise),
- odd lumps or swellings,
- lethargy, floppiness; paucity of movement, excessive sleeping.

Any of these should prompt a thorough re-examination of the baby, and if a deviation from normality is confirmed, the safest course of action is to admit the baby to the neonatal unit and initiate investigation and treatment, including a screen for infection and antibiotic treatment, without delay.

Screening for important neonatal conditions

Developmental dysplasia of the hip

The incidence of developmental dysplasia of the hip (DDH) is about 1–2 per 1000 births, but about 5–20 per 1000 babies have unstable hips in the neonatal period. Girls are affected more often than boys, in a ratio of 5:1. Expert management of DDH diagnosed in the neonatal period can be expected to produce a normal hip, while treatment initiated after the first 6 months of life undoubtedly gives much worse results, even after prolonged and aggressive surgical treatment. Whilst it is not possible to detect all cases using the current screening methods, this should not be used as an excuse for a poor-quality screening programme. The cornerstone of the screening strategy for DDH remains a careful history and clinical examination, using the Ortolani–Barlow manoeuvres. These tests are difficult to describe in words and are best taught by demonstration. Unfortunately, despite initial confidence in the ability of the Ortolani and Barlow tests to detect DDH, the number of cases diagnosed late (0.2 per 1000) has not reduced. Some dislocated hips are not detectable with clinical examination in the newborn period and others may dislocate later, perhaps due to a shallow acetabulum which progresses to dislocation when weight-bearing begins.

Ultrasonography can now be added to clinical examination as a further tool for detecting DDH. Ultrasound can detect clinically stable but anatomically abnormal hips, and show normality in clinically suspect hips. Developmental dysplasia of the hip is commoner following breech presentation, in females, if there is oligohydramnios, and in those with a positive family history. Many hospitals now offer hip ultrasound examinations to selected high-risk groups (Table 22.5); few have the manpower for universal screening.

Hypoglycaemia

Healthy term babies of appropriate weight who are breastfed have lower blood glucose concentrations

Table 22.5 – Screening strategy for using ultrasound in the detection of developmental dysplasia of the hip

- Breech presentation (whether delivered by Caesarean section or vaginally)
- Family history of dysplastic hip
- Any deformity suggesting intrauterine compression, or oligohydramnios
- Clicky hip on clinical examination, or one with restricted abduction
- If sufficient manpower is available, consider firstborn females

than formula-fed babies in the first 2–3 days of life. They also have raised ketone body concentrations and the neonatal brain can use ketone bodies as an alternative fuel. Healthy, normally grown term babies who are breastfeeding well do not need to have their blood glucose concentrations measured for screening purposes. There is no agreement on the lower limit of the normal range in this situation, bedside testing with reagent strips is notoriously inaccurate, and there is no evidence that a lower limit exists below which asymptomatic 'hypoglycaemia' is damaging. Recognition of these facts makes the use of supplementary feeding less likely and encourages breastfeeding.

However, there are undoubtedly babies who are at high risk of developing symptomatic hypoglycaemia and for whom screening is appropriate (Table 22.6). Babies who are at the highest risk are those whose growth has been restricted in utero and those born to diabetic mothers. Occasionally, an apparently healthy term baby has a rare condition such as idiopathic hyperinsulinaemic hypoglycaemia of infancy (formerly called neisidioblastosis) or medium chain acyl coenzyme A dehydrogenase (MCAD) deficiency, which will manifest as symptomatic hypoglycaemia in the first days of life. Very rarely, a healthy baby becomes hypoglycaemic from breast milk insufficiency. In these situations, prolonged symptomatic hypoglycaemia can occur, and this can be brain damaging (see the case history below). A balance needs to be struck between screening for and prevention of symptomatic hypoglycaemia in at-risk infants with recognition of symptomatic hypoglycaemia in infants who are ill, whilst avoiding over-investigation and over-treatment in the normal term baby whose mother is trying to establish breastfeeding.

Table 22.6 – Infants at risk of developing symptomatic hypoglycaemia

Infants with intrauterine growth restriction
Infants of diabetic mothers
Preterm infants
Infants who have suffered fetal distress in labour
Infants who are 'large for dates' – possibility of undiagnosed maternal gestational diabetes

CASE HISTORY

Baby John was born at term to a 35-year-old primigravida who went into spontaneous labour. The admission CTG was normal but later showed reduced baseline variability, and an emergency Caesarean section was carried out. John weighed 2.76 kg (3rd centile) and was in good condition, with Apgar scores of 7[1] and 9[5]. He was transferred to the postnatal ward.

He fed hungrily at first, taking both breast and formula feeds. At the age of about 55 hours, John refused a feed and became floppy. His temperature had fallen to 35.5 °C. He was placed in an incubator but took only 15 mL of formula and remained floppy. His dextrostix was low,

and overnight he remained floppy, cyanosed and intermittently jittery; a 10 per cent dextrose infusion was in place at a rate equivalent to 6 mg/kg per minute. John then developed seizures and required increased amounts of dextrose to maintain his glucose levels.

He has significant disability at follow-up, with visual impairment and developmental delay. MRI of his brain shows changes considered to be characteristic of those seen as a result of hypoglycaemic damage at term. John's parents recently succeeded in obtaining substantial damages on his behalf.

Signs of hypoglycaemia in the newborn are vague and include apathy/floppiness, apnoea and excessive jitteriness (see 'danger signs', above). These non-specific signs can also be due to sepsis. A term baby of normal weight who is sleepy needs help to feed directly from the breast or to be given expressed breast milk or formula from a cup or bottle. However, if the signs are more than just sleepiness, worsen or persist, the baby must be examined fully by a paediatrician, and investigations to exclude sepsis and/or hypoglycaemia should be considered. Checking a glucose level in this situation is not an excuse for omitting a proper examination. Early jaundice, fever, marked floppiness, tachypnoea and poor capillary refill are indications for investigation and treatment. If a low glucose is confirmed, the diagnosis is symptomatic hypoglycaemia until proven otherwise. This is an emergency, and intravenous glucose must be given without delay. Blood samples for true glucose, insulin and ketone body levels should be collected at the same time as commencing an intravenous infusion of 10 per cent dextrose. Boluses of dextrose should be avoided, and restricted to 'mini-boluses' of 3 mL/kg of 10 per cent dextrose to avoid rebound hypoglycaemia.

Hypoglycaemia in at-risk babies (see Table 22.6) should be prevented by screening and supplementary feeding. Small-for-dates babies can require as much as 12 mg/kg per minute to maintain glucose levels. Asymptomatic hypoglycaemia is managed with an increase in feeds in the first instance, with recourse to intravenous treatment only if the baby cannot tolerate feeds, symptoms develop or the hypoglycaemia persists.

Phenylketonuria

Screening for phenylketonuria (1 in 13 000 infants) using dried blood spots collected onto filter paper (the Guthrie test) was introduced in 1969. Milk feeds need to be established first, and midwives collect blood by heel prick on the fifth to ninth day of life, posting the cards to the laboratory.

Hypothyroidism

The same system was expanded to include a screen for congenital hypothyroidism (1 in 3000) from 1981. Audit of the programme shows that it has been extremely successful and picks up far more cases then were suspected clinically at a much earlier stage in life. Virtually all infants with congenital hypothyroidism now start treatment by 28 days of age, and have a better IQ as a result.

Cystic fibrosis and other screens

Certain areas of the UK use the dried blood spot to screen for cystic fibrosis (usually by measuring immunoreactive trypsin) and haemoglobinopathies such as sickle-cell haemoglobin or thalassaemia. Tests are also available for a host of other rare conditions, including maple syrup urine disease, homocystinuria, tyrosinaemia, biotinidase deficiency, galactosaemia, MCAD deficiency, Duchenne muscular dystrophy, fragile X syndrome and congenital adrenal hyperplasia, but none has been implemented in the UK. Widespread screening for neonatal neuroblastoma using VMA levels in urine did not prove cost effective in Canada and seems unlikely to be introduced worldwide, apart from in Japan, where the incidence is particularly high.

Prophylaxis and prevention of disease in the well newborn

Prevention of vitamin K deficiency bleeding (haemorrhagic disease of the newborn)

Vitamin K deficiency bleeding (VKDB) occurs in three forms.

1. Very early VKDB: this is limited to babies whose mothers have taken drugs that interfere with the manufacture of vitamin K-dependent clotting factors, such as antituberculous or anticonvulsant drugs. These mothers should be given extra vitamin K (5 mg daily) in the last month of pregnancy and the babies must be given intramuscular vitamin K prophylaxis.
2. Classical VKDB presents on days 2–7 of life, with bleeding from the umbilical stump, bruising or melaena. The mortality of classical VKDB is low, and the disorder can be prevented by a single dose of vitamin K, given to the baby by any route.
3. Late VKDB occurs virtually exclusively in babies who are breastfed, unless they have liver disease. Small warning bleeds from the gum are a common feature, but the worst problems are associated with the high (50 per cent) chance of intracranial haemorrhage, which can cause permanent neurological handicap.

Late-onset VKDB can be prevented by a single intramuscular dose of vitamin K given at birth, but a single oral dose is ineffective. The UK Department of Health has recently endorsed two alternative regimens: either a single dose of intramuscular vitamin K (Konakion) or repeated oral doses. If oral vitamin K is chosen, the Department of Health recommends that two doses of Konakion MM be given orally in the first week, with a third dose at a month if the baby is breastfed. What is clear is that all infants must be offered vitamin K prophylaxis and there is no longer any place for selective regimens. If parents refuse vitamin K for their baby after counselling, the reasons for the refusal should be clearly documented.

Confirmation of the diagnosis of VKDB is obtained from coagulation tests, which show a normal platelet count and prolonged thrombin and prothrombin times. Treatment is with intravenous vitamin K and fresh frozen plasma.

Screening for group B *Streptococcus* to prevent early-onset disease

Group B *Streptococcus* (GBS) is the most frequent cause of severe early-onset infection in newborn babies, with a 10 per cent mortality and a risk of deafness or cerebral palsy in survivors that may be as high as 40–50 per cent. Early-onset GBS disease is often preventable. There can be no doubt about the effectiveness of intrapartum prophylaxis with high-dose intravenous penicillin (3 g).

The incidence of early-onset GBS disease has declined from about 1.5 to 0.5 cases per 1000 in the USA since the adoption of guidelines proposed by the Communicable Disease Center (CDC; Fig. 22.6). Two alternative strategies exist. In the first, intrapartum antibiotic prophylaxis is offered to women identified as GBS carriers through prenatal screening cultures collected at 35–37 weeks' gestation, and to women who develop premature onset of labour or rupture of membranes before the screening is done. In the second, intrapartum antibiotic prophylaxis is provided to women who have one or more risk conditions at the time of labour or membrane rupture. Screening is not done. Both are in use in different parts of the world, although the US CDC now firmly recommends screening. In the UK, the Health Protection Agency has issued interim guidelines, and the Royal College of Obstetricians and Gynaecologists (RCOG) has a

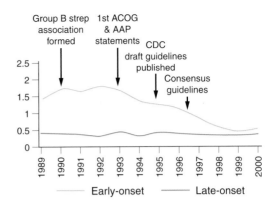

Figure 22.6 Incidence of early-onset and late-onset invasive group B streptococcal disease over time in the USA. (Adapted from CDC. Early-onset group B streptococcal disease, United States, 1998–1999. *MMWR* 2000; **49**:793–6; and Shrag SJ, Zywicki S, Farley MM et al. Group B streptococcal disease in the era of intrapartum antibiotic prophylaxis. *New England Journal of Medicine* 2000; **342**:15–20. Copyright © 2000 Massachusetts Medical society.)

guideline under development. If screening were adopted in the UK, around 30 per cent of all women would require intrapartum antibiotics, and about 7000 women would need to be treated to prevent one neonatal death. There is an interesting contrast with prophylactic corticosteroids, for which the number of women who need to be treated to prevent one death is 23.

Jaundice and prevention of kernicterus

At least two-thirds of all babies develop jaundice in the first week of life, and jaundice is the most common reason for re-admission to hospital at this time. Jaundice in this group reflects the immaturity of the liver's excretory pathway for bilirubin at a time of heightened production. In healthy term infants, bilirubin rises over the first few days, and jaundice is not apparent on the first day of life. Any visible jaundice in the first 24 hours must be urgently investigated, and assumed to be due to haemolysis (rhesus incompatibility, ABO incompatibility, glucose 6-phosphate dehydrogenase (G6PD) deficiency) until proved otherwise. Neonatal 'physiological' jaundice is contributed to by a high neonatal haematocrit, short red cell survival, breastfeeding and an initial absence of gut bacteria. Although neonatal jaundice is usually benign, it is a dangerous fallacy to assume that healthy term newborns are immune from kernicterus

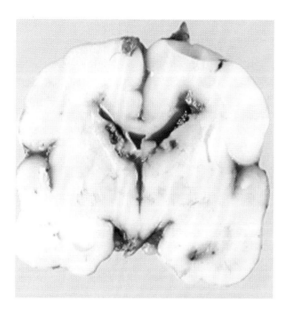

Figure 22.7 Autopsy specimen showing the yellow staining of kernicterus in the basal ganglia of the brain of a baby.

(yellow staining of the basal ganglia by bilirubin; Fig. 22.7). Survivors are severely handicapped by athetoid cerebral palsy, classically with accompanying sensorineural deafness, paralysis of up-gaze and dental enamel dysplasia. The level of unconjugated bilirubin at which kernicterus can occur in well term infants is not known with certainty, but appears to lie somewhere between 425 and 600 µmol/L. A level above 425 µmol/L is reached by only 1 in 770 normal term infants. The risk of kernicterus is probably greater for an infant of 37 weeks' compared to one of 41 weeks' gestation (see the case history below).

The key to successful kernicterus prevention lies in detecting the very few healthy (usually breastfed) babies who are likely to develop a serum unconjugated bilirubin of more than 425 µmol/L, and in paying careful attention to bilirubin levels in moderately preterm babies (34–36 weeks). Babies 'track' for serum bilirubin, so that an infant who is on the 50th centile at 48 hours (136 µmol/L) will not develop a dangerous level unless a new complication develops or he has an undiagnosed haemolytic disease (Fig. 22.8). However, a baby with a similar level at 24 hours is already tracking along the 95th centile and needs a repeat estimation. Such a baby is not be suitable for early discharge unless the parents are willing to return to the hospital for a check to be done.

All those who come into contact with babies in the first week of life need education about the assessment of jaundice. All too often, the early signs of bilirubin encephalopathy (lethargy, irritability, poor suck, shrill cry) are ignored. Assessing the level of jaundice from clinical examination can be difficult, especially in Afro-Caribbean and Asian babies. Various transcutaneous bilirubinometers are under evaluation and may eventually assist in reducing the traffic of blood samples (and babies) to and from maternity hospitals. The dermal zones of Kramer use the fact that jaundice stains the skin from the head to the feet in babies, and when the hands and feet are involved, a level of >300 µmol/L can be anticipated. Babies who are thought to have a bilirubin level of more than

CASE HISTORY: JAUNDICE

Baby Kieran was born normally at 35 weeks' gestation weighing 2.7 kg. His mother had gone into labour following preterm rupture of the membranes. He was in excellent condition at birth, with Apgar scores of 9^1 and 9^5 and a cord pH of 7.34. He required no resuscitation and went to the postnatal ward with his mother.

The midwives noticed jaundice for the first time when he was about 28 hours old. The bilirubin was checked 24 hours later and was 279 µmol/L. On the following day, Kieran was examined by the same doctor, who thought the jaundice was unchanged and discharged him home.

Kieran and his mother were visited at home by midwives, who reassured his young, first-time mother that his jaundice was not serious and no further bilirubin levels were measured. On the eighth day, his concerned parents took him to the local paediatric casualty department, where he was noted to be very jaundiced, cool and feeding poorly. Blood was taken in the accident and emergency department, which revealed a serum bilirubin level of 570 µmol/L. Kieran was admitted to the ward, where the following morning he was noted to be irritable, tense on handling, and to be extending his neck (opisthotonus). An exchange transfusion was done, but Kieran is disabled with deafness and athetoid cerebral palsy. He was awarded substantial damages after a successful claim of medical negligence.

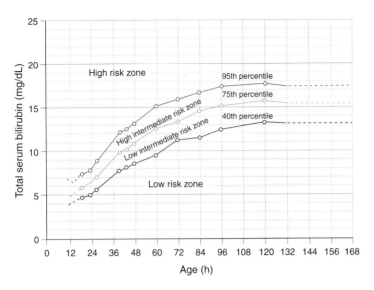

Figure 22.8 Hour specific bilirubin values from more than 13 000 healthy babies. Conversion of mg/dL to μmol/L requires multiplication by 17.1. (From Bhutani VK, Honson L, Sivieri MS, 1999. Predictive ability of a predischarge hour specific serum bilirubin for subsequent significant hyperbilirubinemia in healthy term and near term newborns. Reproduced with permission from *Pediatrics*, vol. 103, pages 6–14, copyright 1999.)

340 μmol/L should have a serum bilirubin estimation carried out. If this level is confirmed, phototherapy should be offered, and at present this requires re-admission to hospital in most areas of the UK. Phototherapy, used correctly, is a remarkably effective treatment and is capable of converting a fifth of the circulating unconjugated bilirubin to harmless photoisomers within a few hours.

Screening for cardiac disease

Early diagnosis of congenital heart disease is important because many of these lesions are now amenable to surgery, and because prostaglandin infusion can be used to keep the ductus arteriosus patent in babies whose lesion is duct dependent. The detection of significant cardiac disease is, like many other screening procedures, bedevilled by false-negative and false-positive results. Innocent murmurs are very common in babies, and yet many babies with seriously malformed hearts have no murmur at all.

Screening begins in the antenatal period, with increasing use of a four-chamber view of the heart as standard at 18–20 weeks. Fetuses whose scan is abnormal are referred for detailed specialized scanning, and many diagnoses are now made this way. However, it is not possible to detect all congenital heart disease with antenatal scanning.

Heart disease in the neonate presents as cyanosis, shock, heart failure, or with the finding of a murmur or absent femoral pulses. Cyanosis can be surprisingly easy to miss, and recently it has been suggested that all babies could be 'screened' with pulse oximetry. Whilst this is not yet of proven value, pulse oximetry is easy to use and should be carried out if there is any doubt about the baby's colour. Innocent murmurs have several features.

- The murmur is mid-systolic, grade 1–2/6 and best heard at the left sternal edge.
- There are no audible clicks.
- The pulses are normal.
- The baby is otherwise well.

Suspicious features mean that the baby should remain in hospital, a chest X-ray and electrocardiogram (ECG) should be done, and an early opinion from a cardiologist obtained. Neither a chest X-ray nor an ECG assists in distinguishing an innocent murmur from one caused by significant heart disease, and they are no longer routinely performed in all babies with murmurs. Slow feeding, grunting, sweatiness and poor weight gain in spite of adequate feeding suggest heart failure and the baby must not be discharged.

Infant feeding

Breastfeeding

Breast milk is the ideal food for babies for the first 4–6 months of life. Human milk contains the carbohydrate lactose, and the proteins casein, α-lactalbumin, immunoglobulin and lactoferrin. Human milk is whey predominant (60:40 whey:casein ratio) and is easily digested. Lactoferrin combines with other anti-infective agents such as lysozyme, and the overall effect is to ensure that breastfed babies are well protected from gastrointestinal and other infections. The fat in human milk is predominantly unsaturated and there are long-chain polyunsaturated fatty acids that may provide important precursors for the infant's nervous system. Cow's milk contains much more protein than human milk (3.5 g/dL versus 1 g/dL), the protein is casein predominant and the whey protein differs from that of human milk (β-lactoglobulin not α-lactalbumin). Casein is the constituent of milk that forms a curd precipitate with acid.

There is a delay of 48 hours before copious milk secretion begins in women. This is unusual; in all animals except guinea-pigs, lactogenesis takes place within hours of parturition. Lactogenesis is initiated by the slowly falling progesterone levels in the presence of a high prolactin concentration. In an attempt to reverse the trend away from breastfeeding, the World Health Organization (WHO) has proposed 'ten steps' as a core item of its Baby Friendly Hospital Initiative (Table 22.7). This programme has been very successful; for example, neonatal infection was reduced from 23 per cent to 3.4 per cent in one Romanian hospital. In the UK, the Department of Health last conducted an infant feeding survey in 2000, and found that there had been an improvement in breastfeeding rates when compared to the 1995 survey. Initial breastfeeding rates were 69 per cent; there was a steep social-class gradient, with 91 per cent of mothers in social class I choosing to breastfeed. Only 46 per cent of teenage mothers were breastfeeding. There is still a high drop-out rate, with a fifth giving up within a fortnight, citing painful nipples and the baby rejecting the breast as reasons.

Formula feeding

Modern formula milks are adjusted (humanized) so that the protein content and the whey:casein ratio are nearer those of human milk. Manufacturers do this by adding demineralized whey (from cheese production) and lactose, but differences in the fatty acid and amino acid composition remain, and formula milk cannot contain any of the anti-infective agents. There is no evidence to support the claim that formulae with a higher casein content are more 'satisfying' for 'the hungry and demanding baby'. Additives are required to emulsify and thicken the milk. Water is required to reconstitute milk powder. Some products sold as 'natural mineral water' contain unacceptably high levels of sodium and nitrate for babies and are unsuitable for re-hydrating dried formula milk.

Unmodified 'doorstep' cow's milk, sheep's and goat's milk are completely unsuitable foods for babies less than a year old. The electrolyte composition is vastly different from that of human milk and they are highly allergenic. Soy formulae have no lactose, the carbohydrate being derived from corn syrup and sucrose. Soy protein is nutritionally inferior to human milk protein and infants grow less well on soy milk. The only reason to use soy formula is if the infant has a cow's milk allergy or requires a lactose-free formula.

Table 22.7 – The WHO ten steps to successful breastfeeding

1. Have a written breastfeeding policy that is routinely communicated to all healthcare staff
2. Train all healthcare staff in the skills necessary to implement this policy
3. Inform all pregnant women about the benefits and management of breastfeeding
4. Help mothers initiate breastfeeding within half an hour of birth
5. Show mothers how to breastfeed and how to maintain lactation even if they are separated from their infants
6. Give newborn infants no food or drink other than breast milk unless medically indicated
7. Practise rooming-in (allow mothers and infants to stay together) 24 hours a day
8. Encourage breastfeeding on demand
9. Give no artificial teats or pacifiers (also called dummies or soothers) to breastfeeding infants
10. Foster the establishment of breastfeeding support groups and refer mothers to them on discharge from the hospital or clinic

Care of the ill term newborn baby

A brief description of a few of the more common and serious illnesses that afflict term newborns follows. For more detail, consult standard texts.

Birth trauma

Birth trauma is fortunately rare in modern neonatal practice, but occasional cases are still encountered.

Erb's palsy

Erb's palsy is caused by damage to the brachial plexus. It is more common in large babies, particularly those whose delivery is complicated by shoulder dystocia. A brachial plexus lesion is revealed by lack of movement in the arm; initially the arm is flaccid. After 48 hours, an upper palsy can be distinguished from a complete palsy. In an upper root palsy (C5, C6, sometimes C7) the arm is internally rotated and pronated, there is no active abduction or elbow flexion (the waiter's tip position; Fig. 22.9). In a complete palsy of upper and lower roots, the arm is flail; there may be a ptosis and a Horner's syndrome due to damage to the stellate ganglion adjacent to C8 and T1. Phrenic nerve palsy should be considered in these cases. Whilst the prognosis of brachial plexus lesions is generally good, with most series reporting an initial

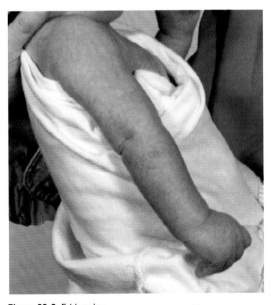

Figure 22.9 Erb's palsy.

recovery rate of 75–95 per cent, a recent study of the long-term effects revealed a surprisingly high incidence of later problems in childhood. The results of surgical nerve repair have improved markedly since the early days, and babies who have no recovery in biceps function by 3 months should be referred to a specialist.

Subgaleal (subaponeurotic) haemorrhage

The subaponeurotic space is potentially very large, lying as it does outside the skull and below the scalp. Babies who bleed into this space can become shocked, and there is a mortality of 20 per cent. The condition is fortunately rare after normal vertex vaginal delivery, but is reported in as many as 6 per 1000 babies delivered by the ventouse. Increasing use of the ventouse apparatus means that early recognition of subgaleal haemorrhage has become more important. The clue to the diagnosis is a boggy swelling of the scalp that crosses suture lines. The baby's head circumference will have increased at least 1 cm from the birth measurement if there is a sizeable subaponeurotic collection. When appropriately recognized and treated with blood transfusion, the long-term prognosis is good.

Transient tachypnoea of the newborn

Transient tachypnoea of the newborn (TTN) is the commonest respiratory disease of term infants, occurring in 4 per 1000. The disease is due to delayed clearance of lung liquid and is much more common after Caesarean section delivery, particularly without labour. At term, the incidence falls between 37 and 40 weeks (Fig. 22.10), and this finding has implications for the timing of elective Caesarean section at term. Fortunately the disease is usually mild, but sometimes requires intubation and ventilation, with the associated risk of complications.

Meconium aspiration syndrome

Meconium aspiration syndrome (MAS) is a disease of post-term pregnancies, with an incidence of about 1:1000 total births in Europe and 2–6 per 1000 in the USA. Meconium can be aspirated before or after birth. The co-existence of asphyxia is the main determining factor in MAS; asphyxia exerts its own detrimental effect on lung function and is associated with the development of persistent pulmonary hypertension, which complicates the treatment of MAS still further. These problems, together with a pre-existing aspiration

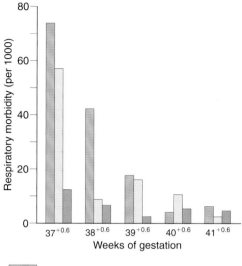

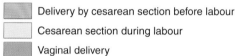

Delivery by cesarean section before labour

Cesarean section during labour

Vaginal delivery

Figure 22.10 Respiratory morbidity (transient tachypnoea of the newborn plus respiratory distress syndrome) at term in infants admitted to the Neonatal Intensive Care Unit, Rosie Maternity Hospital, Cambridge, by each week of gestation and mode of delivery. (From Morrison JJ, Rennie JM, Milton P, 1995. Neonatal respiratory morbidity and mode of delivery at term: influence of timing of elective Caesarean section. *British Journal of Obstetrics and Gynaecology* 102:101–6, with permission.)

of meconium into the airway that is not amenable to even the most aggressive suctioning at delivery, combine to make MAS a very serious neonatal illness.

The fact that some cases cannot be prevented by tracheal toilet should not discourage attempts at preventing meconium entering the airway at birth. Suctioning on the perineum has been shown to be effective in preventing MAS. Meconium in the airway creates a ball-valve effect in which air can be sucked past the obstruction but not exhaled past it, and the substance acts as a chemical irritant to the airways. Any reduction in the load is useful.

Persistent pulmonary hypertension

The term persistent pulmonary hypertension of the newborn (PPHN) is preferable to that of persistent fetal circulation, because the placenta is no longer in the circuit. In this disorder the baby is cyanosed because there is a failure of the usual rapid postnatal fall in pulmonary vascular resistance. There is no parenchymal lung disease, but the pulmonary capillaries are structurally abnormal, possessing excess smooth muscle that persists into smaller branches than usual. PPHN can occur as a primary disorder or as a complication of asphyxia, infection (such as GBS) or pulmonary hypoplasia. The diagnosis should be suspected in a baby who remains hypoxic in 100 per cent oxygen and whose chest X-ray is normal. Echocardiography confirms the right-to-left shunt at atrial and/or ductal level and excludes congenital heart disease from the differential diagnosis. Nitric oxide has recently been confirmed as effective treatment for PPHN and is now the therapy of choice if warmth, artificial ventilation, oxygen and/or alkali therapy do not succeed in correcting the acidosis.

Hypoxic–ischaemic encephalopathy

Seizures are the hallmark of this condition, and hypoxic–ischaemic encephalopathy (HIE) is the commonest cause of early-onset seizures in a term baby. There are many other causes of neonatal seizure, for example meningitis, stroke and hypoglycaemia. A diagnosis of HIE should be considered when there is a combination of:

- fetal distress,
- birth depression (low Apgar score requiring resuscitation),
- metabolic acidosis on cord pH or an early neonatal sample,
- seizures,
- renal impairment (blood in the urine and a low urine output),
- alteration of central nervous system state – the baby is not normally conscious between seizures, but is irritable or lethargic with abnormal primitive reflexes.

The diagnosis should be supported by checking serum creatinine, calcium and glucose, performing a lumbar puncture to exclude meningitis, and carrying out a cranial ultrasound scan. This scan may be normal or show a loss of the gyral pattern with obliterated ventricles, suggesting cerebral oedema. Early electroencephalography (EEG) often confirms electrical seizure activity, and the background pattern can help in prognosis: a normal background, even in the presence of frequent seizures, is reassuring, whereas a very depressed or deteriorating background is an indication of a poor prognosis. An MRI scan, if available, is another investigation that confirms the diagnosis and helps in prognostication.

Management of the preterm infant

The prognosis for preterm infants has improved dramatically over the last 30 years, with survival rates for infants delivered beyond 30 weeks approaching 95 per cent. Neurological handicap, including cerebral palsy, sensori-neural deafness, visual handicap and developmental delay, remains a problem in 10 per cent of survivors below 30 weeks (Fig. 22.11). School failure, poor attention span and behavioural difficulties afflict a further proportion of these children. The future priorities in neonatal intensive care must include achieving more intact survival.

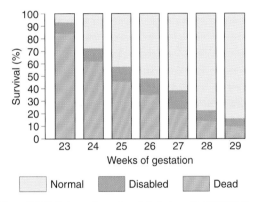

Figure 22.11 Outcome for preterm infants by week of gestation.

The management of many of the complications of prematurity (Table 22.8) is beyond the scope of this chapter, and the reader is directed to standard textbooks. A few of the major conditions are discussed below.

Table 22.8 – Main problems of prematurity

Respiratory distress syndrome
Chronic lung disease
Intraventricular haemorrhage, parenchymal cerebral
 haemorrhage
Periventricular leukomalacia
Infection
Hypoglycaemia
Necrotizing enterocolitis
Patent ductus arteriosus
Jaundice

Respiratory distress syndrome, chronic lung disease

The incidence of RDS is strongly related to gestational age, occurring in virtually 100 per cent of infants delivered at 26 weeks' gestation, 40–50 per cent at 30–31 weeks and about 5 per cent at 35 weeks. RDS is a condition of increasing respiratory distress, commencing at, or shortly after, birth and increasing in severity until progressive resolution occurs among the survivors, usually between the second and fourth day. It is due, at least in part, to insufficiency of pulmonary surfactant. RDS is manifest by respiratory distress (cyanosis, tachypnoea, grunting and recession), and respiratory failure is diagnosed by blood-gas analysis. Diagnosis can be confirmed by an X-ray film showing a ground-glass appearance and air bronchograms, although these radiological features are not pathognomonic of RDS (Fig. 22.12). Antenatal steroids and postnatal surfactant are beneficial. Artificial ventilation remains the mainstay of management, although the modern trend is for 'gentle ventilation', aiming to reduce barotrauma and minimize the risk of chronic lung disease. Chronic lung disease still afflicts as many as 50 per cent of babies weighing <1 kg at birth, and these infants spend many months in oxygen, sometimes only to succumb later to winter viral infections or cor pulmonale.

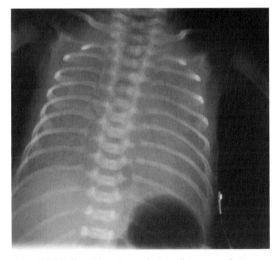

Figure 22.12 Chest X-ray in respiratory distress syndrome.

Preterm brain injury

The neonatal brain is vulnerable to injury, and both intracranial parenchymal haemorrhage and periventricular leukomalacia (PVL) are associated with handicap in childhood. Intracranial haemorrhage is common in preterm infants, and occurs in the germinal matrix region. The germinal matrix is situated in the floor of the lateral ventricle. Bleeding into the germinal matrix often extends into the lateral ventricle of the brain (germinal matrix-intraventricular haemorrhage – GMH-IVH). GMH-IVH can resolve, but is sometimes complicated by persisting enlargement of the lateral ventricles or even progressive hydrocephalus. In these cases the risk of handicap is more than 50 per cent. GMH-IVH can be diagnosed with ultrasound imaging via the fontanelle (Fig. 22.13). Uncomplicated GMH-IVH – that is, bleeding not followed by ventricular dilatation or accompanied by a parenchymal lesion – carries a good prognosis. Only about 4 per cent of ex-preterm infants with no GMH-IVH or an uncomplicated GMH-IVH will develop major neurodevelopmental sequelae. Ventricular enlargement is often a sign of periventricular myelin loss and brain shrinkage, rather than raised intracranial pressure hydrocephalus. Brain growth is an important differentiating feature. The presence of progressive hydrocephalus requiring treatment increases the risk of serious sequelae in preterm infants to about 75 per cent.

Bleeding into the substance of the brain is usually followed by breakdown of tissue into a porencephalic cyst (Fig. 22.13). The outlook for infants with such a cyst can be surprisingly good, but many have a hemiplegia. Periventricular leukomalacia is the term used to describe multiple small cysts that are visualized within the periventricular white matter. MRI scanning later in childhood shows a paucity of myelin in such cases, and the lesion is a very reliable predictor of later cerebral palsy. Cerebral palsy is almost universal in cases with bilateral occipital PVL. Factors that predispose to PVL include prolonged rupture of membranes, chorioamnionitis and neonatal hypocarbia.

Necrotizing enterocolitis

This serious gastrointestinal disease affects 2–5 per cent of preterm infants. Babies who had reversed end-diastolic flow in the umbilical artery and who were growth restricted are at particular risk. The characteristic clinical presentation is of a preterm infant less than 7 days old in whom enteral formula feeding has been commenced. Feeding is accompanied by abdominal distension, increased volume of gastric aspirate, which may be bile stained or bloodstained, and a tender abdomen. Abdominal X-ray may reveal the characteristic signs of intramural gas, a sentinel loop or even gas in the portal tract. Treatment involves omission of enteral feeds and surgery for perforation or failure to respond to medical management. Mortality is about 10–20 per cent and is highest in very preterm infants who develop necrotizing enterocolitis in the first week of life. Long-term complications include stoma requirement, short bowel syndrome and nocturnal diarrhoea.

Key Points

- Ten per cent of all babies require admission to neonatal units, but only 1 per cent require full intensive care.
- All those who attend deliveries should be able to initiate resuscitation with a bag and mask system.
- Survival rates for babies born after 29 weeks' gestation are now around 95 per cent and most will grow and develop normally.

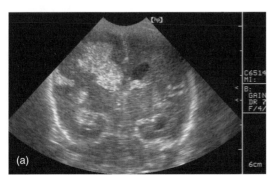 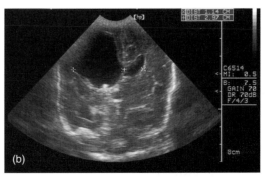

Figure 22.13 Evolution of a right-sided parenchymal lesion (a) into a porencephalic cyst (b) seen on a coronal ultrasound scan. The time interval between the scans was 2 months.

Additional reading and website resources

Guidelines for perinatal care, 5th edn. Washington, DC: American Academy of Pediatrics; American College of Obstetricians and Gynecologists, 2002.

Rennie JM (ed.). *Roberton's textbook of neonatology*, 4th edn. London: Churchill Livingstone, 2004.

Rennie JM, Roberton NRC. *A manual of neonatal intensive care*, 4th edn. London: Arnold, 2002.

Royal College of Paediatrics and Child Health/Royal College of Obstetricians and Gynaecologists. *Resuscitation of babies at birth*. London: BMJ Publishing Group, 1997.

AIDS/HIV treatment information: www.hivatis.org

Baby Life Support charity (support for parents): www.bliss.org.uk

British Association of Perinatal Medicine: www.bapm-London.org.uk

Center for Disease Control and Prevention (USA): www.cdc.gov

Confidential Enquiry into Maternal and Child Health: www.cemach.org.uk

Contact a Family (information on specific disorders): www.cafamily.org.uk

Department of Health (UK Government): www.doh.gov.uk

Group B *Streptococcus* support: www.gbss.org.uk

Health Protection Agency (public health, UK): www.phls.co.uk

National Institutes of Health (US Government): www.nih.gov

OMIM – genetic diagnosis search site: www.ncbi.nlm.nih.gov/Omim

Resuscitation Council (UK): www.resus.org.uk

Statistics (UK Government): www.statistics.gov.uk

Stillbirth and Neonatal Death Society: www.uk-sands.org

UNICEF – world statistics: www.unicef.org

Medico-legal issues

Obstetrics is characterized by rapidly evolving clinical situations; risks to the mother and fetus are considerable, and the potential for misjudgement or mismanagement by the attending doctors and midwives is ever present.

Some mistakes in clinical practice are obvious – such as leaving a swab inside the abdomen at Caesarean section. In contrast, most medicolegal issues are much more contentious. The most significant claims arise from brain damage and cerebral palsy; these are based on the allegation that negligent management resulted in fetal asphyxia and this resulted in brain damage.

As with all medico-legal cases, for the claimant to be successful it needs to be established that:
- there was a breach of duty: this means that the attending staff owed the patient a duty of care and that the standard of care afforded to the patient was below a standard which she could reasonably have expected,
- the injury sustained was caused by the substandard care.

When allegations are made, the case is assessed by experts – on behalf of both the claimant (either and/or the mother and baby) and the defendant (usually the hospital trust).

Breach of duty

Records

The case records and all documentation will be reviewed in detail.
- It is important that case records should be as clear, concise and accurate as possible.
- Every page in the hospital records should have the patient's name clearly stated.

- Every entry in the medical records should be dated and timed.
- Abbreviations should be avoided.
- Entries should be made in dark ink so that photocopying is facilitated.
- Every entry should be signed, with the name printed legibly below.

Cardiotocography tracings

Cases often revolve around the interpretation of intrapartum cardiotocography (CTG) tracings. It is important to obtain good quality CTG tracings. If the recordings of either the fetal heart rate pattern or the tocography tracing are inadequate, every effort should be made to rectify this (for example by repositioning the woman or using a fetal scalp electrode).

Reliance on intermittent auscultation is preferable to the use of an inadequate CTG recording.

Assess and intervene

Good medical practice is based on careful assessment of the clinical situation, followed by instigation of an appropriate management plan. It is important that both the assessment and the management plan are documented. For example, if a fetal heart rate pattern deviates from normal (see Chapter 17), the nature of the abnormality (suspicious/pathological) should be detailed. The management plan consequent upon the fetal heart rate pattern should also be stated. Management options might include continued observation of the fetal heart rate pattern for evidence of further deterioration (either in the baseline rate or fetal heart rate decelerations), fetal blood sampling or an emergency Caesarean section.

Timing of intervention

The timing of any intervention, and whether the timing was appropriate, often becomes an important medicolegal issue. For example, if a decision is taken to perform an emergency Caesarean section, the conventional standard is that the baby should have been delivered within 30 minutes of the decision being taken. This 30-minute time interval is not evidence based, and cannot always be attained.

Appropriate seniority

All procedures should be performed by practitioners with appropriate training and expertise. For example, whilst it could be reasonable for an appropriately trained obstetric senior house officer to perform a non-rotational outlet forceps delivery, if the same individual were to perform a rotational forceps delivery, this could be construed as a breach of duty.

Protocols

Increasingly, obstetric units are introducing guidelines and protocols for the management of most obstetric emergencies. It is important that all staff working in the unit are familiar with the protocols and that these protocols are regularly updated. Deviation from protocols or guidelines does not necessarily constitute breach of duty; however, the reasons for deviating from any protocol should be clearly stated within the medical records.

Training and skills drills

In addition to staff being familiar with the up-to-date protocols, regular programmes of education and training should be in place. For example, all staff working on the labour ward should regularly update their CTG interpretation skills. Many units also perform simulated drills, where staff practise their management of emergencies such as shoulder dystocia, massive obstetric haemorrhage, eclampsia, etc.

Consent

Consent to procedures must be full and informed. The purpose of the procedure and any significant or potential complications should be discussed. The doctor or midwife who is going to perform the procedure should obtain the consent.

Record retention

It is important to keep all documentation for an indefinite period after delivery. Claims are now arising up to 25–30 years after delivery and if the documentation is lost, it is difficult to defend the case.

Causation

In many cases where a child suffers brain damage and develops cerebral palsy, it is accepted that the care afforded was substandard. The argument is then one of causation, i.e. whether the substandard care resulted in the disability. The situation is influenced by the knowledge that only 10–15 per cent of infants born with significant brain damage acquire their disability as a result of the events of labour and delivery. The problem that all obstetricians face is that it can safely be anticipated that all parents who give birth to a child with a neurodevelopmental handicap will seek to ascribe the handicap to issues of management during the labour and delivery.

The American College of Obstetricians and Gynecologists Taskforce on Neonatal Encephalopathy and Cerebral Palsy has recently published the criteria to define an event in labour/delivery sufficient to cause cerebral palsy.

Essential criteria
1. Evidence of a metabolic acidosis in fetal umbilical cord arterial blood obtained at delivery. Ideally, samples are taken from both the umbilical artery and vein. In this situation, metabolic acidosis is defined as a pH < 7 and a base deficit of 12 mmol/L.
2. Early onset of severe or moderate neonatal encephalopathy in infants born at 34 of more weeks' gestation. Encephalopathy is characterized by an altered level of consciousness of the baby and often by seizures. (This criterion applies to babies born at 34 or more weeks' gestation.)
3. The type of cerebral palsy that results from the events of labour/delivery is spastic quadriplegic or dyskinetic cerebral palsy.

4. Other causes of neurodevelopmental handicap, such as trauma, genetic disorders, infectious conditions and coagulation disorders, need to be excluded.

Criteria that suggest that the timing of any injury is close to labour and delivery (within 48 hours)

1. A hypoxic event occurring immediately prior to delivery or during labour.
2. A sudden and sustained fetal heart rate bradycardia or the absence of fetal heart rate variability in the presence of persistent or late variable decelerations. For this criterion to be met, the fetal heart rate abnormality must occur after the hypoxic event, and when the fetal heart rate pattern was previously normal.
3. Apgar scores of 0–3 beyond 5 minutes. The Apgar score is a numerical assessment (out of 10) of the infant's condition, based on heart rate, respiratory effort, muscle tone, reflex response and colour. A low Apgar score after 5 minutes indicates an infant who needs continued resuscitive efforts.
4. Onset of multi-system involvement within 72 hours of birth. In many cases, organ damage such as that to the neonatal kidneys may be temporary.
5. An early imaging study showing evidence of acute non-focal cerebral abnormalities. Ultrasound scans of the baby's head, performed after delivery, can aid assessment of the timing of any injury.

Consideration of issues of causation is often far from straightforward. Different medico-legal expert opinions are obtained – from neonatologists, paediatric neurologists and obstetricians.

Ethics in obstetric practice

The specialty of obstetrics is a hot-bed of ethical dilemmas. New developments in assisted conception, genetic diagnosis and fetal therapy present ethical problems of mind-boggling complexity. Physicians are required to have a sound knowledge of ethical principles in order that their decisions are defensible to their peers, their patients and in a Court of Law. Obstetrics is unique in that the physician is often dealing with two patients, both inextricably linked and whose interests usually, but not always, coincide.

A fundamental understanding of bioethical principles is required to work out pragmatic solutions to these difficult problems. Bioethics is a secular, disciplined study of morality in health care, which is not based on theology or religion or professional consensus, personal conscience or law.

Fundamental to the doctor–patient relationship is the principle of beneficence. It is the core ethical principle of Hippocratic writings: 'Declare the past, diagnose the present, foretell the future; practice these acts. As to disease, make a habit of two things – to help or at least do no harm.'

Beneficence requires the physician to assess objectively the various diagnostic and therapeutic options and to implement those that protect and promote the health-related interests of the patient by securing for the patient the greatest balance of clinical benefits over harm. For centuries, beneficence was the guiding principle for a doctor in clinical decision making. In simple terms, beneficence was the essence of clinical judgement. At the beginning of the twentieth century, it became apparent that beneficence was not enough. Too often, beneficence-based decisions led to paternalism or to the physician over-riding the patient's wishes or intentions.

Beneficence has to be balanced by the principle of respect for autonomy, which accepts that patients have their own perspective on their health-related and other interests and should have the freedom to choose alternatives based on their values and beliefs. The essence of modern bioethics, therefore, is a balance between the beneficence-based obligations and autonomy-based obligations of the physician. In the majority of clinical situations these coincide, but when there is conflict, patient autonomy should prevail unless, in the opinion of the physician, the patient requests a course of action that offends the physician's professional conscience, and under these circumstances he or she must refuse to carry out the patient's request. Occasionally the private conscience of the physician, which is based on his or her up-bringing, personal experience or religious traditions, will justify withdrawal from certain issues, such as termination of pregnancy. Private conscience does not justify the physician being judgemental or denying the transfer of the patient to a colleague whose private conscience is not affected by the issue.

Peculiar to bioethics applied to the pregnant woman is the status of the fetus. The fetus is not a person and has no rights in law. Thus, it could be postulated that the fetus does not have moral status, i.e. the property of a human being to whom obligations are owed. This concept is increasingly being challenged, especially as after 24 weeks' gestation the fetus is independently viable, albeit sometimes with technical support. Modern bioethicists argue that we should grant the independently viable fetus moral status, i.e. that the physician and pregnant woman have beneficence-based obligations to the fetal patient. In other words, physicians should regard the viable fetus as their patient. This may, on rare occasions, cause conflicts when the autonomy-based decision of the mother, as regards her viable fetus, is at odds with the professional judgement of the physician. Some examples and solutions are outlined below.

Case 1

On a routine ultrasound scan at 20 weeks' gestation, a fetus is diagnosed as having a lumbo-sacral spina bifida. The obstetrician looking after the woman has strong religious beliefs that termination of pregnancy is wrong. What is the ethical solution?

Spina bifida is associated with a high risk of infant death or serious handicap. Legally the woman has the right to ask for termination of pregnancy under Section E of the UK Abortion Act: 'there is a substantial risk that if the child were born it would suffer from such physical or mental abnormalities as to be seriously handicapped'. Furthermore, as the fetus is less than 24 weeks' gestation, it is considered pre-viable and does not have the moral status of being a patient unless the woman confers that status, something she is free to withhold. A decision to carry out termination of pregnancy is justified in respect of her autonomy-based decision. The obstetrician can avoid performing this procedure as a matter of personal conscience, but, in terms of professional conscience, is obliged to refer the patient to another obstetrician who has no objections to performing termination of pregnancy.

Case 2

On an ultrasound scan at 34 weeks' gestation, a fetus is found to have the 'double bubble' sign of duodenal atresia. A rapid karyotype from a fetal blood sample taken by cordocentesis reveals that the fetus has trisomy 21. The parents ask for termination of pregnancy. What is the ethical solution?

A fetus at 34 weeks has no rights in law. Nevertheless, it is viable and, therefore, has acquired the moral status of being a fetal patient. Duodenal atresia is a condition that is usually cured by surgery. Down's syndrome is a condition associated with a low IQ, but the child usually has a normal but dependent life. Under Section E of the UK Abortion Act, there is no definition of 'serious abnormality'. To some obstetricians, the case described here would fit the description of serious abnormality and they would recommend that termination of pregnancy would be justified under the Abortion Act and in terms of maternal autonomy. However, on ethical grounds, such a decision would be difficult to justify because Down's syndrome does not necessarily result in a life not worth living. Beneficence-based obligations to the second patient, i.e. the fetus, would not justify causing its death. It would, therefore, be reasonable on ethical grounds to deny maternal autonomy in this case and turn down the woman's request for termination of pregnancy.

Case 3

A woman at 38 weeks' gestation has severe, poorly controlled pre-eclampsia. The fetus is well grown, but has a fetal heart tracing suggesting fetal acidaemia. The cervix is unfavourable, suggesting a long labour is likely. The obstetrician recommends Caesarean section but the woman and her partner refuse to accept this advice. Thus there is conflict between the beneficence-based judgement of the obstetrician and the autonomous decision of the woman.

Theoretically, in this case, it would be possible to obtain a Court Order to carry out Caesarean section against the woman's wishes. The basis for this would be that the life of the fetus (the second patient) is at risk and Caesarean section is the optimal means of saving its life. Caesarean section would also be of benefit to the mother, in that it would reduce her chances of having an eclamptic seizure, renal failure and other consequences of severe pre-clampsia. However, it is generally agreed that obtaining a Court Order to perform Caesarean section would be an unwise step to take. The solution should be to attempt to persuade the prospective parents of the wisdom of performing Caesarean section for the safety of the woman and her unborn child. This persuasion should not be strident or threatening, but carefully reasoned and respectful. If this fails, all attempts should be made to control the pre-eclampsia and recommend to the woman the second best option, which would be induction of labour.

It may be asked why maternal autonomy was over-ridden in Case 2 above and not in Case 3. In Case 2, the woman demanded an action that ethically would be difficult to justify. A decision not to perform a termination of pregnancy can thus be successfully defended. In Case 3, the obstetrician would have to carry out an operation on a woman against her express wishes, with the possible accusation that an assault is being carried out on her body. This would be an unwise course of action and one that would be difficult to defend.

These three cases only touch on the complexity of the ethical considerations that affect day-to-day obstetric decision making. This complexity provides a constant challenge to all healthcare workers in obstetrics, but it is also one of the reasons why obstetrics is such an interesting and exciting specialty.

Index

Compiled by Indexing Specialists (UK) Ltd (www.indexing.co.uk)
Italic page numbers refer to figures, tables and appendices.